Emerging Infections

Emerging Infections

Three Epidemiological Transitions from Prehistory to the Present

Second Edition

Ron Barrett
Associate Professor, Department of Anthropology, Macalester College

Molly K. Zuckerman
Professor, Department of Anthropology and Middle Eastern Cultures, Mississippi State University

Matthew R. Dudgeon
Assistant Professor, Department of Internal Medicine, Emory University School of Medicine

with

George J. Armelagos
Professor Emeritus, Department of Anthropology, Emory University

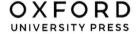

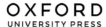

OXFORD
UNIVERSITY PRESS

Great Clarendon Street, Oxford, OX2 6DP,
United Kingdom

Oxford University Press is a department of the University of Oxford.
It furthers the University's objective of excellence in research, scholarship,
and education by publishing worldwide. Oxford is a registered trade mark of
Oxford University Press in the UK and in certain other countries

First Edition published in 2013
Second Edition published in 2024

Published in the United States of America by Oxford University Press
198 Madison Avenue, New York, NY 10016, United States of America

British Library Cataloguing in Publication Data
Data available

Library of Congress Control Number: 2023942630

ISBN 9780192843135
ISBN 9780192843142 (pbk.)

DOI: 10.1093/oso/9780192843135.001.0001

Printed and bound by
CPI Group (UK) Ltd, Croydon, CR0 4YY

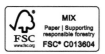

For George

Contents

The Ancient Determinants of Future Infections   **159**

List of Illustrations

Preface

This book emerged from the fateful collision of three remarkable events. The first of these was a major contribution by George J. Armelagos to our understanding of how biology and culture interact to shape the evolution of health and disease. The second was an experiment at Emory University to bridge the fields of biological and cultural anthropology in the training of doctoral students. The third event was a global change in the epidemiology of human infections that began in the last quarter of the twentieth century, although this book will show that its determining factors can be traced to much earlier periods in the human past.

George Armelagos was a leading figure in the field of biological anthropology whose career spanned more than 50 years. He began his journey in the 1960s by studying an ancient Sudanese Nubian population whose naturally mummified remains showed signs of increased malnutrition and disease as people shifted from a lifestyle of mobile foraging to that of sedentary agriculture. Similar discoveries were made in the study of other ancient societies, providing strong evidence for the theory that the first major rise of acute human infections began about 10,000 years ago.

Until these discoveries, it was commonly believed that humans had always struggled with the kinds of infections we experience today, and that their subsequent declines around the time of the Industrial Revolution represented the first major health transition in the history of our species. The research conducted by Armelagos and other anthropologists revealed that this was not the case. The industrial-era decline was actually the second of two major epidemiological transitions, the first being the initial rise of acute infectious diseases as a major cause of death during the Neolithic. Ten thousand years

was a long time for people to suffer from infectious diseases, but it was only 5 or 10 percent of the time that our earlier Paleolithic ancestors had been living on the planet. This prompts us to determine what led to our first emerging infections with the hope that these lessons will help us address the emerging infections that the world is experiencing today.

By the time I first met him in the mid-1980s, George (he was never one for formality) had already contributed this and many other theories to the study of ancient human health, nutrition, and disease. George was also as gregarious, warm hearted, and irreverently funny as he was intelligent. While teaching summer courses at the University of Colorado, George practiced his skills as a gourmet cook while hosting several dinners a week at his temporary home, where we enjoyed much feasting, laughter, and stimulating discussions until well into the night. The discussions were effectively graduate seminars about many of the ideas contained in this book.

At the end of each summer, George would return to his base at the University of Massachusetts. But after building programs there and at the University of Florida, George was eventually recruited to Emory University, where the Anthropology Department was organizing itself around a new vision. At a time when many North American anthropology departments were fractured by differences between subfields and theoretical approaches, Emory sought to bridge some of these divisions through graduate training in biocultural anthropology. While the cultural and biological students continued to focus on their respective fields, they also cross-trained in the other field.

Even more important than its biocultural program, the Emory department fostered a strong ethos of productive engagement with people with diverse ideas and perspectives. The program was ostensibly biocultural, but the wider vision was to train future scholars who would work toward the reintegration of anthropology, which was originally meant to be a holistic discipline. In a similar vein, faculty and graduate students collaborated throughout the campus, which included strong programs in biology, medicine, and public health as well as colleagues at the neighboring Centers for Disease Control (CDC), headquartered on the adjacent campus. It proved to be an ideal environment for the interdisciplinary study of global health issues, especially those concerning infectious diseases.

I entered the Emory program in the early 1990s, around the same time that the world was confronting a major global health challenge: the rise of novel, resurging, and antimicrobial resistant infections. This book will critically examine the determinants and details of these phenomena, but for now it will suffice to say that they were categorized under the heading of emerging and re-emerging infections, and they were a major topic of study and conversation on both the Emory and CDC campuses. Within these conversations, James Lin and I built on George's earlier work to independently propose that these new infectious disease trends constituted a Third Epidemiological Transition.

George generously provided Lin and I with separate opportunities to publish our ideas. Lin, who was then an undergraduate, presented a fine description of the problem. But I wanted to dig a bit deeper into the unique features and underlying determinants of this new transition. With this aim in mind, George created a graduate research group consisting of myself, Chris Kuzawa, and Thom McDade. Each of us brought different strengths to the group: Kuzawa with his emerging work on the developmental origins of health and disease, McDade with his ecological perspective on human immunity, and my own attempt to bridge pathogen biology with medical anthropology. In addition to our respective strengths, all of us shared similar backgrounds in epidemiology, evolutionary theory, and perhaps most importantly, a critical biosocial perspective on human health and disease. Together with George, we collaborated to write the seminal paper that eventually served as the framework for this book.

This book is also the product of many years of teaching. George often developed his ideas in the classroom as well as the laboratory, and I tried to emulate this model when the time came to teach my own courses on infectious disease. Teaching the same topics gave us good reason to stay in contact, and we maintained a close dialog for the next ten years. When we eventually decided to write the first edition of this book, George and I believed that the most important lessons of the Three Transition Theory lie in the human determinants of health and disease, which were fundamentally similar in ancient times to those that are operating today. With this focus on human determinants, we titled the book, *An Unnatural History of Emerging Infections*.

Seven years later, the same human lessons were underscored by the COVID-19 pandemic.

Yet even though the first edition provided lasting tools for the reader to examine *any* future outbreak, a text designed to be more than just another collection of perishable disease facts, it was clear that a major update was needed to address COVID-19 and other more recent infections as well as the latest developments in several scientific fields. Unfortunately, George had since passed away, and the quality and spirit of the project called for more collaborators. So in the same collaborative spirit, I allied with two other professors who had also been trained in the Emory Program: Molly Zuckerman, a biological anthropologist and former student of George's who conducts research on the evolution and ecology of past diseases; and Matt Dudgeon, a biological anthropologist and practicing physician who is currently caring for patients with COVID-19 and other infections. Together, we have expanded the text by more than 50 percent, and although its framework and major arguments are largely unchanged, we revised this edition to the point that it now deserves a new title. As with the first edition, we hope that this book will contribute to an improved understanding of, and future solutions to these ancient and recurring challenges.

Ron Barrett
April 30, 2023

Acknowledgements

This book is the culmination of many years of work with many talented people. In particular, we would like to thank Chris Kuzawa and Thom McDade, who were co-authors on the seminal article that led to this book. Credit also goes to James Lin for independently noting that the current infectious disease trends constitute a Third Epidemiological Transition. Special thanks to Kristin Harper, who contributed to our later thinking about these transitions, and to the students in our infectious disease courses for their many questions and insights as the framework developed. We are very grateful to those who closely read and provided expert advice on selected chapter drafts: Mark Cohen and Scott Legge on the ancient materials; John Eyler on the historical materials; and Robin Shields-Cutler on the microbiological materials, as well as our other three anonymous reviewers. Thanks as well to Katherine Bjork, Peter Brown, Ian Buffit, Eric Carter, Steve Hackenberger, Joe Lorenz, Debra Martin, Richard Meidl, Emily Mendenhall, Bill Moseley, Mark Nichter, Lene Peterson, Merrill Singer, Allen Swedlund, Dennis VanGerven, and David Woolsey for their input, reflections, and support. We received valuable editorial support from the Greg Birch, the Croftville writers circle, Addie Engebretson, Audrey Eyler, Steve Schack, and especially Amy Barrett, who worked on nearly every chapter draft. Houston Partridge, Larra Diboyan, and Rachael Oyondoyin assisted with references. Sierra Malis and Aisha Reynolds assisted with figures. Dennis VanGerven and Gwen Robbins Shug permitted us to use their images in this book, and Justin Gibbens captured the concept in his brilliantly provocative cover art. We were delighted to work with an excellent editorial team at Oxford University Press: Helen Eaton, Lucy Nash, Muhammed Ridwaan, G. Kari Kumar, Charles Bath, Katie Lakina, and especially Ian Sherman, who went above and beyond his duties to shepherd both editions to completion. Finally, we are very grateful to our family and spouses: Derek Anderson, Amy Barrett, and Elissa Meites for their love and support. Special thanks to Jean Dudgeon, who continues to inspire many people in the world.

Introduction

We ask the God of Plague: "Where are you bound?"
Paper barges aflame and candlelight illuminate the sky.
Mao Zedong (1958). *Farewell to the God of Plague*[1]

What defines an *emerging* infectious disease? Assuming we know enough to say a disease is infectious, which can be difficult to ascertain, we could also say it was emerging if the disease had only recently appeared in the human population and the number of cases was increasing beyond some agreed-upon metric. This technical definition, however, does not sufficiently address the ominous connotations of an *emerging* threat: that its appearance was somehow unexpected, a dangerous enemy that came out of nowhere. Framing our problems as emergencies can be an effective way to garner our attention. Yet once we begin to address the problems, any sinister associations should not interfere with scientific reason.

The biomedical sciences have long since rejected the early theories of spontaneous generation, which claimed that living organisms regularly arise on their own from non-living matter. Nevertheless, we often attribute more independence than we should to these same organisms when they are implicated in human disease outbreaks. We respond to them by selectively examining the molecular and microscopic determinants of infectious diseases without giving at least as much consideration to their social and environmental determinants. This selective attention has left us blindsided by outbreaks of Ebola virus disease (EBV), drug-resistant tuberculosis (MDRTB; XDRTB), and of course, the highly pathogenic coronavirus infections (severe acute respiratory syndrome (SARS); Middle East respiratory syndrome (MERS); and COVID-19). These infections took us by surprise when we should have been preparing for them a long time ago. We are also left wondering about future outbreaks that we should be preparing for right now.

We cannot predict the future with certainty or precision, but we can learn from the history and prehistory of human disease and apply lessons learned from these to the prevention, detection, and control of whatever infections come our way. With the aim of discovering these lessons, this book will examine the human determinants of infectious diseases during three major health transitions that occurred between the Paleolithic and the present day. This examination will include evidence from many fields, ranging from archeology, ethnography, and history to clinical medicine, evolutionary biology, and human ecology. Each of us, the authors, is an anthropologist with training in at least two of these fields and cross-training in most of the others. All of us share a multidisciplinary approach to the problem of human infectious disease.

Synthesizing a wide array of evidence and perspectives, we will demonstrate that, despite the unique biosocial characteristics of each and every infection, the outbreaks of the last 11,000 years have been largely determined by human activity patterns according the same recurring themes: changing modes of subsistence, shifting populations, environmental disruptions, and socioeconomic disparities. These themes have consistently arisen throughout the world during this vast stretch of time, a period known as the Anthropocene. Seen from this broader perspective, they can be found among Paleolithic foragers, Neolithic farmers, and nineteenth-century

Emerging Infections. Second Edition. Ron Barrett, Molly K. Zuckerman, Matthew R. Dudgeon, with George J. Armelagos, Oxford University Press.

factory workers alike. They loom even larger among those of us who are presently trying to live and survive in the twenty-first century.

0.1 From emerging infections to emerging awareness

Microbes are the ultimate critics of modernity.[2] Lacking any thought or culture, they can nevertheless adapt to our latest technologies by the simple means of genetic mutation and rapid reproduction. Bacteria, viruses, and other microparasites have evolved to operate in almost any human environment: in our ovens and refrigerators, in our heating ducts and air-conditioning vents. Some thrive in the industrial excrement of our oil spills, car mufflers, and smokestacks. Others thrive in the human body itself. No matter how many personal hygiene products we use, there will still remain ten times the number of bacterial cells than human cells in our bodies.[3] Even within the human cells, we find about 8 percent of our DNA is composed of sequences from ancient viral infections (Johnson 2019).[4] Despite our reigning "civilizations," it is the microbes, not the humans, who are the colonial masters of the living world.

Outnumbered and outgunned, we should not be surprised by our inability to control pathogens, the particular subset of microbes that contribute to infectious disease. Yet for many years, this unfortunate reality did not prevent authorities from making optimistic pronouncements about the imminent demise of human infections.[5] Sir Frank Macfarlane Burnet, the pioneering Australian virologist and Nobel laureate, famously described the middle of the twentieth century as "the end of one of the most important social revolutions in history, the virtual elimination of the infectious diseases as a significant factor in social life" (Mcfarlane Burnet 1962: iii). As president of the American Association of Medical Colleges, Robert Petersdorf predicted that there would be little role for infectious disease specialists in the next century, unless, as he put it, they would "spend their time culturing one another" (Petersdorf 1986: 478). Such statements reflected a clinical consensus that most major human infections would be eradicated by the beginning of the twenty-first century, and that attention and resources would be better focused on

eliminating the so-called chronic diseases of civilization such as cancer, diabetes, and heart disease. Many health policies shifted accordingly, as did funding for the prevention and control of infectious diseases.

Odds notwithstanding, the medical community had reasons to be optimistic. Infectious diseases had been steadily declining in the affluent world since the beginning of the Industrial Revolution, and similar trends could be seen in many low- and middle-income nations in the decades before and after the Second World War (Riley 2005). By 1977, smallpox had been completely eradicated from the human race. The success of this program was a major inspiration for efforts toward the global eradication of malaria, polio, tuberculosis (TB), and other major infections (Henderson 1980). After penicillin, new antibiotic molecules had been discovered every decade until the end of the 1970s (Amyes 2001). The revolutionary new field of molecular biology promised even smarter medicines, informed by the genetic sequences of disease-causing microbes and their human hosts. In the face of these developments, one might understandably conclude that pathogens were on the eve of extinction.

Yet while medical leaders were dissuading would-be infectious disease specialists, the AIDS pandemic was already well underway. The AIDS virus was among more than 80 newly identified human pathogens discovered between 1980 and 2005, including Legionella, Ebola, Marburg, and highly pathogenic strains of *V. cholera* and *E. coli* (Woolhouse and Gaunt 2007). International support had declined for major disease eradication programs, as had domestic support for public health programs aimed at the prevention and control of infections among the poorest segments of the richest nations. In low- and middle-income nations, an ever-growing division between rich and poor impeded recent gains in infectious disease mortality (Armelagos et al. 2005). With global poverty as a reservoir, infections once thought to be under control returned instead to cross borders and haunt the affluent as "re-emerging" diseases. Tuberculosis (TB) was a prime example of this re-emergence. Long considered a receding plague of poverty, TB made a major comeback in world's wealthiest nations (Farmer 1997). Moreover, it did so at time when these wealthy nations were experiencing their first increases in infectious disease mortality after more than a century of decline (Jones et al. 2008).

Worse still, these new and recurring diseases demonstrated increasing resistance to antimicrobial drugs. Since the early days of penicillin, bacteria had been steadily evolving resistance to antibiotics within a few years of their development and use (Zaman 2020). Although researchers continued to develop new-generation drugs, these substances were no more than clever modifications of less than two dozen truly unique molecules, and the rate of new discoveries had declined precipitously (Amyes 2001; World Health Organization 2017). Meanwhile, an increasing number of serious infections were showing resistance to more than one type of drug, TB among them (Kim et al. 2005). It appeared that the rates of microbial evolution had outpaced the technological revolutions of their human hosts and that we were rapidly moving toward a post-antibiotic era.

With increasing awareness of these developments, optimism turned to concern in the 1990s. During this time, health professionals coined the phrase "emerging and reemerging infections" to describe significant increases in new, recurring, and drug-resistant diseases. The phrase became the namesake of several conferences, a major publication by the Institute of Medicine, and an academic journal produced by the US Centers for Disease Control and Prevention (Lederburg et al. 1992; Satcher 1995). These projects pointed to factors of globalization and shortcomings in public health policies and programs. They also shared a common aim of increasing public awareness, spurring new research, and rekindling previously neglected health initiatives. Yet unlike the medical optimists of the previous decades, their primary aim was practically achievable.

It is unrealistic to expect that humankind will win a complete victory over the multitude of existing microbial diseases, or over those that will emerge in the future. . . . Still, there are many steps that scientists, educators, public health officials, policymakers, and others can and should be taking to improve our odds in this ongoing struggle. With diligence and concerted action at many levels, the threats posed by infectious diseases can be, if not eliminated, at least significantly moderated.

(Lederburg et al. 1992: 32)

Despite good intentions, fear got the better of reason as the concept of emerging infections spread to the popular media. Films such as *Outbreak* and bestselling books such as *The Hot Zone* focused public attention on a few novel diseases with putative origins in exotic foreign lands (Preston 1994). They cast gruesome images of people bleeding from all orifices and rotting to death, while emphasizing that, in this interconnected world, any infection was only a plane flight away (see Figure 0.1). Perhaps more damaging, these stories promoted high-tech and military-style interventions over basic public health measures as the most effective approach for controlling these diseases. Unfortunately, the military approach was popular among policy-makers as well, and more so after the anthrax attacks of 2001, when resources for preventing known disease threats were diverted to biosecurity programs aimed against unknown and unlikely threats such as smallpox (Barrett 2006; Cohen et al. 2004). By framing the problem as emerging and re-emerging infections, the medical community succeeded in raising public awareness about a global health issue, but important lessons were misunderstood or lost in translation.

However well-intended, the terms "emerging" and "re-emerging" are prone to misunderstanding, especially when they convey false perceptions that the problem of human infections is new, or that their appearance is sudden and spontaneous. Neither is the case. To begin with, not all newly identified pathogens are actually new to human populations—HIV and legionella being two prominent examples. Physicians first became aware of AIDS in 1981 when an unusual cluster of patients appeared in US hospitals with either a rare form of cancer or a pneumonia rarely found in younger adults (CDC 1981). Researchers identified HIV a few years later, and soon developed a test for the virus. They subsequently tested preserved blood samples from patients who had died of similar opportunistic diseases, revealing HIV infections going back to 1959 (Zhu et al. 1998). Similarly, after Legionnaire's disease made its debut at an American Bicentennial convention, retrospective studies of preserved tissue samples revealed that the *Legionella* bacterium was responsible for at least 2,000 deaths that had been previously diagnosed as non-specific

(a)   (b)

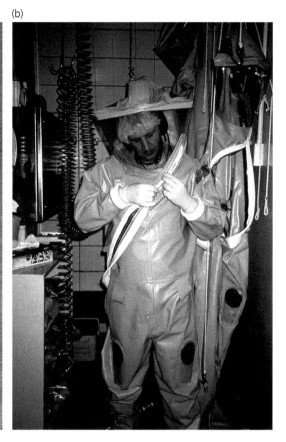

Figure 0.1 Biosecurity then and now. The illustration on the left is an engraved copper plate of a Seventeenth Century plague doctor wearing a protective suit. The beaked mask contained materials designed to filter out "bad air." The contemporary photograph on the right is a technician donning positive-pressure biohazard suit before entering one of the U.S. Centers for Disease Control's (CDCs) maximum containment laboratories. While conveying safety concerns, such images can also spread unnecessary alarm, stigmatize populations, and distort public perceptions of risk.

Sources: a: Welcome Collection Galleries. https://wellcomeimages.org/indexplus/image/L0025221.html b: Brian W.J. Mahy (Date unknown). U.S. Centers for Disease Control and Prevention.

pneumonias (Meyer 1983). Because of examples like these, biologists and health officials typically use the phrase "newly *identified* pathogen" more often than "new pathogen" when describing novel infections.

Furthermore, the term "re-emerging infections" is only relevant for diseases that were previously assumed to be under control. These assumptions are usually made in affluent societies that have long since benefited from declining infectious disease rates. The concept of re-emergence makes little sense in poor societies where the same infections had never declined in the first place. Case in point,

smallpox had declined for two centuries in Western Europe and North America until it became a rare disease in these regions after the Second World War. Nevertheless, the infection still persisted in low-income countries, particularly those in South Asia and Sub-Saharan Africa. With the permeability of national borders and social boundaries, smallpox periodically (and predictably) returned to the affluent West in the form of 53 limited outbreaks over the next 30 years before its final eradication (Barrett 2006). Back then, these outbreaks were known as "re-importation" epidemics. Today, they are better known as "re-emerging" infections.

Returning to the original question, when does an infection qualify as an *emerging* or *re-emerging* infection? Some public health workers joke that it is when the first White person gets it. Cynical though it is, the joke reflects a global situation in which pathogens are freely transmitted between nations and societies, but the solutions to these problems are often segregated and contained (Farmer 1996). Incubating in poverty, wealthy societies can afford to deny attention and sufficient resources to certain diseases—that is, until these same diseases make a surprise return to their communities. Such is the situation today, which is less about emerging pathogens and more about an emerging awareness among their human hosts of long-standing problems that were never sufficiently addressed in the first place.

0.2 Epidemiologic transitions

The current phenomenon of emerging and re-emerging infections is the result of shifting health and population patterns known as epidemiological transitions (Barrett et al. 1998). Currently, we are experiencing the latest of three major epidemiological transitions that occurred between the Late Paleolithic and today. The First Transition was linked to a major shift in human lifestyles from mobile foraging to sedentary living and intensive agriculture beginning around 11,000 years ago (Armelagos and Harper 2009). The Second Transition coincided with the Industrial Revolution beginning in a handful of Western European and North American countries in the late eighteenth century, and continuing in different forms among low- and middle-income countries before and after the Second World War. The Third Transition began in the last quarter of the twentieth century and it is still occurring today (Barrett et al. 1998).

Abdel Omran first introduced the concept of the epidemiological transition as a theoretical model to explain how changing disease patterns affected major population changes associated with the Industrial Revolution (Omran 1971). This model built on another model, that of demographic transition alone, that had previously been used to describe the shift from high birth and death rates (fertility and mortality, respectively) to low birth

and death rates in wealthier nations undergoing industrial economic development (Caldwell 1976). This was an important observation, but the Demographic Transition Model simply pointed to associations between economic and population changes. It did not address their underlying causes (see Figure 0.2).

Omran sought to address this shortcoming by demonstrating how changes in large-scale epidemiological patterns affected population change. His goal was to focus attention "on the complex change in patterns of health and disease and on the interactions between these patterns and the demographic, economic, and sociological determinants and consequences" (Omran 1971: 510). It was an ambitious attempt to bring together experts from different disciplines to understand the underlying determinants of a major shift in the health patterns of large human populations.

To demonstrate his model, Omran collected historical population data from as many countries as he could gather. However, because the wealthier countries had more complete and reliable data, he mainly focused on Europe and North America in what is often referred to as the Western or Classic Transition Model. With less data, Omran also attempted to formulate a Delayed Transition Model for low- and middle-income countries that had undergone modest forms of this transition in later years. We will return to these delayed transitions later in the book. For now, we will focus on Omran's better-known Classic Model.

Omran divided the Classic Epidemiological Transition into three stages, the first of which he called *The Age of Pestilence and Famine*. This age was characterized by populations in which high fertility rates were offset by high mortality rates—families gave birth to many children, but many of these children also died from infectious diseases and under-nutrition. For instance, in seventeenth-century Sweden, a country now known for its excellent health statistics, birth rates ranged from five to ten per family, but at least a third of these infants died before the age of one, and half the remaining children did not survive to adulthood (McKeown 1988). These days, it would be difficult for any parent with reasonable means to imagine the loss of even a single child, much less three or more.

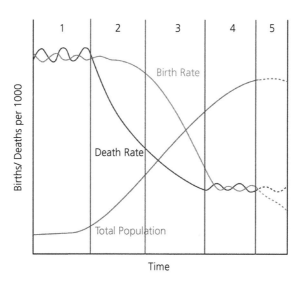

Figure 0.2 Mortality decline in affluent nations around the time of the Industrial Revolution. This decline resulted in population increases despite declining fertility rates. While demographic transition theorists described this phenomenon earlier, Omran's Classic Epidemiological Transition specifically linked these changes to declining infectious diseases. Note that this figure includes the five stages in Omran's original formulation of the Classic Transition Model.

Source: en:User:Charmed88 via Wikimedia commons.

But for many centuries these tragedies were all-too-common, even within the world's most affluent countries.

Following this tragic baseline, Omran described an *Age of Receding Pandemics*, beginning in Western Europe around the middle of the eighteenth century. Here, countries began to experience modest declines in the endemic or day-to-day infections that had been typically present in their populations. More importantly, they also experienced significant declines in the frequency of unusually large epidemics or pandemics, such as the smallpox, plague, and typhus outbreaks that sporadically appeared every few decades and swept away millions of lives in their wake. These changes brought an increase in life expectancy of birth from 40 to 50 years of age. Of course, major infectious epidemics did not recede altogether. The industrial world continued to experience major disease events. Overall levels of endemic infections remained quite high as well, but with a noticeable leveling of the disease spikes that characterized centuries past. If we were to liken infection to a body of water, one could say that the seas were calmer, even if overall water levels were high compared to the present day.

The Age of Degenerative and Manmade Diseases is the third and final stage of Omran's Classic Epidemiological Transition. This brought major overall declines in infectious disease mortality from the late nineteenth to mid-twentieth centuries. Life expectancy rose dramatically during this period, as much as 30 years in many countries. But life expectancy is a special kind of average that can be easily misinterpreted. In this case, increased life expectancy did not mean that adults were living to older ages so much as children were surviving to adulthood, primarily because of declining infections. In place of these infections, chronic degenerative diseases such as cancer and heart disease became the major causes of death in the affluent industrialized world. This Classic Transition was largely responsible for the optimism in the 1960s and 1970s regarding the future demise of human infections.

Omran's theory has been criticized for its emphasis on unilinear and universal change, ignoring race and gender differences, and its assumption that industrial development is the primary engine for health and demographic change (Salomon and Murray 2002). We share these concerns, but we prefer to address them in more fundamental terms and with an eye toward improving the model. As Omran intended, the Classic Transition does help to explain complex interactions between economics, demographics, and disease rates.

That said, the model has two important shortcomings. The first is historical: the concept of a single epidemiological transition suggests that pre-industrial societies have always suffered from high rates of infectious diseases, which is not the case. For the majority of our evolutionary history, human beings lived in small, scattered, and highly mobile groups that primarily fed themselves by foraging the wild plants and animals around them. These lifestyles were not conducive to the spread of acute and virulent infections. It was only after we began living in larger and more permanent settlements, relying on domesticated plants and animals as primary food sources, that the deadlier infections became a major human problem—this was actually our first major epidemiological transition.

Even with recognition of delayed transitions in low- and middle-income nations, the second major shortcoming of Omran's model is that it primarily addresses economic improvements in already affluent societies; this implies that poorer societies would eventually experience similar improvements once they become sufficiently modernized. Although many poorer societies underwent some degree of transition in the decades following the Second World War, these declines were more modest than in their affluent counterparts, and more dependent on antimicrobial medications facing an increasing threat of drug-resistant infections (Riley 2005). At the same time, these countries were experiencing the challenges of aging populations and chronic degenerative diseases, a situation that could be characterized as the worst of all worlds.

Far from a single, universal, or unilinear event, these epidemiological transitions have arisen in various forms and trajectories in different societies and historical periods. Yet with the rapid globalization of these different societies, humankind is now converging into a single disease ecology, one that involves a convergence of disease patterns as well as the transmission of pathogens across populations and national boundaries. This convergence represents a Third Epidemiological Transition, characterized by the accelerated and directional evolution of human transmissibility, increased virulence, and drug resistance among infectious pathogens. Globalization notwithstanding, the underlying determinants of this latest transition are much the same as first. Although industrial technologies have accelerated and expanded our impact, the same human activities have shaped and reshaped the evolution of human infections for the last 11,000 years.

0.3 Organization of this book

This book is organized according to the three epidemiological transitions, each of which are addressed in a section comprising two chapters. In Chapter 1, we begin with a Paleolithic baseline of overall human health that most likely preceded later increases in acute infectious diseases. This baseline consists of mobile foraging lifestyles and their health implications during 99.995 percent of our evolutionary history. While there is much debate about the particulars of these lifestyles and their supporting evidence, there is general agreement that the basic parameters of nomadic foraging could not sustain the kinds of infections commonly seen in settled agricultural societies. We know that nutritional states are closely linked to immunological states. Among contemporary[6] foragers, survival and wellbeing depends on the ability to obtain a diverse range of wild food sources. This diversity, in turn, tends to result in richly varied diets: ones that are high in lean protein and fiber, low in unhealthy cholesterols and fat, and more likely to cover all the human micronutrient requirements. The same principles apply to foraging then and now. Although Paleolithic foragers probably faced other subsistence challenges, they were less likely to experience the under-nutrition commonly seen in their agriculturally based descendants, and by extension, they were less susceptible to infectious diseases overall.

Additionally, foraging does not usually entail the same duration of contact with wild animals as farming does with domesticated animals. Prolonged contact increases opportunities for spillover, the entry of animal-based pathogens (zoonoses) into human populations. If and when they make this leap, those pathogens that produce acute and virulent diseases require large, dense, and highly interconnected human host populations in order to sustain person-to-person transmission. This would have been difficult in the small, and sparsely distributed groups that characterized ancient foraging societies. Finally, it should be noted that while known foraging societies are by no means free of social inequalities and conflict, they do not display the same degrees of social hierarchy and material disparities that are commonly seen in state-level societies. The latter often include impoverished communities who often become vulnerable entry points and reservoirs for pathogens.

In Chapter 2, we move from the Paleolithic to the Neolithic and other later periods, when human populations began to rely on intensive agriculture for their subsistence. We consider the health consequences of these shifts based on evidence obtained from the human remains of ancient societies as they were undergoing their agricultural transitions. Comparing the skeletons and mummies of people who lived at different stages of this transition, we find strong indications that the foraging groups were significantly healthier than their agricultural descendants. This evidence appears in the context of diminished food variety, increased size and density of populations, and the appearance of burial differences indicative of social stratification. Taken as a whole, these findings strongly support the theory that lifestyle changes surrounding the transition to primary agriculture resulted in increased nutritional and physical stress, and increased risk for infectious diseases.

Agriculture begat the First Epidemiological Transition, which was characterized by a major increase in the size of human populations and a major increase in human infections. The populations increased as fertility outpaced mortality, even though mortality was significantly higher than it was before. The mortality increase was primarily due to a rise in acute infectious diseases, the first truly emerging infections in the long prehistory of the human species. From its many origins, primary agriculture spread throughout the world as agrarian societies displaced, replaced, or assimilated their foraging neighbors. These societies also transformed the environments around them in

irreversible ways. Some may argue that the pervasiveness of these changes, along with many technological developments, speak to the success of agriculture. But even if we were to define success by these criteria, it came at a terrible cost to human health over the next 100 centuries.

Moving ahead to the Industrial Revolution, Chapter 3 examines the decline of infectious diseases in the affluent societies of Europe and North America from the late eighteenth to the early twentieth centuries, focusing in particular on the well-documented health and policy changes that occurred in England and Wales. Declining infections profoundly affected the demography of these societies by increasing the survival of children to adulthood and older ages. As a result, populations grew steeply as overall mortality fell precipitously; this occurred despite losses from declining fertility and an increasing prevalence of non-infectious diseases. These changes constituted the affluent version of the Second Epidemiological Transition.

The Second Transition gave rise to the biomedical optimism that was prevalent in the decades prior to the so-called emerging and re-emerging infections of today. Much of this optimism was based on a popular belief that Germ Theory, and its subsequent medical developments, had turned the tide in the battle against infectious diseases. With closer historical analysis, however, we will find that, as with primary agriculture, the early adoption of Germ Theory was neither simple nor sudden, and it would be decades before microbiological discoveries had a substantial epidemiological impact. Indeed, the majority of infectious disease declines occurred prior to the discovery of effective antibiotics and most of the vaccines we use today. Until these discoveries, the chief determinants of declining infections were improved nutrition and living conditions, and the better distribution of these essentials across social groups. These improvements addressed the same ancient factors that brought these infections to the human species thousands of years earlier.

Chapter 4 examines the Second Transition in poorer societies from a critical perspective that helps explain the so-called re-emerging infections of today. In the years following the Second World War, many poorer nations saw declining rates of infectious disease mortality. These declines, however, were more modest than those of their wealthier neighbors. They were also more closely tied to the use of antimicrobial medicines, a troubling issue given the recent rise in drug-resistant infections. At the same time, low- and middle-income countries have experienced comparable increases in chronic, non-infectious diseases along with rising proportions of older people. This poor version of the Second Transition could be characterized as a "Worst-of-All-Worlds" Syndrome.

At this point, we introduce the concept of syndemics: outbreaks involving synergistic interactions between multiple physical diseases, both infectious and non-infectious, that occur in the context of multiple social diseases such as poverty, racism, and all forms of violence. With syndemics in mind, we must consider that the First and Second Epidemiological Transitions were not linear progressions, and as demonstrated by the Second Transition in poorer societies, they were not universally experienced throughout the world. Today accelerated globalization is rapidly connecting all of these health and social problems, thus converging them into a single disease ecology. These trends characterize the Third Epidemiological Transition of today, the by-products of which include the increasing entry and spread of genuinely new pathogens in the human population, and increasing drug resistance in many of our long-standing infectious diseases. with many syndemic interactions between them. A situation connecting all our societies and converging on of societies is currently bringing these incomplete trends into collision, resulting in a Third Epidemiological Transition characterized by the entry of new pathogens to the human species, and the evolution of virulence and antimicrobial resistance in many of the old pathogens that had previously been ignored.

Chapter 5 applies very old lessons to newly identified or newly virulent pathogens. Given that the majority of these infections are evolutionary descendants of zoonotic infections, we consider the manner and conditions required for the spillover and onward transmission of these pathogens in human populations. Here, we re-encounter the same major themes of the Neolithic but with mechanized tools and larger, denser, and more extensively connected populations. Large-scale commercial agriculture and resource extraction enterprises are disrupting previously uninhabited environments and increasing the interface between humans and wild animals, especially higher risk disease vectors such as bats and non-human primates. Commercial agriculture is also increasing the densities and stress levels of our domestic livestock, which are also in contact with wild species, and the international trade in live animals is moving them across countries and continents. These and other practices increase the risk that our meat supplies will become major incubators and reservoirs for novel human infections.

In many instances, human conditions resemble those of our food animals. The majority of our species now resides in dense urban environments, and most of the world's urban residents live in poverty. Urbanization is often associated with decreased fertility, which eventually leads to higher proportions of older people. As we discussed earlier, this aging trend is occurring in poorer societies as well as richer ones. The distinction is the elderly poor and their families tend to live in more densely packed urban spaces with higher levels of industrial pollution and diminished access to clean water and sanitation. These populations face much higher risks for respiratory and diarrheal diseases. Add mosquitos, violence, substance abuse, and the stress these produce, and then connect these populations within a day's travel to everyone else in the world. These conditions are ideal for the entry and incubation of new pathogens in human populations.

Many of these same conditions are also driving the evolution of drug-resistant pathogens. Chapter 6 explores whether this evolution will inevitably lead to a post-antimicrobial era. For as long as their existence, microbial species have evolved chemical defenses and countermeasures against one another. Aside from some dye-based chemicals, most of the effective antimicrobial drugs are either facsimiles or derivatives of these natural defenses. But just as naturally, many microbial pathogens have evolved countermeasures to resist one or more of these drugs within a few years of their discovery. Far from conquering these pathogens, antimicrobial drugs have accelerated the arms race. Even more alarming, the evolution of microbial resistance has been outpacing the discovery of new antimicrobials. There may soon become a time when the treatable infections we have come to ignore become untreatable and potentially deadly, just as they were less than a century ago.

Focusing on the human determinants, we will examine how the overuse and misuse of these drugs can drive the evolution of resistance. With regards to the problems of human consumption, the most effective solutions are not likely to be simple matters of education and behavioral change. We must also consider the economies of time and money for patients and healers, especially in settings where other resources are lacking. With regards to animal consumption, common practices in commercial agriculture play an even greater role, especially with regard to the use of antibiotic growth factors.

Finally, we will examine some of the synergistic interactions that occur between infectious and non-infectious diseases, especially as they occur in otherwise vulnerable host populations. Given the trends, we are likely to see more novel infections in the coming years, and most our antimicrobial medicines may eventually become obsolete. Yet even if they do, we should recall that our modes of living have had far greater impact on the prevention and control of infectious diseases than all our pharmaceuticals combined.

There was a time when a "social disease" solely referred to a sexually transmitted infection. But the primary lesson of this book is that all of our infections, past and present, are essentially social diseases insofar as they have been largely driven by collective human practices.

Notes

1. Purportedly, Mao Zedong was inspired to write this poem after reading a newspaper announcement that schistosomiasis had been eradicated from Yukiang Valley. The disease, however, was not eradicated. Although the Chinese government has made significant progress toward the control of this parasitic infection, it still remains endemic in at least some regions of the country (Gross 2016).

2. For the purposes of this book, we use the term "microbe" (a contraction of "microbiological organism") in the more expanded sense to include viruses and prions as well as other microscopic parasites. Some authors exclude these entities insofar as viruses and prions do not independently engage in their own reproduction or metabolism.

3. There are approximately 10^{13} human cells and 10^{14} bacterial cells in a human adult body. Yet because they are much smaller, the total biomass of these bacterial cells is little more than a mere kilogram.

4. These are known as Human Endogenous Retroviral sequences (HERVs). Most HERVs are "junk" sequences that no longer code for functional genes. That said, a few active HERV genes have been identified that contribute to the cellular regulation of important human tissues as well as producing human diseases (Johnson 2019).

5. Some readers who are well-versed in the history of public health may wonder why we do not use the oft-cited quote by William H. Stewart, Surgeon General of the United States (1965–1969): "It is time to close the book on infectious diseases and declare the war against pestilence won." Our reason is that the quote is apocryphal. No one has found an original source for it, Stewart himself does not recall making this statement, and it would have been contrary to other warnings he gave about the ongoing challenges of controlling human infectious diseases (Spellberg and Taylor-Blake 2013).

6. Archaeologists and paleoanthropologists often use the word "contemporary" to distinguish present-day or recently historical people (and their cultures) from those in the deep past. Applying this usage, contemporary foragers are people today and in recent centuries whose cultural traditions are primarily geared toward the hunting, fishing, and gathering of wild foods. We are not referring to urban hipsters who dumpster dive and steal vegetables from other people's yards.

References

Amyes, Sebastian. 2001. *Magic Bullets, Lost Horizons: The Rise and Fall of Antibiotics*. New York: Taylor & Francis.

Armelagos, George J., Peter J. Brown, and Bethany Turner. 2005. "Evolutionary, historical and political economic perspectives on health and disease." *Social Science & Medicine* 61: 755–765.

Armelagos, George J., and Kristin N. Harper. 2009. "Emerging Infectious Diseases, Urbanization and Globalization in the Time of Global Warming." In *The Blackwell Companion to Medical Sociology*, edited by William C. Cockerham, 289–311. Hoboken: Wiley Publishing.

Barrett, Ronald. 2006. "Dark winter and the spring of 1972: Deflecting the social lessons of smallpox." *Medical Anthropology* 25 (2): 171–191.

Barrett, Ronald, Christopher W. Kuzawa, Thomas McDade, and George J. Armelagos. 1998. "Emerging Infectious Disease and the Third Epidemiological Transition." In *Annual Review Anthropology*, edited by W. Durham, 247–271. Palo Alto: Annual Reviews Inc.

Caldwell, John C. 1976. "Toward a restatement of demographic transition theory." *Population and Development Review* 2 (3/4): 321–366.

CDC. 1981. "Kaposi's Sarcoma and pneumocystis pneumonia among homosexual men—New York City and California." *Morbidity and Mortality Weekly Report* 30: 305–308.

Cohen, H.W., R.M. Gould, and V.W. Sidel. 2004. "The pitfalls of bioterrorism preparedness: The anthrax and smallpox experiences." *American Journal of Public Health* 94 (10): 1667–1671.

Farmer, P. 1996. "Social inequalities and emerging infectious diseases." *Emerging Infectious Diseases* 2 (4): 259–269.

Farmer, P. 1997. "Social scientists and the new tuberculosis." *Social Science & Medicine* 44 (3): 347–358.

Gross, Miriam 2016. Farewell to the God of Plague: Chairman Mao's Campaign to Deworm China. Univ of California Press.

Henderson, Donald A. 1980. "Smallpox eradication." *Public Health Reports* 95 (5): 422–426. https://doi.org/10.1038/npg.els.0003994

Johnson, Welkin A. 2019. "Origins and evolutionary consequences of ancient endogenous retroviruses." *Nature Reviews Microbiology* 17: 355–370.

Jones, K.E., N.G. Patel, M.A. Levy, A. Storeygard, D. Balk, J.L. Gittleman, and P. Daszak. 2008. "Global trends in emerging infectious diseases." *Nature* 451 (7181): 990–993.

Kim, Jim Yong, Aaron Shakow, Kedar Mate, Chris Vanderwarker, Rajesh Gupta, and Paul Farmer. 2005. "Limited good and limited vision: multidrug-resistant tuberculosis and global health policy." *Social Science & Medicine* 61 (4): 847–859.

Lederburg, J., R.E. Shope, and S.C. Oaks. 1992. *Emerging Infections: Microbial Threats to Health in the United States*. Washington, DC: Institute of Medicine, National Academy Press.

Mcfarlane Burnet, F. 1962. *Natural History of Infectious Disease*. Cambridge UK: Cambridge University Press.

McKeown, T. 1988. *The Origins of Human Disease*. Oxford: Basil Blackwell.

Meyer, R.D. 1983. "Legionella infections—A review of 5 years of research." *Reviews of Infectious Diseases* 5 (2): 258–278. <Go to ISI>://WOS:A1983QN73500009.

Omran, A.R. 1971. "The epidemiologic transition: A theory of the epidemiology of population change." *Millbank Memorial Fund Quarterly* 49 (4): 509–538.

Petersdorf, Robert G. 1986. "Training, cost containment, and practice: Effect on infectious diseases." *Review of Infectious Diseases* 8 (3): 478–487. https://doi.org/10.1093/clinids/8.3.478

Preston, Richard. 1994. *The Hot Zone*. New York: Random House.

Riley, James C. 2005. "Estimates of regional and global life expectancy, 1800–2001." *Population and Development Review* 31 (3): 537–543. https://doi.org/https://doi.org/10.1111/j.1728-4457.2005.00083.x

Salomon, Joshua A., and Christopher J.L. Murray. 2002. "The epidemiological transition revisited: Compositional models by age and sex." *Population and Development Review* 28 (2): 205–228.

Satcher, D. 1995. "Emerging infections: Getting ahead of the curve." *Emerging Infectious Diseases* 1 (1): 1–6.

Spellberg, Brad, and Bonnie Taylor-Blake. 2013. "On the exoneration of Dr. William H. Stewart: debunking an urban legend." *Infectious Diseases of Poverty* 2 (3). http://www.idpjournal.com/content/2/1/3

World Health Organization 2017. Antibacterial agents in clinical development: an analysis of the antibacterial clinical development pipeline, including tuberculosis. No. WHO/EMP/IAU/2017.11. World Health Organization.

Woolhouse, Mark, and Eleanor Gaunt. 2007. "Ecological origins of novel human pathogens." *Critical Reviews of Microbiology* 33: 231–242.

Zaman, Muhammad H. 2020. *Biography of Resistance: The Epic Battle Between People and Pathogens*. New York: HarperCollins.

Zhu, T, B.T. Korber, A.J. Nahmias, E. Hooper, P.M. Sharp, and D.D. Ho. 1998. "An African HIV-1 sequence from 1959 and implications for the origin of the epidemic." *Nature* 391 (6667): 594–597.

PART 1

The First Epidemiological Transition

CHAPTER 1

Our Paleolithic Baseline

*Man selects only for his own good; Nature only for
that of the being which she tends.*
Charles Darwin (1859: 83)

The early twenty-first century has seen rapid
advancements in biotechnology, ranging from gene
therapy and nanomedicine to robotic surgery and
AI diagnostics. At the same time, emerging threats
from some of the Earth's most ancient forms
of life are outpacing discoveries of vaccines and
antimicrobials—medicines that we have come to
rely on for day-to-day survival. These threats are
emerging just as our global networks of transport and trade are enabling the spread of these
pathogens to every corner of the globe. Our future
may glow with the promise of new technologies
but it may not be long before our technological responses to infectious diseases may be little different than those we employed in centuries
past.

That said, our past may hold future solutions to
these problems. Newer technologies are helping us
to gain insight into the earliest stages of human prehistory. There we can learn important lessons from
the lifestyles of our Paleolithic ancestors, who somehow managed to evade many of the more acute
and devastating infections we experience today. As
we will see, these lessons go far beyond simple
lifestyle recommendations and recipes for another
fad diet. Rather, they are fundamental adaptations to the biological, physical, and social environments in which our human ancestors lived for more
than 300,000 years. Indeed, many of these adaptations were employed by our proto-human ancestors (hominins) for several million years before we
became biologically "modern" human beings.

Humans are imaginative and narcissistic primates, so we should not be surprised that speculations about our hominin ancestors pre-date any
supporting scientific evidence. Such speculations
were popular among Enlightenment philosophers
of Europe. In Thomas Hobbes' seventeenth-century
treatise, *Leviathan*, the author argued for a central-
ized state to prevent the negative consequences of
what he hypothesized to be humanity's earliest,
"natural" form of social organization, the "war of
all against all." With this agenda in mind, Hobbes
described our ancestors as living in "continual fear
and danger of violent death," an existence which he
summarized as "solitary, poor, nasty, brutish, and
short" (Hobbes 1651). A century later, Jean Jacques
Rousseau issued a strong rebuttal in his *Discourse
on Inequality*, asserting that "natural man" was free
and living in "celestial and majestic simplicity, as
created by the 'divine Author'" (Rousseau 1754).
Shaped by political philosophy rather than empirical evidence, neither of these views were scientifically valid.

Despite the accumulation of scientific evidence
in subsequent years, the ghosts of Hobbes and
Rousseau continue to haunt twentieth-century
anthropological debates about ancient and contemporary foraging societies, groups often referred
to collectively as "hunter-gatherers." Some have
described them as an "original affluent society,"
based on observations of egalitarianism and lighter
workloads among certain contemporary groups
(Sahlins 1972). Others paint a bleaker picture,

Emerging Infections. Second Edition. Ron Barrett, Molly K. Zuckerman, Matthew R. Dudgeon, with George J. Armelagos, Oxford University Press.
© Ron Barrett, Molly K. Zuckerman, Matthew R. Dudgeon (2024). DOI: 10.1093/oso/9780192843135.003.0002

pointing to archaeological and ethnographic evidence of violence, food shortages, and gender inequality (Kaplan 2000). As in most academic debates, the answers probably lie somewhere between these extremes. And as with most human issues, they are probably subject to considerable variation.

We hope to avoid these pitfalls by presenting a basic pattern of Paleolithic living supported by multiple lines of evidence. These include direct evidence from archaeological and bioarchaeological studies of ancient, pre-agricultural societies, as well as biomolecular evidence from ancient sites and contemporary living organisms. They also include indirect evidence from ethnographic studies of contemporary foraging societies whose modes of subsistence, settlement, and social organization are probably similar to those of our Paleolithic past. These studies demonstrate how foraging modes of subsistence often produced the dietary diversity needed to maintain health and support immunity against infections. They also demonstrate how small, highly mobile, and geographically dispersed populations probably impeded the human-to-human transmission of acute or virulent pathogens. Finally, these studies strongly suggest how a more equitable distribution of essential resources in foraging band-level societies increased the physical resilience of people who might otherwise serve as initial targets and hosts for new infections.

As we will see, Paleolithic living was not a panacea for all problems and all diseases. Ancient foraging societies probably faced higher rates of parasitic infections and exposure to natural toxins than many settled societies today. Yet when we compare the lifestyles of this Paleolithic baseline to the major changes that occurred with the intensification of agriculture around the time of the Neolithic, we will understand better why our ancient foraging ancestors probably experienced fewer and less severe infectious diseases than did their farming descendants. Our present-day lifestyles are radically different from those of our Paleolithic past but the same broad factors of subsistence, settlement, and social organization still determine our risks for infectious diseases today, though they come at greater velocities and with global effects.

1.1 Evolutionary discordance and syndemics

We are examining a time frame that begins with a biological process, the emergence of biologically modern humans,[1] and ends with a cultural process, the emergence(s) of agriculture as the primary means of human subsistence. The earliest skeletons that closely resemble present day humans date to about 300,000 years ago while the earliest signs of intensive agriculture date to around 11,000 years ago. Between them lies a very long time period, and it should be noted that, in strictly archaeological terms, it spans from the Middle Paleolithic to the beginning of the Neolithic.[2] Most of our focus is on the Late Paleolithic and the period between the Paleolithic and the Neolithic (Epipaleolithic, Mesolithic), but these distinctions are not as important as the similarities and differences between human populations today and those of our pre-agricultural past.

Biologically, we are not so different from our prehistoric ancestors who once hunted on the African savanna. If a group of Late Paleolithic people were dressed in contemporary garb and instantly transported to the present day, they would easily blend in, appearance-wise, with the variety of people who frequent any international airport or train station. This is because the rate of mammalian evolution is too slow to see major anatomical changes in 50,000 years. Minor changes can and do arise, however, and genetic studies have found many instances of relatively rapid microevolution in response to selective pressures from regional environmental conditions. For humans, the rates of these minor changes may actually have increased in the last 20,000 years (Sabeti et al. 2006). We will address some of these microevolutionary issues later, but for now, it should be noted that the minor physiological differences that they have produced are well within the variation we would expect to find within human populations today. More importantly for this chapter and the next, microevolution does not account for the rapid change in mortality from disease that occurred when ancient foragers shifted to agricultural modes of living.

Cultural change occurs more frequently than genetic change. It can also spread more rapidly throughout our species. To demonstrate this, we need only consider how quickly most societies have changed, for better and worse, when the Internet and smartphones became widely available. Major health events can also produce rapid cultural transitions; it took less than a year for the world to change in response to the COVID-19 pandemic. Add another 10,000 years and we find that the descendants of fewer than 10 million mobile foragers settled down and expanded to a population of 8 billion people who are almost entirely dependent on agriculture. Our lifestyles have radically changed since the Paleolithic. Today, more than half the world's population lives in urban environments and billions of us shop for food produced industrially and brought to us by machines moving about in globally connected markets. All these changes occurred with little alteration to our biological makeup. We have essentially become "stoneagers living in the fast lane" (Eaton et al. 1988).

The mismatch between our cultural and biological makeup is known as evolutionary discordance.[3] This biocultural discrepancy has wide-reaching implications for human health in general and infectious diseases in particular. To begin with, it helps explain our susceptibility to the most prevalent chronic non-infectious diseases that increase our risk of dying *from* infectious diseases. For example, chronic non-infectious diseases have had a profound impact on COVID-19 mortality (Villalobos et al. 2021). While the details are still unfolding, a recent meta-analysis of COVID-19 patients reveals that the hazard of infection-related mortality increases 63 percent among people with cancer, 94 percent with diabetes, 210 percent with hypertension, and 360 percent with chronic kidney disease (Ng et al. 2021).

Past outbreaks of other coronaviruses show similar patterns. We find similar risk factors for infection during the 2002–2004 severe acute respiratory syndrome (SARS) pandemic,[4] adding chronic obstructive pulmonary disease (COPD) to the previous list of comorbid conditions (Booth et al. 2003; Chen et al. 2005; Leung et al. 2004). Among the first 47 cases of Middle East respiratory syndrome (MERS) in 2012, which was first documented in 2012, 45 had at least one pre-existing medical condition, the most common being diabetes, hypertension, and chronic heart and kidney diseases (Assiri et al.

2013). Yet although these coronavirus infections may be new, associations between infectious and non-infectious diseases have been known since the early 1930s, when unusually high indicators of tuberculosis (TB) were found in autopsies and X-rays of patients with diabetes (Root 1934). Since the 1990s, there has been a re-emerging interest in TB–diabetes comorbidity and its association with the rising prevalence of both diseases. This research reflects a recent emphasis by biomedical researchers on the relationships between comorbid infectious and non-infectious diseases (Cadena et al. 2019).

Associations between non-infectious and infectious diseases extend beyond simple matters of comorbidity, a clinical term that merely describes the presence of more than one medical condition in a patient. In recent years, the term syndemics has been used to describe the synergistic interactions between two or more co-occurring health conditions within a population. These synergies produce higher morbidity and mortality than the sum of their separate effects (Singer and Claire 2003; Weaver et al. 2016). Focusing on the root causes of these synergistic epidemics, medical anthropologists usually include social determinants such as poverty, violence, bigotry, and population displacement as health conditions in and of themselves (Mendenhall and Singer 2020). Syndemics mean that risk isn't just a feature that individual patients have but is instead a product of the interacting social, biological, and physical conditions that each resides within in their communities (Mendenhall and Singer 2020).

Non-infectious diseases can further the risk of infectious diseases by suppressing people's immune systems, putting sick patients in close contact with each other via frequent and lengthy hospital stays, and having them treated with repeated rounds of antimicrobials that further the evolution of drug-resistant pathogens. These kinds of proximate interactions reach syndemic proportions when they are further driven by large-scale social forces (Mendenhall and Singer 2020). When combined in a syndemic, the multiplied effects of these social and clinical factors produce a large reservoir of susceptible hosts for the entry, proliferation, and further spread of infectious diseases in human populations (Poteat et al. 2020).

Thinking in terms of prevention, many of us understand that chronic non-infectious diseases are strongly linked to our modern modes of living: our diets, our activities (or lack thereof), and the modified environments around us. Professionals and pundits tell us how these so-called lifestyle factors are bad for our health. For example, they tell us that cholesterol-rich diets can lead to heart disease through the accumulation of plaques in our arterial walls. They tell us that for many of us, an excess of processed, sugar-rich foods can lead to adult-onset (type 2) diabetes by overwhelming our body's ability to metabolize glucose. And they also tell us how physical exercise helps us to maintain optimum blood pressure and overall weight. But while we may understand the "hows" of healthy living, few of us understand *why* certain lifestyles are better or worse for human health.

To answer these "why" questions, we must begin with the fact that our present-day lifestyles are very different from those of our early human ancestors. Anthropologists commonly refer to these earlier lifestyles as environments of evolutionary adaptation (EEAs), and many propose that our EEAs hold the keys to human health. For thousands of centuries, Paleolithic humans, whose anatomy and physiology were very similar to our own today, lived as mobile foragers on the patchy forests of Africa and the temperate zones of Europe and Asia.

Prior to this, our hominin (pre-human) ancestors lived under similar conditions for another 3 million years or more. This means that 99.995 percent of our evolutionary history has been spent with our bodies adapting to mobile foraging lifestyles (see Figure 1.1). Therefore, because of the comparatively slow pace of genetic change, it would take more than 1,000 generations for our bodies to catch up, genetically speaking, to adapt fully to the cultural and ecological changes that have occurred in only a few millennia since the intensification of agriculture. In the meantime, we must contend with the hazards of the calorie-rich but nutrient-poor diets, physical inactivity, exposure to industrial pollution, and chronic stresses that typically characterize our current modes of living.

Not surprisingly, popular health messages for avoiding these hazards are essentially prescriptions for living more like our Paleolithic ancestors (Eaton et al. 1985, 1988). But although some of these messages have scientific validity, such as reducing how much processed food you eat, this chapter is not simply focused on diet and exercise; nor is it focused on individual lifestyles. Our aim is to examine broad categories of adaptive strategies and lifestyles among Paleolithic human populations, the ways in which these adaptations decreased the risk of developing some diseases and increased the risk

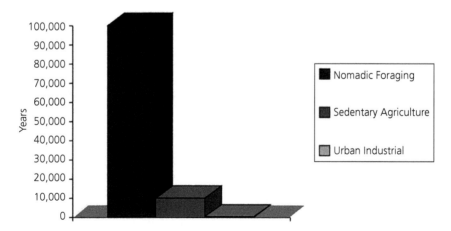

Figure 1.1 Histogram comparing the approximate number of years that humans spent engaged in nomadic foraging, sedentary agriculture, and urban industrial modes of living.

Source: Ron Barrett

of others, and the potential lessons this knowledge holds for adapting better to our world today.

1.2 Mobile foraging: Then and now

Reconstructing ancient lifestyles requires the consideration of evidence obtained by many different methods in multiple fields and disciplines, each having its own particular strengths, biases, and limitations. The most direct evidence comes from archaeological and bioarchaeological studies of ancient human remains, human artifacts, plant and animal remains, and other physical traces from surrounding environments. Biomolecular studies of these ancient materials (or archaeogenetics) can yield direct evidence of the organisms themselves, while further genomic analysis and modeling can yield indirect evidence of their broader relationships and evolutionary trajectories.

That said, these ancient materials can also pose significant methodological challenges. One major challenge is the degradation of these materials over long periods of time. These taphonomic processes involve physical and chemical changes that are mediated by the characteristics and contents of their surrounding environments. Under some of these conditions, plant, animal, and human remains will decompose quickly and are thus lost to time. Even recovered biomolecules like DNA and some proteins are often degraded to the point that analyses may be incomplete and highly challenging. Furthermore, because these taphonomic processes increase over time, our views of the Paleolithic can be biased by the more complete evidence at later rather than earlier periods (Bherensmeyer et al. 2000; French 2016).

Not surprisingly, the material remains of mobile foragers have tended to be geographically scattered. This is the case with animal and plant remains, and it is especially so with human remains. It would have been impractical for mobile societies to transport their dead over long distances in order to dispose of them in collective locations. Consequently it is very rare to find collective, ceremonial burials before the end of the Paleolithic, and with a few possible exceptions in the Mesolithic, no actual cemeteries appear until the Neolithic (Munro and Grosman 2010; Terberger et al. 2016). This is not to say that Paleolithic foragers did not have well-developed funerary traditions or other ritualized means of body disposal such as cremation and "sky" burials, only that the material evidence for these possible traditions is thus far unavailable until the Neolithic.

An additional challenge is that small, mobile forager Paleolithic bands rarely altered their environments in ways that left lasting traces in the archaeological record. Their habitations were designed to last for seasons, perhaps years, but not millennia, and they generally accumulated only those possessions that they could easily carry with them. Their possessions were most likely to have been made of degradable organic materials such as wood, bone, animal hides, and various plant materials not likely to be preserved in the archaeological record. Mobile foraging does not lend itself to accumulated possessions and a great deal of waste.

In contrast, present-day industrial agricultural societies are leaving behind mountains of garbage for future archaeologists. The United States alone produces 292 million tons of solid waste a year, with 22 percent of its foodstuffs going directly into the trash (US Environmental Protection Agency 2018). Perhaps more than our libraries and museums, this discarded waste will say a great deal about our industrial agricultural lifestyles. Not so with Paleolithic foragers, who possessed little and wasted even less. What little Paleolithic waste that has been found in the archaeological record is food garbage in the form of animal bones; these provide important clues about diet and subsistence behavior during this time period (Stiner and Bar-Yosef 2005).

Despite their paucity, cooking hearths and trash pits known as middens have provided important evidence about Paleolithic lifestyles. These sites contain the charred and butchered bones of wild as opposed to domestic animals, indicating that they obtained their animal protein through hunting game rather than from animals that they had domesticated. They also reveal that for many populations, marine and aquatic resources, like shellfish, gradually became critical components of Paleolithic diets (French 2016). Additionally, the emerging field of paleogenomics, aided by the development of high throughput, next-generation DNA sequencing, is independently tracing the timelines for the genetic divergence of wild and domesticated animal species (McHugo et al. 2019). Biochemical and even genetic evidence has been found in ancient human fecal remains, known as coprolites, which can reveal information about past diets, parasite loads, and environments, as well as human health in general (Camacho et al. 2018; Shillito et al. 2020).

Plant remains also provide a rich source of data for understanding Paleolithic diets and lifestyles. There is an entire subfield of archaeology, known as paleoethnobotany (in New World studies) or archaeobotany (in Old World studies), that examines the relationships between human populations and plants by examining the particular characteristics of ancient pollen, spores, and other tiny organic particles (Salamini et al. 2002; Vanderwarker et al. 2016). By examining the morphology and chemical composition of these particles, paleoethnobotanists can explore when plants gradually shifted certain characteristics from their wild to domesticated forms. These early shifts occurred during the Upper Paleolithic in some regions and in the Mesolithic and Epipaleolithic in other regions. Yet on the whole, these floral and faunal data confirm that, until about 11,000 years ago, humans primarily obtained their food by hunting wild animals and gathering wild plants. There may have been instances of small-scale horticulture or plant cultivation, as we often see in many contemporary foraging societies, but these activities were not of the duration and scale to produce detectable environmental changes.

Then and now, the foraging lifestyle is not conducive to large and densely clustered human populations. In the African patchy forests where the earliest humans lived, current foraging societies require an average of about one square mile per person to obtain an adequate diet from their local environment (Lee 1990). Such spacing requires that human beings live in small, widely scattered groups, which is also supported by the archaeological record. With the exception of ancient coastal fishing communities, most archaeological discoveries reveal cohabitating groups of no more than 30 to 40 people, which is similar to the median group size of contemporary foraging populations (Binford 2001; Kelly 2013; Marlowe 2005). That said, day-to-day cohabitation does not preclude larger networks of relationships,

and many contemporary smaller groups have complex and shifting interactions with one another, and the groups themselves change over time. This suggests that Paleolithic foragers consistently lived in small, scattered groups, but it is also likely that they temporarily convened into larger groups on a regular basis.

To sustain a successful foraging lifestyle, Paleolithic foraging societies had to maintain geographic dispersal over many thousands of years, so they must have somehow curbed their population growth, intentionally or unintentionally, and somehow balanced their birth rates and their death rates. A range of theories have been proposed to explain this, many of which are not exclusive of one another. Birth spacing may have been achieved through a combination of postpartum abstinence and lactational amenorrhea due to traditions of prolonged breastfeeding (Stallings et al. 1996). For example, the San mothers of the Kalahari often breastfeed their children until four years of age (Lee 1979). Selective female infanticide may have sometimes been used (Kimbrough et al. 2021) or population growth could have been checked by consistently very high rates of child mortality. A combination of Paleolithic archaeological evidence and ethnographic data from select contemporary foraging societies suggests that approximately 30 percent of infants died before the age of one year, while approximately 50 percent of children died before the age of 15—one out of every two children died before reaching maturity (Volk and Atkinson 2013). In some societies, periodic catastrophes could have resulted in major population declines, thereby checking the population growth (Gurven and Davison 2019). Paleolithic societies could have also dealt with increasing population size through subsequent group divisions and migration to other territories (Pennington 2001).

It should be noted that even for the populations and decades that have been reliably surveyed, we also do not always see constant population sizes among contemporary foraging societies (Gurven and Davison 2019). The Paleolithic spans a much longer period of time and includes much greater variation in the Earth's climate, which is likely to have led to fluctuations in birth and death rates in different populations, and thus regional fluctuations in human population levels over the course of many millennia (Page and French 2019). Indeed, these fluctuations may have driven some populations toward primary, permanent agriculture.

In addition to food remnants and artifacts there is a great deal to be learned about the health of Paleolithic foragers from their skeletons and teeth. Chapter 2 will examine this skeletal evidence in some detail for the purpose of comparing the overall health of human societies before and after the transition from foraging to agriculture. In the meantime, we can examine ethnographic data from contemporary foraging societies with cultural adaptations analogous to those ancient past and synthesize these data with basic archaeological information about ancient subsistence and demography.

Ethnographic studies of contemporary foraging societies present their own set of unique challenges. Chief among them is environmental and cultural representation. All human societies were foraging prior to the Neolithic. However, by the mid-nineteenth century, primary foragers[5] were almost non-existent, comprising less than 0.001 percent of the world's population (Pennington 2001). By the mid-1990s, it was estimated that of the few remaining foraging societies, no population was consuming an entirely wild diet. Today, if we use the criteria that members of a foraging society must consume a diet of over 90 percent wild foods, no society would meet this requirement (Apicella and Crittenden 2015). Instead, almost all foraging populations consume a mixed diet that includes varying degrees of farmed foods, wild foods, and possibly nutritional subsidies (Crittenden and Schnorr 2017; Headland and Blood 2002). As such, we might regard contemporary foragers to be exceptional cases, especially when we consider that many of their local environments are in remote or inhospitable locations, places that are impractical for modern settlement (Volk and Atkinson 2013). From this perspective, today's mobile foraging is not what it used to be; at least, not precisely.

As suggested by the mixed diets, none of today's remaining foraging societies could be considered pristine in the sense of being untouched by the industrialized world (Crittenden and Schnorr 2017; Headland and Blood 2002). It is important to note that most recent or contemporary forager societies have exchange relationships with their sedentary neighbors (Crittenden and Schnorr 2017; Headland and Blood 2002). We also should not assume that every foraging group has been living continuously as foragers in the same manner. For example, the !Kung San, an extensively studied foraging society in the southern African Kalahari, had already experimented with pastoralism long before they met their first anthropologist (Lee 1990). Likewise, the Punan of Borneo probably shifted from agriculture to foraging in order to trade forest products with the Chinese (Hoffman 1986).

Other contemporary foraging societies may still be mobile and dependent on wild resources but have nevertheless adopted many cultural elements from industrialized agricultural societies (see Figure 1.2) (Headland and Blood 2002). For example, members of the Martu, Australian indigenous societies in western Australia, prefer to use LED headlamps when they hunt at night and employ iPods to listen to Lady Gaga (Bird 2010). And among the Hadza, another extensively studied contemporary foraging society in northern Tanzania, musicians make visits to town to collaborate with members of urban Chaka communities on fusion-rap recordings (Kweka 2017). These shifting patterns and cultural contacts have sparked debates among anthropologists about the extent to which contemporary foragers are culturally representative of our prehistoric ancestors (Ames 2004; Guenther 2007).

Yet even when we recognize these limitations, there are basic characteristics of subsistence, population structure, and social organization for which contemporary foraging societies may serve as proxies for Paleolithic living. Mindful of the gross and sometimes ethnocentric generalizations that have been made about foraging societies in the earlier years of anthropological scholarship, we can still make conservative and carefully contingent claims about *some* cultural similarities in the adaptive strategies of these groups when they are based on well-grounded empirical research. These claims are necessarily made at lower resolution than those of finer-grained and context-specific ethnographic studies, yet the two approaches can complement one another, and diversity aids our analysis when

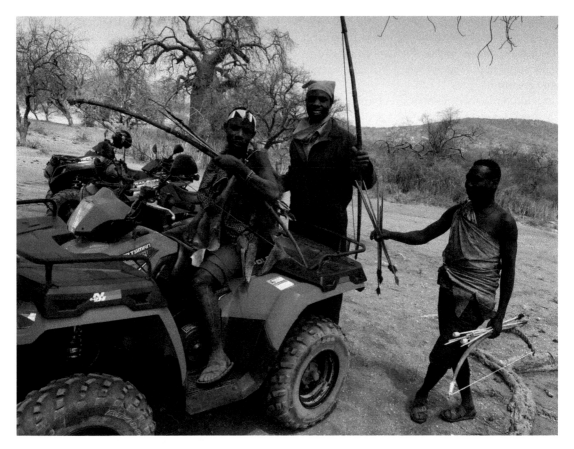

Figure 1.2 Photograph of contemporary Hadza foragers using all-terrain vehicles (ATVs) for hunting. The use of contemporary technology belies the notion that primary foraging societies are somehow "pristine," and thus living in conditions that are identical to the Paleolithic past.

Source: Kiretono (2015). Wikimedia commons. CCA-SA 4.0 International. https://commons.wikimedia.org/wiki/File:Traditional_Meets_Modern.jpg

even modest similarities are shared across very different societies. Triangulating these findings with archaeological and biological data, we can begin to understand how these adaptations would have affected the disease landscapes of our ancient foraging ancestors.

1.3 Subsistence, nutrition, and activity

Anthropologists have collected detailed data on the subsistence activities and nutritional intake of foraging societies in nearly every human-occupied natural environment in the world (Crittenden and Schnorr 2017). Additionally, there is a great deal of biomedical research on the many links between nutrition and immunity. Tragically, the latter is

supported by an overwhelming number of clinical and epidemiological observations about the consequences of malnutrition, both under-nutrition and over-nutrition (e.g., obesity), for human morbidity and mortality to all manner of diseases. Combining these lines of evidence reveals the ways in which the subsistence strategies employed by foraging societies can function to increase or decrease the risk of both infectious and non-infectious diseases.

Closely tied to human immunity, adequate nutrition has always been our chief line of defense against infectious diseases. Conversely, malnutrition is the primary cause of immunodeficiency worldwide (Katona and Katona-Apte 2008). Malnutrition includes deficiencies of micronutrients, which are essential vitamins and minerals such as zinc and calcium, as well as macronutrients, such as carbohydrates, fat, and protein. Over the human life course, malnutrition can greatly impact the competence of the immune system to protect against invading pathogens. A large reason for this is that the immune system demands a significant amount of metabolic energy, if only to muster defenses against the range of pathogens that we encounter on a daily basis, even in the safest of human environments. For example, in their inactive state, white blood cells (leukocytes), immune cells that play key roles in protecting the body against infection, consume about 22 percent of our basal metabolic energy; this can increase to 50 percent in the case of a significant infectious disease like a blood-borne infection (Straub et al. 2010). Combined with these demands, the hypermetabolism of other vital tissues can more than double energy requirements, even before including the additional demands of fever and physical activities such as shivering (Miles 2006).

During a severe infection, the immune system needs immediate glucose, stored in the form of glycogen, to produce and mobilize immune cells specific to the antigens of the infecting pathogen as well as other signaling molecules. The human body initially meets these demands by becoming hyperglycemic until its glycogen stores are depleted; then it turns to fats, ketones, and, as a last resort, the proteins of muscle cells (Ullrey 2005). Suffice to say, it is necessary to have an adequate margin of stored metabolic energy to avoid the latter stages and survive a major infectious disease. This margin is also necessary for preventing a major infection in the first place.

With metabolic energy in mind, we turn to protein-energy malnutrition (PEM) (a.k.a. protein-energy under-nutrition (PEU)), which describes the overall imbalance or lack of macronutrients to energy requirements (protein and/or energy). Even in its milder phases, PEM is associated with decreased antibody production, thymus and lymph node reduction, and diminished function of phagocytes, cytokines, and t-lymphocytes, all of which are needed to mount an effective immune response to pathogens. Studies show that otherwise healthy individuals with only moderate PEM have immune indicators, such as arginase deficiency, that are

comparable to those found in people living with HIV who have low T-lymphocyte counts bordering on full-blown AIDS (Cloke et al. 2010; Takele et al. 2016). Thus it is not surprising that PEM is associated with opportunistic infections commonly found in AIDS patients, tuberculosis being a major example (Saag et al. 2018; Shaible and Kaufman 2007).

Micronutrients are also essential to healthy immune function, and their deficiencies can profoundly affect innate as well as adaptive (i.e., acquired) host defenses (Gombart et al. 2020). For example, iron deficiency, the most common form of anemia worldwide, has widespread effects throughout the immune system and it interferes with the differentiation and growth of protective epithelial tissues, such as in the respiratory tract. Consequently, iron deficiency is associated with the breakdown of cell membranes, such as in the skin, the respiratory tract, and the gastrointestinal tract. Vitamin A deficiency is similarly associated with the breakdown of epithelial barriers to pathogen entry. For these reasons, even minor deficiencies in nutrients can lead to major infections (Gombart et al. 2020).

Prior to industrial-era systems of agricultural food production, supplementation, and distribution, dietary diversity was the only way to achieve the breadth of intake necessary to avoid nutritional deficiencies and thus maintain immunological competence. From tropical to temperate environments, anthropologists have found that most contemporary forager societies have highly diverse diets in comparison to agriculturalist societies in the same regions, and they are even more diverse than some industrialized societies (Cordain 2002; Crittenden and Schnorr 2017). This diversity is well illustrated in the !Kung San of the southern African Kalahari desert, who regularly hunt 34 different species of animals, and occasionally hunt another 24 species (Lee 1990). The San identify 14 edible fruits and nuts, 15 edible berries, 41 roots and bulbs, and another 17 vegetables that even urbanized Westerners might find in their salads.

Although extensively studied, the !Kung San represent only one example of human foraging diversity. Prior to their forced settlement, the Ache of Paraguay hunted 56 animal species and gathered another 44 plant species, as well as honey, within their tropical forest environments (Hill and Hurtado 1996). Studies of the Anbarra in Australia, the Efe in Central Africa, and the Hadza in east Africa reveal similarly diverse diets (Jenike 2001). The dietary diversity of these foraging societies represents behavioral and social adaptations to their environments. Their dietary breadth greatly increases the likelihood that members of these societies will meet the nutritional requirements for health in general, and immunological competence in particular (Turner and Thompson 2013). Indeed, analyses of nutrition status among the !Kung San and several indigenous Australian groups, show that they were well within healthy ranges (Metz et al. 1971; O'Dea 1996).

Linking these cultures of dietary diversity to our environment of evolutionary adaptation, we should not be surprised to find evidence that our species has evolved physiological "incentives" for seeking a variety of foods (Ó Gráda 2009; Rolls et al. 1982). These include neural mechanisms for shifting food interest with food quantity, biocultural relationships between specific foods, emotions, and associative memories, and genetically mediated variations in taste perception, the latter most likely arising in the Late Upper Paleolithic and Neolithic (Turner and Thompson 2013).

In addition to meeting nutritional requirements, dietary diversity has other adaptive advantages. Chief among them is behavioral flexibility in the face of changing environmental conditions. Droughts, floods, and crop diseases can have devastating effects on agricultural societies that depend on only a few food types for their subsistence. We have seen this with the Irish Potato Famine as well as the Ethiopian and Chinese famines of the nineteenth century (Ó Gráda 2009). Although these events were influenced by important political and socio-economic factors, their impact was greatly exacerbated by reliance on only one or a few different food sources. Societies that can obtain a variety of foods under different conditions are better protected against the potential hazards of these environmental crises, especially when they can resort to a range of alternative "famine foods" during severe shortages. Finally, the ability to forage a variety of foods allows greater migratory flexibility for mobile groups that may need to travel through relatively scarce regions to arrive at more plentiful destinations (Hawkes and O'Connell 1992).

Within their diverse menus, foragers commonly eat foods that are high in protein, high in fiber, and low in saturated fats. Much of this is accomplished through a diet proportionally higher in plant-based foods than animal-based foods (Crittenden and Schnorr 2017). Large-scale surveys of foraging societies completed in the mid-twentieth century indicate that for most foragers, especially those living in warm climates (e.g., temperate environments), the median diet is composed of approximately 53–65 percent gathered plant foods and 26–35 percent hunted foods, with fished foods often making up the difference; furthermore red meat from wild animals is much leaner than domestic varieties (Eaton et al. 1988; Marlowe 2005, 2010). These estimates are averaged across seasons, within which substantial variation could occur. Nevertheless but most non-circumpolar foragers consumed largely plant-based diets (Marlowe 2010).

Biomolecular evidence from Paleolithic archaeological sites can also reveal information on past human diets. While Paleolithic human coprolites are scarce, calcified human dental plaque, or dental calculus recovered from human teeth is nearly ubiquitous in the archaeological record. Calculus not only preserves biomolecules from human tissues but also from microbes present in the oral cavity (oral microbiota), as well as organic debris from dietary intake and any environmental material that enters the mouth (Hendy et al. 2018; Warinner et al. 2015). As such, these data can yield a wealth of biomolecular data on human diets, overall health, and surrounding conditions. It is therefore noteworthy that dental calculus recovered from Middle to Upper Paleolithic skeletons supports archaeological evidence that these individuals were eating plant based diets, filled with complex carbohydrates that came from unprocessed plants rather than processed grains (Hardy et al. 2015).

Overall, we can estimate that most Paleolithic foragers consumed around six times the fiber of the average American today, while the latter consumes almost twice the calories from dietary fat as the average forager (Eaton and Eaton 2000). Interestingly, studies also reveal that the gut microflora of some present-day foragers, such as the Hadza, are uniquely better adapted to these higher fiber diets than are those of present-day consumers of industrial diets (Schorr et al. 2014). Additionally, Biometric studies of societies that engage almost exclusively in foraging for subsistence typically find them to be thinner and with higher aerobic capacities than people in industrial societies. Consequently, they have significantly lower prevalences of diabetes, heart disease, and several forms of cancer (Cordain et al. 2002).

Many readers may be familiar with the popular Paleo Diet movement. This movement has its origin in the work of two physician-anthropologists, who applied the concept of evolutionary discordance to extol the benefits of a diet similar to those of our Paleolithic ancestors (Eaton and Konner 1985). These recommendations were expanded into a health advice book entitled *The Paleolithic Prescription* (Eaton et al. 1988). Fourteen years later, an exercise physiologist built on these and other contributions, including his own collaboration with one of the *Paleolithic Prescription* authors, to publish *The Paleo Diet* (Cordain 2002). It too was informed by evolutionary discordance and solid analysis of evidence from multiple disciplines, but the popularity of this book also led to contributions from many others who were not so scientifically inclined. Thus began diet books for vegans and household pets, gourmet recipes and high-cost specialty food items, as well as lifestyle programs for parenting, office politics, and sexual relations. For better and for worse, the original ideas underlying evolutionary discordance have evolved from a specialized suffix ("Paleo") to a household buzzword for healthy lifestyles in the twenty-first century.

To be clear, our Paleolithic ancestors did not have a singular formula for diet and healthy living any more than the recommendations of the previously cited authors. Instead, the previous authors promoted a set of general parameters that are still common to a wide variety of contemporary foraging societies (Konner and Eaton 2010). Given the diversity of environments in which contemporary foragers live, we should not be surprised to find similar variation in their respective diets. Indeed, it could be argued that adaptive flexibility in the face of diverse environmental conditions is probably the best way to generalize the wide variety of Paleolithic and contemporary foraging strategies.

It would be impossible for most of us to eat *exactly* how Paleolithic people did, even if we try to eat lean proteins, fruits, vegetables, seeds, and nuts that approximate the ancient proportions. Unless everything we eat comes from foraged wild plants and animals, then everything we would buy at the store will be the product of thousands of years of domestication and most likely connected to an industrial production system. But with high contemporary interest in Paleolithic diets and lifestyles, we would argue that most safe and sensible diets are at least as similar to a Paleolithic diet as they are to one another. We could summarize them with another popular recommendation: "Eat food. Not too much. Mostly plants" (Pollan 2007). However, for the sake of authenticity, we may wish to add some wild game to the list.

It should also be noted that subsistence foraging also comes with significant drawbacks and challenges. Being a successful full-time forager requires considerable skill and experience. This includes a detailed knowledge of plants, animal behavior and tracking, land navigation, and weather patterns. Hunting and gathering also requires a significant investment in bodily energy. An adult !Kung San female, for example, who is typically twice as efficient at obtaining food as her hunting male counterparts, expends an average of 2,500 calories over two hours while gathering 23,000 calories worth of food (Lee 1990). Compare this with the modern suburban shopper within our industrial agricultural system, who may expend 100 calories over the 20 minutes it takes to obtain the same 23,000 calories. Of course, this does not count the effort needed to earn the money for the food, which could range from 150–400 calories per hour, depending on whether the shopper sits at a desk or performs heavier tasks in an urban environment. Yet even by conservative estimates, the !Kung San forager expends about seven times more energy than the shopper to extract the same amount of calories.

Foraging also involves a great deal of uncertainty. Although most foragers have a broad range of available food sources, they may face seasonal shortages of edible plants and wild game, forcing them to range over longer distances in search of better opportunities (Hawkes and O'Connell 1992); notably though, recent foragers are much less likely than agriculturalists to experience famine (Berbesque et al. 2014). Large-game hunting entails high levels of physical risks in the pursuit and killing of animals, including the risk of falling prey to other carnivorous animals. Even plant foods may entail significant risks; many wild food staples, like wild cassava, contain high percentages of cyanide-like substances and other toxins specifically harmful to the liver, gut, and central nervous system (Johns 1996). Although many societies have developed processing methods for reducing these toxins, gathering and eating them can still be risky. Government-approved foods on store shelves in our present-day industrial societies may not always be nutritious, or even proper "food" per se, but they rarely pose the same risks for poisoning as plants found in the wild.

Lastly, foraging lifestyles often pose a high risk of exposure to parasites, a broad category of organisms that include single-celled (non-bacterial) protozoans, helminthic worms, and small arthropods that live within or upon our bodies at our expense.[6] Many of these parasites are considered "heirloom" pathogens insofar as they originated in Africa during human and hominin evolution and have affected us for so many millennia that we share a long coevolutionary history (Harper and Armelagos 2013; Kliks 1990; Sprent 1969). Much like our prized family heirlooms, these species have been "in our possession" for a very long time. Heirloom pathogens can be identified by their shared presence in both humans and non-human primates such as chimpanzees (Mitchell 2013). They can also be identified based on evidence of their presence at both human and hominin archaeological sites in Africa, where there is genomic evidence of a long period of coevolution between the parasites and their hosts (Harkins and Stone 2015).

Many heirloom parasites have been recovered from human coprolites, mummies, pelvic soil from burials, and latrines recovered from archaeological sites (Mitchell 2013). Their presence is indicated by microscopic evidence, such as the presence of identifiable parasite eggs, as well as microbial DNA in the case of protozoa. Notably, the prevalence of eggs and DNA traces in Paleolithic coprolites indicates that ancient foragers were often afflicted with pinworms, roundworms, and tapeworms, as well as

head and body lice (Mitchell 2013; Reinhard et al. 2013). (Figure 1.3). They were also afflicted with some lower-virulence pathogens that cause chronic infections, like *Helicobacter pylori*, a common cause of stomach ulcers, and in the Americas, the non-venereal subspecies of *Treponema pallidum* responsible for yaws (Harper et al. 2008; Linz et al. 2007; Moodley et al. 2012).

Immune mechanisms that underlie atopic[7] conditions, such as a variety of common allergies and certain forms of asthma found in many contemporary societies, suggest that parasitic infections were a major selective force in our evolutionary history. Presently, about 400 million people experience allergic rhinitis (a.k.a. hay fever), 300 million experience some form of allergic asthma, 200 million people experience at least one food allergy, and about 10 percent of the human population is allergic to at least one biopharmaceutical (American Academy of Allergy, Asthma, & Immunology 2021; World Allergy Organization 2013). These allergies, also known as atopic conditions, are overreactions of the immune system to substances that would otherwise be minimally harmful or not harmful at all. The overreactions are mediated by a class of antibodies known as immunoglobulin E (IgE). For a time, it seemed that IgEs had no other function other than to cause allergies, but later research found they are a key defense against parasitic infections, targeting the same proteins found on many helminthic species, and the infections themselves activate the same immune cells, specifically TH-2 cytokines, eosinophils, and mast cells associated with atopic conditions (Fitzsimmons et al. 2014). These parasite-specific immune defenses are shared with other mammalian species, indicating that they were present throughout hominin evolution and, given their energetic cost, they would have gradually deteriorated over time, like the human appendix, if parasites were not a major problem in our Paleolithic environments.

These common pathways also support what is known as the Hygiene Hypothesis, which proposes that exposure to parasites, organic contaminants, and possibly other minimally pathogenic microorganisms, such as in the oral microflora, is essential for developmentally training the immune system during childhood growth and development

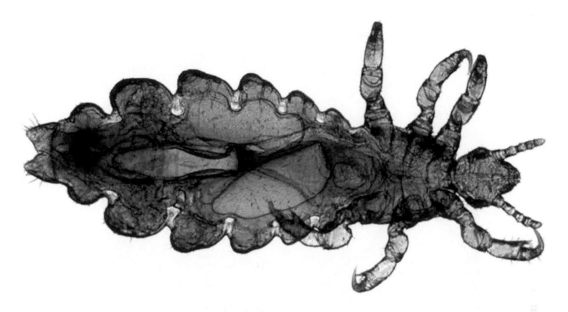

Figure 1.3 Female body louse (*Pediculus humanus var. corporis*) magnified 39 times by a scanning electron microscope (SEM). Lice were likely heirlooms that we inherited from our non-human primate ancestors. Following the Neolithic, this and other lie species would become vectors of more acute and virulent diseases such as typhus.

Source: Janice Haney Carr (2006). U.S. Centers for Disease Control and Prevention. Public domain. https://phil.cdc.gov/Details.aspx?pid=9243

(Strachan 1989). In other words, our immune systems require a certain level of "dirt" to develop, without which it may be predisposed to dysregulation, thereby inducing the hyper-reactions associated with atopic conditions. This explains why the prevalence of allergies is increasingly high among populations living in well-developed urban areas that are often much cleaner than poor and rural areas of the world (Gage 2005). When organisms to which our immune systems have long become accustomed—our "old friends"—are removed, as in the case of overly clean environments, human immune systems may be predisposed to dysregulation. If so, then this would suggest that our immune systems are evolutionarily better adapted to the higher parasite exposure of our Paleolithic ancestors than the more sanitized environments of affluent urban living.

Informed by growing research in the human microbiome, this hypothesis has been expanded to include the immunological training provided by diverse populations of microflora in the mouth and gut among our old friends. Notably, the hygiene hypothesis may also explain the high and growing

prevalence of chronic inflammatory and autoimmune conditions (CIDs) in high-income industrial populations, though researchers are cautious to note that these latter diseases are often mediated by complex genetic and environmental variables that are independent of the atopic mechanisms discussed above (Rook 2012).

In contrast to the heirloom species, souvenir pathogens are those acquired by human populations after the ancient migrations out of Africa (Kliks 1990; Sprent 1969). Humans acquired these pathogens as they moved into new environments, much like a traveler acquiring a souvenir from a journey. Most souvenir pathogens are zoonotic, meaning that their primary hosts were non-human animals (Mitchell 2013). Among foraging societies without any domesticated animals (e.g., horses, dogs), souvenir infections would have occurred through incidental exposures such as insect and animal bites, contact with animal urine and feces, and the preparation and consumption of infected meat. In the Paleolithic, these souvenir pathogens are likely to have included African trypanosomiasis (a.k.a. sleeping sickness), tetanus, scrub typhus,

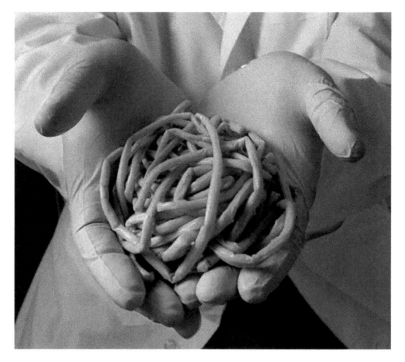

Figure 1.4 Mass of *Ascaris lumbricoidis* worms that had been passed by a child in Kenya. Humans first acquired these helminth (i.e. worm) infections during ancient migrations to new environments. *Ascaris* worms are typically transmitted in egg-form via fecal-oral route.

Source: Photograph by James Gathany. Provided by Henry Bishop, U.S. Centers for Disease Control and Prevention. Public domain. https://phil.cdc.gov/Details. aspx?pid=9813

relapsing fever, trichinosis, avian or ichthyic tuberculosis, leptospirosis, and schistosomiasis (Cockburn 1971; Froment 2001; Harper and Armelagos 2013). But although these pathogens were probably endemic to Paleolithic foragers, most existed as chronic infections that people could live with and carry around for long periods of time, or else they were primary zoonoses with little to no human-to-human transmissibility (see Figure 1.4).

Paleolithic foragers probably experienced their greatest risk of acquiring souvenir pathogens when butchering wild animals, an issue we will return to later in the book when we discuss the potential role of so-called bushmeat hunting in the present-day introduction of new pathogens to human populations. But although ancient foragers probably faced the same exposure risks as hunters today, we will see in the next Section that the small and scattered nature of these highly mobile groups would have prevented the kind of widespread transmission characteristic of today's densely settled and globally interconnected populations.

1.4 Population and transmission dynamics

Although the global human population today is exponentially larger and more interconnected than it was during the Upper Paleolithic, the same principles of size, density, and mobility affect the transmission of infectious diseases. Those diseases with short time periods between infection and the onset of debilitating symptoms generally require large and dense human host populations in order to sustain ongoing transmission. Measles is a prime example of this principle. A pathogen which diverged from the recently eradicated bovine rinderpest around 5,000 years ago, the measles virus is so contagious that 90 percent of unvaccinated people can contract the disease simply by sharing the same room with an infected person (Furuse et al. 2010).

To quantify the infectivity of measles transmissibility, we can employ an epidemiological measure known as the basic reproduction number (R_0 or "R-naught"), that denotes the average number of people infected by a single case in a (theoretical) population in which everyone is susceptible and equally in contact with one another. It should first be noted that calculations of R_0 can vary based on different underlying assumptions; these can only crudely approximate the socio-environmental as well as biological factors involved in actual disease transmission (Delamater et al. 2019). That said, retrospective data from previous outbreaks can give us reasonable R_0 estimates for particular places and moments in time: 1.5 for Ebola in West Africa in 2014–2016; 3.5 for SARS in southern China in 2002–2003; and in the years just prior to its eradication, 4.5 for smallpox in India (van der Driessche 2017). In comparison, a 1960s measles outbreak in Ghana had a reproduction number of 14.5, which falls within a general estimate of 12–18 for this infection.

Yet even with its high transmissibility and capacity for further spread, measles rarely persists in small, relatively isolated, unvaccinated communities when they are exposed to the virus. For example, a classic longitudinal study that followed 19 native Caribbean island communities over 15 years found that measles outbreaks were self-limited in unvaccinated populations of less than 500,000 people (Black 1980). Similar outcomes were observed for measles outbreaks in the Faro islands, the common cold on the Norwegian island of Spitsbergen, and poliomyelitis among isolated communities of northern Indigenous Alaskans. When initially exposed, all these communities were highly susceptible to these acute infections, but ongoing transmission was limited by populations sizes and densities and, more precisely, the rates at which people came into contact with one another (Black 1980).

This is not to say that small, insular populations are free of viruses. Another classic study found many isolated native Amazonian groups with antibody titers for herpes and Epstein-Barr viruses that were comparable to suburban populations in the eastern United States (Black 1975). The key here

is that the herpes and Epstein-Barr viruses usually persist as chronic infections with recurring symptoms that are usually relatively mild. Like the heirloom and souvenir parasites of Paleolithic foragers, these chronic viruses can be carried for long periods of time and thus do not require frequent transmission in order to maintain themselves in human populations.

Even in larger and more socially connected societies, an infectious disease epidemic can extinguish itself when the initial onset of the disease is too rapid and the symptoms too severe to sustain human to human transmission. This was the case for 13 outbreaks of Ebola Virus Disease (EVD) that had occurred in Sub-Saharan Africa over a period of 28 years prior to the 2013–2016 epidemic (CDC 2021). All these prior outbreaks were severe, with case mortality ranging from 37 percent to 88 percent, but not one of them resulted in more than 500 known infections without any effective treatments or vaccines at the time. These epidemics essentially "flashed out" in those populations.

It is highly probable that the sudden and terrible nature of EVD posed a limit on its transmission. Like the HIV virus, the Ebola virus is largely transmitted by blood and body fluids, though fomite (object) transmission is also possible (Jacob et al. 2020). Yet for HIV, people can unknowingly transmit the virus for years before serious symptoms appear, and even these may not be easily recognized or attributed to the virus. In contrast, Ebola progresses to a highly debilitating and often recognizable condition known as the "wet symptoms" in about eight to ten days. In the rural areas where the virus appeared, this would have been a narrow window for person-to-person transmission.

The 2013–2016 Ebola epidemic was very different. It resulted in far more cases and deaths than all previous epidemics combined: more than 28,000 cases and 11,000 deaths if we only count Guinea, Liberia, and Sierra Leone (CDC 2021). Why was this epidemic so large? One possibility is that it involved a more infectious variant than in prior epidemics. The RNA genome of the Ebola virus is especially prone to mutation, and as such, nearly every epidemic entails new genetic variants. We are still awaiting further research to determine whether any coding differences led to actual traits that could increase human-to-human transmissibility during this particular epidemic (Dudas et al. 2017; Holmes et al. 2016; Kelly et al. 2018). Chapter 5 explores these issues in further detail.

Without excluding the potential contribution(s) of viral evolution, we can be certain of one major difference: the 2013–2016 epidemic involved denser and more mobile host populations than the previous epidemics. This was the first epidemic that was concentrated in urban centers, and these centers were had increased their population densities by almost threefold in the last 50 years (Alexander et al. 2015). West Africa has long been known for its interregional mobility, and there are denser road networks in Guinea, Liberia, and Sierra Leone than in the Central African countries where the previous epidemics had occurred. Correlating known Ebola cases with road density, one study found that the district-level risk of infection increased 3.7 percent for every 10 meters of road per square kilometer (Gomez-Barroso 2017).

Foraging societies offer a stark contrast to the densely clustered and fast-moving populations of urbanized agriculturally based societies. A comparative study of 478 foraging cultures revealed a median local group size of 30 people, usually composed of a few family units organized as a band or camp, and a median population density of 10 people per square kilometer (Marlowe 2005). There can be considerable variation in these numbers, especially when fishing and pastoral communities in northern temperate zones are included. Yet if we focus only on a subsample of 175 societies that live in warmer climates and travel solely on foot, then the median group size further decreases to 26 people, though the overall population density increases to a whopping five people per square kilometer. Compare this with the majority of the world population, which lives in urban centers of at least 50,000 people at a minimum density of 5,000 inhabitants per square kilometer (Ritchie and Roser 2019).

The tendency of present-day foraging societies to live in small and scattered groups makes sense when we consider the time and energy required to obtain sufficient food resources for a given community. Most of these societies engage in what is known as "central place foraging" in which they camp in resource-rich locations (a.k.a. dense food

patches) and disperse radially for hunting and gathering activities (Kelly 2013). Depending on the characteristics of the local environment—such as the availability and predictability of resources, and the risks and energy involved in obtaining them—a larger group usually requires a much larger foraging radius to feed itself. Yet at some point, there is a limit to this radius in terms of the cost-benefit trade-off between the time and energy expended on food acquisition and the energy obtained from the food itself. In this way, particular environments and subsistence activities constrain the maximum size of foraging groups.

This kind of analysis is informed by a more general framework known as Optimal Foraging Theory. This theory considers the most evolutionarily advantageous pattern of human or animal food-acquisition behaviors while balancing factors such as energy, risk, and time (Pyke 1984). These are very practical considerations, applicable to a variety of human subsistence issues, and we will see this framework again when we examine the origins of plant domestication (Piperno 2017). That said, it should also be noted that specific hypotheses generated from Optimal Foraging Theory do not always prove to be accurate, and its explanations are often insufficient to address the great complexity of human–environmental interactions.

We see this complexity when considering the density of foraging populations in relation to the primary biomass, the total mass of plant material, as a proxy measure for the carrying capacity of local subsistence environments (Marlowe 2005). Initially, there is a tendency for population densities to increase with primary biomass, but the densities level off at a certain point. After this, local group sizes tend to persist independent of biomass, suggesting that social relationships may also be a determining factor, an issue we will address in the next section.

We also need to account for mobility and contacts between foraging groups. Even though most foragers co-reside in small groups, their external networks of social relations can extend considerably (Bird et al. 2019). If the rates of inter-group exchange are high enough, some foraging societies might even approximate the conditions of larger populations, at least in terms of contacts for disease transmission. Ethnographic studies also reveal a great deal of social fluidity within these groups, with families and subgroups breaking off and reforming because of shifting subsistence opportunities, interpersonal conflicts, or changes in adult sex ratios (Kelly 2013). But these fission–fusion dynamics often occur over the course of months and years, which is longer than the incubation periods of most acute infectious diseases.

We can reasonably assume that inter-group contact would be infrequent for people traveling on foot, and thus the opportunities for inter-group infection would also be infrequent. If a Paleolithic forager contracted a highly transmissible disease like measles, it would quickly spread to the rest of the group with devastating consequences. But if it took several weeks before the infected group came into contact with other groups and so forth, then there would be little opportunity for onward transmission to the broader population. Moreover, if the disease is severe enough to restrict mobility then, with the possible exception of forays for outside assistance, the group as a whole would be immobilized until the last person either recovers from their infection or dies.

Pedestrian mobility may be too slow for intergroup transmission of acute and virulent infectious diseases. Furthermore, movements over the course of months or seasons reduce environmental exposure to pathogens in any given area, which could prevent infections from occurring in the first place. In the aforementioned cross-cultural study, contemporary foraging societies move an average of seven times per year (Marlowe 2005). Such mobility is important for tracking the movements of animal prey, taking advantage of changing resource opportunities, and avoiding shortages as well as the total depletion of local microenvironments. Mobility can also reduce the amount of time spent in a given micro-environment, where zoonotic pathogens might otherwise evolve the ability to infect human hosts over time. We will return to this issue in later chapters when examining the evolutionary dynamics of new and drug resistant pathogens.

Lastly, the mobility of foraging societies reduces the accumulation of waste and water that could serve as growth media for pathogens and their vectors. Waste inevitably accumulates, even in the best maintained camps. Burying food waste and feces outside camps would still attract insects and animals to the general area. Food stores would attract animal vectors within or closer to the perimeter and human habitation. The size of these stores would likely be proportional to the period of residence, and longer storage periods would increase the risk of food contamination. Housing itself can provide niches for arthropods and rodents. Moving locations, even on a seasonal basis, would significantly reduce these accumulations and their associated risks for infection.

1.5 Social organization and inequalities

In the introductory chapter, we discussed the epidemiological problems posed by socioeconomic inequalities in a globally connected world. If political borders and social boundaries are permeable to pathogens but impermeable to resources for their prevention and control, then the higher rates of infection among impoverished and vulnerable people will inevitably result in more infections for everyone. We saw this with smallpox, which continued to re-infect high-income countries after the Second World War until it was eventually eliminated in low-income countries and then eradicated[8] in the late nineteenth century (Barrett 2006). Today high-income countries must continue their polio vaccination programs because the disease still persists in low-income countries from South Asia to Sub-Saharan Africa (Polio Global Eradication Initiative 2021). And at the time of this publication, the COVID-19 pandemic is becoming globally endemic with new variants emerging from poorer societies that do not have enough vaccines for their populations (Dyer 2021).

Inequalities are also driving the evolution of antimicrobial resistant infections. Chapter 5 examines these dynamics in some detail, but for now it will suffice to consider the threat posed by multidrug-resistant (MDRTB) and extensively drugresistant tuberculosis (XDRTB). Prior to the development of antibiotics, TB was one of the chief causes of infectious disease mortality worldwide, causing an estimated 1 billion deaths over the last 200 years (Paulson 2013). We may see these numbers again if the disease becomes incurable due to widespread drug resistance. Some of the world's poorest countries carry the greatest burdens of MDRTB and XDRTB, with the highest risk factors being poverty and healthcare underutilization along with under-nutrition, incarceration, displacement, and comorbidity with HIV and diabetes (Dheda et al. 2017; Pradipta et al. 2018; WHO 2020). It will only be a matter of time before these so-called hot spots and reservoir populations become launching points for the global spread of an incurable and deadly infection. TB is but one of many diseases that is developing drug resistance in vulnerable populations.

We have examined nutritional and population factors that protected Paleolithic populations against acute infections. These would have included diseases such as smallpox, polio, and the pathogenic coronaviruses afflicting present-day societies. TB, however, can persist as both a dormant and chronic infection, so it is not surprising to discover evidence that human-infective strains probably arose 75,000 years ago (Cardona et al. 2020). But a TB infection is not the same as TB disease. This distinction is illustrated by today's global burden of latent TB infection, which is estimated to affect 24 percent of the world population, while only about 10 million of these people actually become sick with the disease (Houben and Dodd 2016; WHO 2020). Ten million is an alarming and unacceptable number, but it is far fewer than the 1.9 billion cases that would occur if every TB infection progressed to full-blown disease. As with many infections, pathogen exposure alone is insufficient to cause actual TB disease. The pathogen must also find the right host and environmental conditions, and these are strongly mediated by poverty and other health disparities. This disparity principle would have also applied to the parasitic and chronic infections that occurred in Paleolithic foraging societies.

Socio-economic disparities are far less prevalent in contemporary foraging societies than in state-level societies. Across a tremendous diversity of cultures and surrounding environments, most present-day foragers are characterized by relatively egalitarian social structures and extensive sharing practices (Binford 2001; Kelly 2013; Marlowe 2005). There are several explanations for this phenomenon. Small groups do not require formal leadership, so it is common to find that group decisions are made by some kind of consensus, though depending on the culture, the decision-making body may be restricted according to gender and age (Lee and Daly 1999). Individuals who assert too much authority often find themselves ignored or abandoned by the local group, and any major conflicts between competing factions are typically resolved by splitting into separate groups (Marlowe 2010).

Foraging societies also tend to have few divisions of labor or specializations that could form class distinctions, though once again, those associated with gender and age are common (Kelly 2013). Indeed, over-specialization may even be hazardous, given the flexibility needed to obtain a variety of resources as environments change by season and year, or as the group moves from place to place. Also, mobility itself poses a limit on the accumulation of material resources when no-one can possess more than can be consumed or carried on foot. With few total possessions, there cannot be many material distinctions between people (Flannery and Marcus 2012).

Contemporary foragers often have strongly held rules and beliefs about the sharing of food, work, and territory. Even when skilled foragers wastefully pursue rare food sources as displays of prowess, a phenomenon known as *costly signaling*, the social message conveys a promise of future generosity when the wealth is widely shared (Bird and Smith 2005). This does not mean that everyone shares alike, however, or that people do so without obtaining some benefit or advantage; rather, sharing often occurs without expectation of specific or immediate returns, but with a general expectation that returns will come, even if they take a different form, occur at a later time, pass through a different channel, or benefit a relative rather than one's self. Borrowing a concept from evolutionary biology, anthropologists refer to these interactions as reciprocal altruism (cf. Trivers 1971).

Sharing can offer many practical benefits for foragers. It can increase dietary diversity, as when foragers pool, exchange, or redistribute different kinds of food. It can also serve as a kind of risk insurance in the face of indeterminate resources, such as when a successful hunting party shares its meat with an unsuccessful party on one day, and then receives meat from that party on another day when the fortunes are reversed (Kelly 2013). The insurance principle can also apply to longer-term risks. For instance, when the Ache were living as foragers, individuals from families considered to be highly generous received more food from the larger group when they were sick or injured than those from families who were considered to be less generous (Gurven et al. 2000). Similarly, the Hadza avoid sharing with people who have been stingy in the past by moving away from them altogether, which can have dire consequences for day-to-day subsistence as well as for long-term health (Marlowe 2010). Health and wellbeing are strong motives for generosity.

This is not to suggest that foraging lifestyles are free of all inequalities and conflicts. As previously discussed, there are often cultural instances of gender inequalities, such as men obtaining better cuts of meat, or women doing a disproportionate share of the work (Endicott 1999). Some groups also experience high levels of interpersonal violence, which can be a significant reason for group fissions and relocations (Gurven and Kaplan 2007). Yet even when faced with these challenges, most foraging societies are far more egalitarian and equitable in their distributions and duties than their agricultural counterparts.

Finally, when comparing these ethnographic observations with the archaeological record, it is notable that material evidence of social differences does not appear until the Neolithic (Flannery and Marcus 2012. By extension, we could also predict that the concomitant health benefits and disease risks would also be more equitably distributed in ancient foraging groups than in their agrarian descendants, offering an additional layer of health protection. We will test this prediction in the next chapter.

Notes

1. *Homo sapiens sapiens.*
2. The Paleolithic begins with the first evidence of human material culture (stone tools) approximately 3 million years ago, and ends with the first evidence of agricultural intensification approximately 12,000 to 10,000 years ago. The Paleolithic is divided into the Early (c. 3 million to 300,000 years ago), Middle (300,000 to 50,000 years ago), and the Upper or Late Paleolithic (c. 50,000 to 12,000 years ago). The Epipaleolithic (in the Near East) and the Mesolithic (southeastern Europe) represent periods between the Upper Paleolithic and the Neolithic. The Neolithic began approximately 12,000 years ago, with the beginning of agricultural intensification, and ended approximately 6,000 years ago.
3. This is also referred to as genetic discordance or mismatch hypothesis.
4. Although some have termed the SARS outbreak a pandemic due to its international impact, others have rightfully noted that there were not enough cases to warrant the term. The distinctions between epidemics and pandemics are not clear, so the latter is operationally defined by health officials.
5. Defined as those who consumed 100 percent of their diet from wild foods (Lee and Devore 1968).
6. Biologists commonly use the term "parasite" in two distinct ways. The first way is used theoretically to describe a general set of relationships and interactions between species that are detrimental to one or both participants. In this sense, any pathogen is a parasite by definition. The second way is used taxonomically to describe the three categories of pathogens we discuss and distinguish them from bacteria and viruses. Although parasites are not part of the Lineal taxonomy, this category is commonly used in the fields of parasitology and infectious disease medicine.
7. "Atopic" means sensitivity to allergens.
8. Elimination of disease occurs when its incidence has been reduced to zero in a geographical area through deliberate efforts, like vaccination. Eradication of a disease occurs when its incidence has been permanently reduced to zero, meaning that intervention measures are no longer needed.

References

Alexander, Kathleen A., Claire E. Sanderson, Madav Marathe, Bryan L. Lewis, Caitlin M. Rivers, Jeffrey Shaman, John M. Drake et al. 2015. "What factors might have led to the emergence of Ebola in West Africa?" *PLoS neglected tropical diseases* 9 (6): e0003652.

American Academy of Allergy Asthma & Immunology. 2021. "Allergy statistics."

Ames, K.M. 2004. "Supposing hunter-gatherer variability." *American Antiquity* 69 (2): 364–374. https://doi.org/10.2307/4128427

Apicella, C.L., and A.N. Crittenden. 2015. "Hunter-Gatherer Families and Parenting." In *The Handbook of Evolutionary Psychology*, edited by D. Buss, 578–597. New Jersey: John Wiley & Sons.

Assiri, Abdullah, Jaffar A. Al-Tawfiq, Abdullah A. Al-Rabeeah, Fahad A. Al-Rabiah, Sami Al-Hajjar, Ali Al-Barrak, Hesham Flemban et al. 2013. "Epidemiological, demographic, and clinical characteristics of 47 cases of Middle East respiratory syndrome coronavirus disease from Saudi Arabia: A descriptive study." *Lancet Infectious Diseases* 13 (9): 752–761. https://doi.org/10.1016/S1473-3099(13)70204-4

Barrett, R. 2006. "Dark winter and the spring of 1972: Deflecting the social lessons of smallpox." *Medical Anthropology* 25 (2): 171–191.

Behrensmeyer, A.K., S.M. Kidwell, and R.A. Gastaldo. 2000. "Taphonomy and paleobiology." *Paleobiology* 26 (4): 103–147. https://doi.org/10.1666/0094-8373(2000)26[103:Tap]2.0.Co;2

Berbesque, J.C., F.W. Marlowe, P. Shaw, and P. Thompson. 2014. "Hunter-gatherers have less famine than agriculturalists." *Biology Letters* 10(1): 20130853. https://doi.org/10.1098/rsbl.2013.0853

Binford, Louis. 2001. *Constructing Frames of Reference: An Analytical Method for Archaeological Theory Building Using Hunter-Gatherer and Environmental Data Sets*. Berkeley: University of California Press.

Bird, Rebecca. 2010. Personal communication. May 2010.

Bird, Rebecca Bliege, Brooke Scelza, Douglas W. Bird, and Eric Alden Smith. 2012. "The hierarchy of virtue: mutualism, altruism and signaling in Martu women's cooperative hunting." *Evolution and Human Behavior* 33 (1): 64–78.

Bird, R.B., and E.A. Smith. 2005. "Signaling theory, strategic interaction, and symbolic capital." *Current Anthropology* 46 (2): 221–248.

Black, Francis L. 1975. "Infectious diseases in primitive societies." *Science* 187: 515–518.

Black, Francis L. 1980. "Modern Isolated Pre-Agricultural Populations as a Source of Information on Prehistoric Epidemic Patterns." In *Changing Disease Patterns and Human Behavior*, edited by N.F. Stanley and R.A. Joske, 37–54. London: Academic Press.

Booth, C.M., L.M. Matukas, G.A. Tomlinson, A.R. Rachlis, D.B. Rose, H.A. Dwosh, S.L. Walmsley et al. 2003. "Clinical features and short-term outcomes of 144 patients with SARS in the greater Toronto area." *Journal of the American Medical Association* 289 (21): 2801–2809. https://doi.org/10.1001/jama.289.21.JOC30885

Cadena, J., S. Rathinavelu, J.C. Lopez-Alvarenga, and B.I. Restrepo. 2019. "The re-emerging association between tuberculosis and diabetes: Lessons from past centuries." *Tuberculosis* 116: S89–S97. https://doi.org/10.1016/j.tube.2019.04.015

Camacho, M., A. Araujo, J. Morrow, J. Buikstra, and K. Reinhard. 2018. "Recovering parasites from mummies and coprolites: an epidemiological approach." *Parasites & Vectors* 11. https://doi.org/10.1186/s13071-018-2729-4

Cardona, P.J., M. Catala, and C. Prats. 2020. "Origin of tuberculosis in the Paleolithic predicts unprecedented population growth and female resistance." *Scientific Reports* 10 (1). https://doi.org/10.1038/s41598-019-56769-1

CDC. 2021. *History of Ebola Disease Outbreaks: Cases and Outbreaks of Ebola Disease by Year*. Centers for Disease Control and Prevention. https://www.cdc.gov/vhf/ebola/history/chronology.html. Accessed: 11/16/2023. Last Updated: August 30, 2023.

Chen, K.T., S.J. Twu, H.L. Chang, Y.C. Wu, C.T. Chen, T.H. Lin, S.J. Olsen et al. 2005. "SARS in Taiwan: An overview and lessons learned." *International Journal of Infectious Diseases* 9 (2): 77–85. https://doi.org/10.1016/j.ijid.2004.04.015

Cloke, T.E., L. Garvey, B.S. Choi, T. Abebe, A. Hailu, M. Hancock, U. Kadolsky et al. 2010. "Increased level of arginase activity correlates with disease severity in HIV-seropositive patients." *Journal of Infectious Diseases* 202 (3): 374–385. https://doi.org/10.1086/653736

Cockburn, T.A. 1971. "Infectious disease in ancient populations." *Current Anthropology* 12 (1): 45–62.

Cordain, L., S.B. Eaton, J. Brand Miller, N. Mann, and K. Hill. 2002. "The paradoxical nature of hunter-gatherer diets: meat-based, yet non-atherogenic." *European Journal of Clinical Nutrition* 56(Suppl 1): S42–S51.

Cordain, Loren. 2002. *The Paleo Diet: Lose Weight and Get Healthy by Eating the Food You Were Designed to Eat*. New York: John Wiley.

Crittenden, A.N., and S.L. Schnorr. 2017. Current views on hunter-gatherer nutrition and the evolution of the human diet. *American Journal of Physical Anthropology* 162: 84–109. https://doi.org/10.1002/ajpa.23148

Darwin, Charles. 1859. *On the Origin of Species by Means of Natural Selection*. London, UK: J. Murray.

Delamater, P.L., E.J. Street, T.F. Leslie, Y.T. Yang, and K.H. Jacobsen. 2019. "Complexity of the basic reproduction number (R0)." *Emerging Infectious Diseases* 25 (1): 1–4.

Dheda, K., T. Gumbo, G. Maartens, K.E. Dooley, R. McNerney, M. Murray, J. Furin et al. 2017. "The epidemiology, pathogenesis, transmission, diagnosis, and management of multidrug-resistant, extensively drug-resistant, and incurable tuberculosis." *Lancet Respiratory Medicine* 5 (4): 291–360. https://doi.org/10.1016/s2213-2600(17)30079-6

Dudas, G., L.M. Carvalho, T. Bedford, A.J. Tatem, G. Baele, N.R. Faria, D.J. Park et al. 2017. "Virus genomes reveal factors that spread and sustained the Ebola epidemic." *Nature* 544 (7650): 309. https://doi.org/10.1038/nature22040

Dyer, O. 2021. "Covid-19: Variants are spreading in countries with low vaccination rates." *British Medical Journal* 373. https://doi.org/10.1136/bmj.n1359

Eaton, Stanley Boyd, and Stanley Boyd Eaton III. 2000. "Paleolithic vs. modern diets–slected pathophysiological implications." *European journal of nutrition* 39: 67–70.

Eaton, S. Boyd, and Melvin Konner. 1985. "Paleolithic nutrition. A consideration of its nature and current implications." *New England Journal of Medicine* 312 (5): 283–289.

Eaton, S. Boyd, Marjorie Shostak, and Melvin Konner. 1988. *The Paleolithic Prescription: A Program of Diet & Exercise and a Design for Living*. New York: Harper & Row.

Endicott, Karen L. 1999. "Gender relations in hunter-gatherer societies." In *The Cambridge Encyclopedia of Hunter-Gatherers*, edited by Catherine Panter-Brick, Robert Layton, and Peter Rowley-Conwy, 411–418. Cambridge UK: Cambridge University Press.

Fitzsimmons, Colin, Franco Falcone, and David Dunne. 2014. "Helminth allergens, parasite-specific IgE, and its protective role in human immunity." *Frontiers in Immunology* 5 (51): 1–12.

Flannery, Kent, and Joyce Marcus. 2012. *The creation of inequality: how our prehistoric ancestors set the stage for monarchy, slavery, and empire*. Cambridge, MA: Harvard University Press.

French, J.C. 2016. "Demography and the Palaeolithic archaeological record." *Journal of Archaeological Method and Theory* 23 (1): 150–199. https://doi.org/10.1007/s10816-014-9237-4

Froment, Alain. 2001. "Evolutionary Biology and Health of Hunter-Gatherer Populations." In *Hunter-Gatherers: An Interdisciplinary Perspective*, edited by Catherine Panter-Brick, Robert Layton, and Peter Rowley-Conwy, 236–266. Cambridge UK: Cambridge University Press.

Furuse, Yuki, Akira Suzuki, and Hitoshi Oshitani. 2010. "Origin of measles virus: Divergence from rinderpest virus between the 11th and 12th centuries." *Virology Journal* 7 (1): 52–55.

Gage, Timothy B. 2005. "Are modern environments really bad for us?: revisiting the demographic and epidemiologic transitions." *American Journal of Physical Anthropology* 128 (S41): 96–117.

Gombart, A.F., A. Pierre, and S. Maggini. 2020. "A review of micronutrients and the immune system-working in harmony to reduce the risk of infection." *Nutrients* 12 (1). https://doi.org/10.3390/nu12010236

Guenther, M. 2007. "Current issues and future directions in hunter-gatherer studies." *Anthropos* 102 (2): 371–388.

Gurven, Michael D., and J. Davison Raziel. 2019. "Periodic catastrophes over human evolutionary history are necessary to explain the forager population paradox." *Proceedings of the National Academy of Sciences* 116 (26) 12758–12766. https://doi.org/10.1073/pnas.1902406116

Gurven, Michael, and Hillard Kaplan. 2007. "Longevity among hunter-gatherers: A cross-cultural examination." *Population and Development Review* 33 (2): 321–365. https://doi.org/10.1111/j.1728-4457.2007.00171.x

Gurven, M., W. Allen-Arave, K. Hill, and M. Hurtado. 2000. "'It's a wonderful life': Signaling generosity among the Ache of Paraguay." *Evolution and Human Behavior* 21 (4): 263–282. https://doi.org/10.1016/s1090-5138(00)00032-5

Hardy, Karen, Jennie Brand-Miller, Katherine D. Brown, Mark G. Thomas, and Les Copeland. 2015. "The importance of dietary carbohydrate in human evolution." *The Quarterly review of biology* 90 (3): 251–268.

Harper, Kristin N., and George J. Armelagos. 2013. "Genomics, the origins of agriculture, and our changing microbe-scape: time to revisit some old tales and tell some new ones." *American journal of physical anthropology* 152: 135–152.

Harper, K.N., P.S. Ocampo, B.M. Steiner, R.W. George, M.S. Silverman, S. Bolotin, A. Pillay et al. 2008. "On the origin of the treponematoses: a phylogenetic approach." *PLoS Neglected Tropical Diseases* 2: e148

Hawkes, K., and J.F. O'Connell. 1992. "On optimal foraging models and subsistence transitions." *Current Anthropology* 33 (1): 63–66.

Hendy, Jessica, Christina Warinner, Abigail Bouwman, Matthew J. Collins, Sarah Fiddyment, Roman Fischer, Richard Hagan et al. 2018. "Proteomic evidence of dietary sources in ancient dental calculus." *Proceedings of the Royal Society B: Biological Sciences* 285 (1883): 20180977.

Headland, T.N., and D.E. Blood. 2002. *What Place for Hunter-Gatherers in Millennium Three?* Dallas: SIL International

Hill, Kim R., and A. Magdalena Hurtado. 1996. *Ache Life History: The Ecology and Demography of a Foraging People.* Hawthorne: Aldine de Gruyter.

Hobbes, Thomas. 1651. *Leviathan, or, the Matter, Forme, & Power of a Common-Wealth Ecclesiasticall and Civil.* London: Printer for A. Cooke.

Hoffman, Carl L. 1986. *The Punan: Hunters and Gatherers of Borneo.* Ann Arbor: UMI Research Press.

Holmes, E.C., G. Dudas, A. Rambaut, and K.G. Andersen. 2016. "The evolution of Ebola virus: Insights from the 2013–2016 epidemic." *Nature* 538 (7624): 193–200. https://doi.org/10.1038/nature19790

Houben, Rein MGJ, and Peter J. Dodd. 2016. "The global burden of latent tuberculosis infection: a re-estimation using mathematical modelling." *PLoS medicine* 13 (10): e1002152.

Jacob, S.T., I. Crozier, W.A. Fischer, A. Hewlett, C.S. Kraft, M.A. de La Vega, M.J. Soka et al. 2020. "Ebola virus disease." *Nature Reviews Disease Primers* 6 (1): 31. https://doi.org/10.1038/s41572-020-0147-3

Jenike, Mark R. 2001. "Nutritional ecology: diet, physical activity and body size." *Hunter-gatherers: An interdisciplinary perspective,* edited by Catherine Panter-Brick, Robert H. Layton and Peter Rowley-Conwy, 205–238. Cambridge: Cambridge University Press.

Johns, Timothy. 1996. *The origins of human diet and medicine: Chemical ecology.* Tucson, AZ: University of Arizona Press.

Kaplan, D. 2000. The Darker Side of the "Original Affluent Society." *Journal of Anthropological Research* 56: 301–24.

Katona, P., and J. Katona-Apte. 2008. "The interaction between nutrition and infection." *Clinical Infectious Diseases* 46 (10): 1582–1588. https://doi.org/10.1086/587658

Kelly, J.D., M.B. Barrie, A.W. Mesman, S. Karku, K. Quiwa, M. Drasher, G.W. Schlough et al. 2018. "Anatomy of a hotspot: Chain and seroepidemiology of Ebola virus transmission, Sukudu, Sierra Leone, 2015–16." *Journal of Infectious Diseases* 217 (8): 1214–1221. https://doi.org/10.1093/infdis/jiy004

Kelly, Robert L. 2013. *The Foraging Spectrum: Diversity in Hunter-Gatherer Lifeways.* Washington DC: Smithsonian Institution Press.

Kimbrough, E.O., G.M. Myers, and A.J. Robson. 2021. "Infanticide and human self domestication." *Frontiers in Psychology* 12. https://doi.org/10.3389/fpsyg.2021.667334

Kliks, M.M. 1990. "Helminths as heirlooms and souvenirs: a review of New World paleoparasitology." *Parasitology Today* 6 (4): 93–100.

Konner, M., and S. Boyd Eaton. 2010. "Paleolithic nutrition twenty-five years later." *Nutrition in Clinical Practice* 25: 594–602

Kweka, John (Chaga). 2017. Personal communication. October, 2017.

Lee, R.B. 1968. *The !Kung San: Men, Women, and Work in a Foraging Society.* Cambridge: Cambridge University Press.

Lee, Richard B. 1979. *The !Kung San: Men, Women, and Work in a Foraging Society.* Cambridge UK: Cambridge University Press.

Lee, Richard B., and Richard Daly. 1999. "Foragers and Others." In *The Cambridge Encyclopedia of Hunter-Gatherers,* edited by Richard B. Lee and Richard Daly, 1–19. Cambridge UK: Cambridge University Press.

Leung, G.M., P.H. Chung, T. Tsang, W. Lim, S.K.K. Chan, P. Chau, C.A. Donnelly et al. 2004. "SARS-CoV antibody prevalence in all Hong Kong patient contacts." *Emerging Infectious Diseases* 10 (9): 1653–1656. https://doi.org/10.3201/eid1009.040155

Linz, B., F. Balloux, Y. Moodley, A. Manica, H. Liu. P. Roumagnac, D. Falush et al. 2007. "An African origin for the intimate association between humans and Helicobacter pylori." *Nature* 445: 915–918.

Marlowe, Frank W. 2005. "Hunter-gatherers and human evolution." *Evolutionary Anthropology* 14: 54–67.

Marlowe, Frank W. 2010. *The Hadza Hunter-Gatherers of Tanzania.* Berkeley: University of California Press.

McHugo, G.P., M.J. Dover, and D.E. Machugh. 2019. "Unlocking the origins and biology of domestic animals using ancient DNA and paleogenomics." *BMC Biology* 17 (1). https://doi.org/10.1186/s12915-019-0724-7

Mendenhall, Emily, and Merrill Singer. 2020. "What constitutes a syndemic? Methods, contexts, and framing from 2019." *Current Opinion in HIV and AIDS* 15 (4): 213–217.

Metz, J., D. Hart, and H.C. Harpending. 1971. "Iron, folate, and vitamin B12 nutrition in a hunter-gatherer people: A study of the !KungBushmen." *American Journal of Clinical Nutrition* 24, 229–242.

Miles, J.M. 2006. "Energy expenditure in hospitalized patients: Implications for nutritional support." *Mayo Clinic Proceedings* 81 (6): 809–816. https://doi.org/10.4065/81.6.809

Mitchell, Piers D. 2013. "The origins of human parasites: exploring the evidence for endoparasitism throughout human evolution." *International Journal of Paleopathology* 3(3): 191–198.

Moodley, Y., B. Linz, R.P. Bond, M. Nieuwoudt, H. Soodyall, C.M. Schlebusch, S. Bernhoft et al. 2012. "Age of the association between Helicobacter pylori and man." *PLoS Pathology* 8.

Munro, Natalie D., and Leore Grosman. 2010. "Early evidence for feasting at a burial cave in Israel." *Proceedings of the National Academy of Sciences* 107 (35): 15362–15366.

Ng, W.H., T. Tipih, N.A. Makoah, J.G. Vermeulen, D. Goedhals, J.B. Sempa, F.J. Burt et al. 2021. "Comorbidities in SARS-CoV-2 patients: A systematic review and meta-analysis." *Mbio* 12 (1). https://doi.org/10.1128/mBio.03647-20

O'Dea, Kerin. 1996. "Body weight and the risk of diabetes in Aborigines." *Aboriginal and Islander Health Worker Journal* 20 (3): 5–7.

Ó Gráda, Cormac. 2009. *Famine: A Short History*. Princeton: Princeton University Press.

Page, Abigail, and Jennifer French. 2019. "Reconstructing prehistoric demography: What role for extant hunter-gatherers?" *Evolutionary Anthropology* 29: 332–335.

Paulson, T. 2013. "A mortal foe." *Nature* 502 (7470): S2–S3. https://doi.org/10.1038/502S2a

Polio Global Eradication Initiative. 2021. "Polio now." https://polioeradication.org/polio-today/polio-now/

Pennington, Renee. 2001. "Hunter-gatherer demography." *Hunter-gatherers: An interdisciplinary perspective*: 170–204.

Piperno, Dolores R. 2017. "Assessing elements of an extended evolutionary synthesis for plant domestication and agricultural origin research." *Proceedings of the National Academy of Sciences* 114 (25): 6429–6437.

Pollan, Michael. 2007. *The omnivore's dilemma: A natural history of four meals*. New York, NY: Penguin.

Poteat, Tonia, Gregorio A. Millett, Laron E. Nelson, and Chris Beyrer. 2020. "Understanding COVID-19 risks and vulnerabilities among black communities in America: the lethal force of syndemics." *Annals of Epidemiology* 47: 1–3. https://doi.org/10.1016/j.annepidem.2020.05.004

Pradipta, Ivan Surya, Lina Davies Forsman, Judith Bruchfeld, Eelko Hak, and Jan-Willem Alffenaar. 2018. "Risk factors of multidrug-resistant tuberculosis: A global systematic review and meta-analysis." *Journal of Infection* 77 (6): 469–478. https://doi.org/10.1016/j.jinf.2018.10.004

Pyke, Graham H. 1984. "Optimal foraging theory: a critical review." *Annual review of ecology and systematics* 15 (1): 523–575.

Reinhard, Karl J., Luis Fernando Ferreira, Françoise Bouchet, Luciana Sianto, Juliana MF Dutra, Alena Iniguez, Daniela Leles et al. 2013. "Food, parasites, and epidemiological transitions: a broad perspective." *International Journal of Paleopathology* 3 (3): 150–157.

Ritchie, Hannah, and Max Roser. 2019. "Urbanization." *Our World in Data*. https://ourworldindata.org/urbanization

Rolls, B.J., E.T. Rolls, and E.A. Rowe. 1982. "The Influence of Variety on Human Food Selection and Intake." In *The Psychobiology of Food Selection*, edited by L.M. Baker, 101–122. Westport: AVI.

Rook, Graham AW. 2012. "Hygiene hypothesis and autoimmune diseases." *Clinical reviews in allergy & immunology* 42: 5–15.

Root, H.F. 1934. "The association of diabetes and tuberculosis." *New England Journal of Medicine* 210: 1–13. https://doi.org/10.1056/NEJM193401042100101

Rousseau, J. J. 1754. A Discourse on a Subject Proposed by the Academy of Dijon: What is the Origin of Inequality among Men, and is it Authorized by Natural Law? Translated by G.D.H. Cole, public domain. Rendered into HTML and text by Jon Roland of the Constitution Society. <http://www.constitution.org/jjr/ineq.htm>, last accessed October 31, 2001.

Saag, L.A., M.P. LaValley, N.S. Hochberg, J.P. Cegielski, J.A. Pleskunas, B.P. Linas, and C.R. Horsburgh. 2018. "Low body mass index and latent tuberculous infection: a systematic review and meta-analysis." *International Journal of Tuberculosis and Lung Disease* 22 (4): 358. https://doi.org/10.5588/ijtld.17.0558

Sabeti, P.C., S.F. Schaffner, B. Fry, J. Lohmueller, P. Varilly, O. Shamovsky, A. Palma, et al. 2006. "Positive natural selection in the human lineage." *Science* 312 (5780): 1614–1620. https://doi.org/10.1126/science.1124309

Sahlins, Marshall. 1972. *Stone Age Economics*. Chicago, IL: Aldine.

Salamini, F., H. Ozkan, A. Brandolini, R. Schafer-Pregl, and W. Martin. 2002. "Genetics and geography of wild cereal domestication in the Near East." *Nature Reviews Genetics* 3 (6): 429–441. https://doi.org/10.1038/nrg817

Schnorr, Stephanie L., Marco Candela, Simone Rampelli, Manuela Centanni, Clarissa Consolandi, Giulia Basaglia, Silvia Turroni et al. 2014. "Gut microbiome of the Hadza hunter-gatherers." *Nature Communications* 5(1): 1–12.

Schaible, Ulrich E., and Stefan H. E. Kaufmann. 2007. "Malnutrition and infection: complex mechanisms and global impacts." *PLoS medicine* 4(5): e115.

Shillito, L.M., J.C. Blong, E.J. Green, and E.N. van Asperen. 2020. "The what, how and why of archaeological coprolite analysis." *Earth-Science Reviews* 207. https://doi.org/10.1016/j.earscirev.2020.103196

Singer, Merrill, and Scott Clair. 2003. "Syndemics and public health: Reconceptualizing disease in bio-social context." *Medical Anthropology Quarterly* 17 (4): 423–441.

Sprent, J. F. A. 1969. "Evolutionary aspects of immunity in zooparasitic infections." *Immunity to parasitic animals* 1.

Stallings, J.F., C.M. Worthman, C. PanterBrick, and R.J. Coates. 1996. "Prolactin response to suckling and maintenance of postpartum amenorrhea among intensively breastfeeding Nepali women." *Endocrine Research* 22 (1): 1–28.

Stiner, Mary C., and Ofer Bar-Yosef. 2005. *The faunas of Hayonim Cave, Israel: A 200,000-year record of Paleolithic diet, demography, and society*. No. 48. Harvard University Press.

Strachen, David. 1989. "Hay fever, hygiene, and household size." *British Medical Journal* 299 (6710): 1259–1260.

Straub, R.H., M. Cutolo, F. Buttgereit, and G. Pongratz. 2010. "Energy regulation and neuroendocrine-immune control in chronic inflammatory diseases." *Journal of Internal Medicine* 267 (6): 543–560. https://doi.org/10.1111/j.1365-2796.2010.02218.x

Takele, Y., E. Adem, M. Getahun, F. Tajebe, A. Kiflie, A. Hailu, J. Raynes, et al. 2016. "Malnutrition in Healthy Individuals Results in Increased Mixed Cytokine Profiles, Altered Neutrophil Subsets and Function." *PloS One* 11 (8). https://doi.org/10.1371/journal.pone.0157919

Terberger, Thomas, Andreas Kotula, Sebastian Lorenz, Manuela Schult, Joachim Berger, and Bettina Jungklaus. 2016. "Standing upright to all eternity—The Mesolithic burial site at Groß Fredenwalde, Brandenburg (NE Germany)." *Quartär* 62: 133–153.

Trivers, Robert L. 1971. "The evolution of reciprocal altruism." *The Quarterly review of biology* 46 (1): 35–57.

Turner, Bethany L., and Amanda L. Thompson. 2013. "Beyond the Paleolithic prescription: incorporating diversity and flexibility in the study of human diet evolution." *Nutrition Reviews* 71 (8): 501–510. https://doi.org/10.1111/nure.12039

Ullrey, Duane E. 1993. "Nutrition and predisposition to infectious disease." *Journal of Zoo and Wildlife Medicine*: 304–314.

US Environmental Protection Authority. 2018. "National overview: Facts and figures on materials, wastes and recycling." US Environmental Protection Authority. https://www.epa.gov/facts-and-figures-about-materials-waste-and-recycling/national-overview-facts-and-figures-materials#:~:text=The%20total%20generation%20of%20municipal,25%20million%20tons%20were%20composted. Webpage accessed 07/19/2023.

van der Driessche, Pauline. 2017. "Reproduction numbers of infectious disease models." *Infectious Disease Modeling* 2: 288–303.

VanDerwarker, A.M., D.N. Bardolph, K.M. Hoppa, H.B. Thakar, L.S. Martin, A.L. Jaqua, M.E. Biwer et al. 2016. "New World paleoethnobotany in the new millennium (2000–2013)." *Journal of Archaeological Research* 24 (2): 125–177. https://doi.org/10.1007/s10814-015-9089-9

Villalobos, Fernández, N.V., J.J. Ott, C.J. Klett-Tammen, A. Bockey, P. Vanella, G. Krause, and B. Lange. 2021. "Effect modification of the association between comorbidities and severe course of COVID-19 disease by age of study participants: A systematic review and meta-analysis." *Systematic Reviews* 10 (1): 194. https://doi.org/10.1186/s13643-021-01732-3

Volk, Anthony A., and Jeremy A. Atkinson. 2013. "Infant and child death in the human environment of evolutionary adaptation." *Evolution and Human Behavior* 34 (3): 182–192.

Warinner, Christina, Camilla Speller, Matthew J. Collins, and Cecil M. Lewis Jr. 2015. "Ancient human microbiomes." *Journal of human evolution* 79: 125–136.

Weaver, L.J., R. Barrett, and M. Nichter. 2016. "Special section on comorbidity: Introduction." *Medical Anthropology Quarterly* 30 (4): 435–441.

WHO. 2020. *World Tuberculosis Report*. Geneva: World Health Organization.

World Allergy Association. 2013. *Whitebook on Allergy: 2013 Updates*. World Allergy Association.

CHAPTER 2

Agriculture and the First Emerging Infections

I have placed a curse on the ground. All your life you will struggle to scratch a living from it. It will grow thorns and thistles for you, though you will eat of its grains. All your life you will sweat to produce food, until your dying day.
Genesis 3:17–19

It was the greatest change in human living since the beginning of our species, transforming our societies and our planet more than all the political upheavals, scientific discoveries, and paradigm shifts that followed. The "Agricultural Revolution" first occurred about 11,000 years ago, when our ancestors began shifting from foraging to agriculture: settling into semi-permanent residences and domesticating plants and animals as their primary means of subsistence (Armelagos et al. 1991; Kujit and Goring-Morris 2002). This shift from mobile foraging to sedentary (i.e., settled) farming would eventually lead to a massive increase in the human population from less than 10 million people to 8 billion and still growing today. It would also reshape much of the biosphere, transforming wilderness into crop fields and grazing ranges that now account for more than 38 percent of the Earth's land mass (UN FAO 2020). Agriculture also triggered a cascade of major cultural changes: emerging states and colliding empires, emerging industries and social stratification. And tragically, this major change in human living produced our first emerging infections by increasing our exposure and susceptibility to new and acute microbial diseases until they became the primary cause of human mortality.

Although costly, there is little doubt that agriculture also conferred benefits for those societies who adopted this new mode of living. Domestic cereal grains are a rich source of carbohydrates, basic calories packed into preservable seeds that can be accumulated and stored for leaner seasons. Domestic animals offer reliable, though not always abundant, protein returns. For these reasons, raising animals for food and farm labor is like putting money in a bank for later withdrawal. Farming and animal husbandry can provide an abundance of food energy for expanding populations that in turn allow for larger-scale collective endeavors and labor specialization for greater productivity and technical development (Gehlsen 2009). With their larger populations, greater surpluses, and more permanent structures, agrarian societies often have considerable military advantages over their foraging neighbors.

That said, each of these benefits is a double-edged sword. Although cereal grains are packed with carbohydrates, they are often lack other important nutrients. These nutritional shortcomings posed a significant health challenge to early agrarian societies that focused on producing a narrower range of plants and animals than are typically obtained through foraging. The subsequent reduction in dietary diversity poses a greater risk for nutritional deficiencies, even when overall food energy is sufficient. Domestic food production not only fuels growing populations, it also requires more people to meet the heavy labor demands of farming. These larger populations require additional regulation, which is often addressed by the establishment

Emerging Infections. Second Edition. Ron Barrett, Molly K. Zuckerman, Matthew R. Dudgeon, with George J. Armelagos, Oxford University Press.
© Ron Barrett, Molly K. Zuckerman, Matthew R. Dudgeon (2024). DOI: 10.1093/oso/9780192843135.003.0003

of formal leadership classes. Along with further specialization and greater opportunities for differential accumulation, these class distinctions create new layers of social hierarchy and economic difference. Finally, despite the military advantage held by agrarian societies, their dependence on permanent territory is more likely to extract the price of violence at very large scales (Flannery and Marcus 2012).

Determining that its costs far outweighed its benefits, a popular science article written by Jared Diamond asserts that the "Agricultural Revolution" was "the worst mistake in the history of the human race"(Diamond 1987). Drawing on bioarcheological evidence, including findings from one of us (Armelagos), Diamond expands his argument in *Guns, Germs and Steel* with particular attention to the health consequences of ancient agriculture in Neolithic populations (Diamond 1998).[1] We agree with the general direction of this particular argument, and needless to say, we concur with at least some of Diamond's sources. However, we would not go so far as to claim that agriculture was humanity's worst mistake. As with its Paleolithic predecessor, the Neolithic presents a complex picture of ancient adaptations that defy any simple conclusion.

With complexity in mind, our aim in this chapter is to determine the major consequences of the shift to primary agriculture for human health and the proximate determinants of these effects. For these purposes, it is helpful to consider explanations for why such a radical change in human living occurred in the first place, and subsequently, why it spread to nearly every corner of the world. The global shift to agriculture left many skeletons behind, and researchers can use the tools of bioarcheology and paleopathology to estimate the health and disease states of ancient people. With this evidence, we can compare the health of more than a dozen societies before and after they made the shift to agriculture as a primary means of subsistence. Combined with other material evidence, these comparisons show how changes in subsistence, settlement, and social organization created opportunities for the evolution and spread of acute infectious diseases in growing human populations. In popular parlance, these could be considered our first emerging infections. In scientific terms, the impact of these emerging infections on human health and demography constituted the First Epidemiological Transition (Barrett et al., 1998).

2.1 The origins and spread of plant and animal domestication

The "revolution" did not happen all at once, nor did it spread globally from a single source. The earliest known instance of primary plant domestication occurred approximately 12,000 to 10,000 years ago[2] in southwest Asia (a.k.a. the Near East) between the Tigris and Euphrates rivers, a region that archaeologists commonly describe as the Fertile Crescent; this same region would later see the rise of Mesopotamia and the present-day countries of the Persian Gulf (Bellwood 2005). This first instance was once famously known as the "Neolithic Revolution," but evidence points to the independent adoption of primary agriculture in East Asia, Central Africa, Melanesia, and the Americas occurring at different periods up to 2,000 years ago (Kelly 2019; Price and Bar-Yosef 2011). Instead, it was a series of cascading changes in human living, and as we will see, none of these changes occurred overnight (see Figure 2.1). For this reason, it is more accurate to describe it is a global transition or shift rather than a revolution in the punctuated sense of the term.

Research into agricultural origins is very dynamic, generating a steady publication of new findings and theories that often lead to vigorous debates (Larson et al. 2014; Piperno et al. 2017). As such, the map shown in Figure 2.1 is but one snapshot of an emerging picture, and theories vary as to the total number of centers for the independent origins of primary domestication. Determining the total number of centers, however, is less important than understanding the reasons for this major cultural transition. For this, we must draw on our knowledge of the Paleolithic and compare it with what we can learn about the Neolithic (in the broader sense of the term). And as with the Paleolithic, we must triangulate findings from an array of different methods and fields: archeology, bioarcheology, and ethnography, as well as the agricultural and biological sciences.

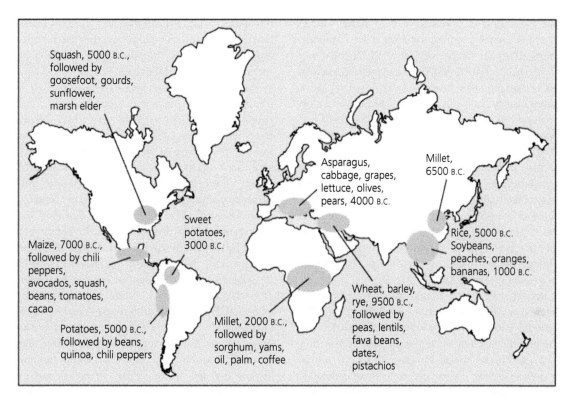

Squash, 5000 B.C., followed by goosefoot, gourds, sunflower, marsh elder

Asparagus, cabbage, grapes, lettuce, olives, pears, 4000 B.C.

Millet, 6500 B.C.

Sweet potatoes, 3000 B.C.

Rice, 5000 B.C. Soybeans, peaches, oranges, bananas, 1000 B.C.

Maize, 7000 B.C., followed by chili peppers, avocados, squash, beans, tomatoes, cacao

Wheat, barley, rye, 9500 B.C., followed by peas, lentils, fava beans, dates, pistachios

Potatoes, 5000 B.C., followed by beans, quinoa, chili peppers

Millet, 2000 B.C., followed by sorghum, yams, oil, palm, coffee

Figure 2.1 Geographic centers for the independent domestication of major food plants, based on an analysis by Robert Kelly (2019).

Source: Robert Kelly (2019). The Fifth Beginning: What Six Million Years of Human History Can Tell Us About Our Future. Berkeley: University of California Press.

As we discussed in Chapter 1, humans have long been engaged in small-scale horticulture, but there is no evidence of intensive agriculture or primary reliance on domesticated food sources at any point during the Early or Middle Paleolithic. During these periods, the archeological record includes many tools for hunting and butchering, but residues from hearths and kitchen middens (refuse heaps) reveal only the remains of wild rather than domesticated animals (French 2016). The same can be said for Early and Middle Paleolithic plant residues; their pollen, spores, and phytoliths are from wild rather than domesticated varieties (Salamini et al. 2002; Vandarwarker et al. 2016). Thus far, we can reasonably conclude that, prior to around 11,000 years ago, there was none of the sustained and intensive agriculture that would have led to large-scale plant and animal domestication.

The archeological record began to radically change toward the very end of the Paleolithic,

after which domestication intensified and spread throughout the world in less than 12,000 years. Given the scope of this change, it is puzzling why humans did not make the transition earlier. Some naïvely argue that domestication never occurred to people before the Neolithic; it became the sensible choice once the connection between seed and plant was discovered. Others argue more moderately for a stepwise accumulation of knowledge, with each step occurring under particular environmental conditions, until people eventually reached a threshold in which they saw the greater benefits of agriculture and adopted the process as a primary means of subsistence (Braidwood, 1967). Such propositions may reflect a kind of "Neolithic chauvinism," but they are nevertheless worth consideration, if only for the purpose of ruling them out.

Although there is no evidence of intensive agriculture prior to the Neolithic, archeological findings include evidence of small-scale seed harvesting and the processing of flours from wild plant sources in at least some populations during the Late Paleolithic (Groman-Yaroslavski et al. 2016; Jovanovic et al., 2021; Kelly 1995). In these places, such as the Levant in southwestern Asia, archaeological evidence clearly shows that domestication was a slow process, preceded by centuries to millennia of pre-domestication levels of plant cultivation (Brown et al. 2009). Even in the absence of such evidence in other populations, we can make reasonable inferences about level of knowledge for this undertaking based on ethnographic studies of contemporary foragers in a variety of environments. These studies demonstrate that successful and sustainable foraging practices require extensive knowledge of the biology, behavior, and life cycles of particular flora and fauna (Berkes 2008).

Recognizing that this expertise is a form of ethnoscience, many ecologists have used the phrase Traditional Ecological Knowledge (TEK) to describe the broad corpus of indigenous research, teaching, and learning by which foraging and horticultural societies develop objectively accurate and detailed understandings of their local environments over time. To confirm the importance of this knowledge for wellbeing and survival, one study measured levels of environmental knowledge among individuals within Tsimané of the Amazon in Bolivia, the Baka of the Congo Basin in Central Africa, and the aforementioned Punan in Borneo, relatively isolated societies who engage in various combinations of foraging and farming (Reyes-García et al. 2016). In these groups, detailed environmental knowledge was positively associated with hunting success and self-reported health.[3] Although some horticultural knowledge may have influenced health outcomes, it is notable knowledge of gathered medicinal plants alone made significant health contributions. We will examine the medicinal roles of traditional plants and foods later in this chapter and again in Chapter 6.

If we can reasonably assume that effective foraging has always been a "high-TEK" endeavor, then such knowledge would have been sufficient to begin the process of domestication. Indeed, most contemporary foraging societies engage in some degree of horticulture for *secondary* subsistence, and as we stated earlier, there is evidence of small-scale

harvesting prior to the Neolithic.[4] Humans already had the requisite knowledge and they were already engaging in the initial practices. Something else must have prompted the shift.

Archeologists have proposed a variety of plausible theories to explain why societies shifted from primary foraging to primary agriculture. Most of these theories emphasize environmental or demographic determinants, with innovation playing a secondary role as the process became further intensified.[5] Environmentally oriented theories often begin by pointing out the importance of rising temperatures at the end of the last ice age (Bar Yosef 2011; Binford 1968; Flannery 1969; Richerson et al. 2001). But although the warmer climate was necessary for many modes of farming, it does not explain the absence of these modes between earlier periods of glaciation. Smaller scale climate changes, such as extended droughts, could have desiccated foraging areas, thereby concentrating people, plants, and animals into small oases of cultivation. Within these oases, archaeologist V. Gordon Childe famously argued that the "propinquity" of plants and animals would make domestication inevitable, since intensive interaction between people and candidate species would lead to a greater understanding of their exploitation as food sources (Childe 1936). In places less impacted by these events, alternative theories have rejected oases as being especially conducive to domestication. Instead, they have focused on how domestication probably originated within the natural ranges of wild candidate species. For example, the earliest known domestication of like goats, sheep, and wheat, was probably fostered by changing conditions along the "hilly flanks" surrounding the Fertile Crescent and Levant regions of the Middle East, rather than oases and riverine areas of the lowlands (Braidwood 1967).

Demographically oriented theories often point to the destabilization and expansion of human populations, not to the degree that would later happen with agriculture, but enough to pressure societies beyond their capacities to sustain effective and peaceful foraging (Binford 1969; Cohen 2009; Flannery 1969). The reasoning follows that, under the warmer, wetter environmental conditions at the end of the Late Pleistocene, foraging populations gradually but steadily expanded into a set of habitable regions until they could no longer migrate. Such theories can explain the archaeological evidence for surges of animal exploitation in places and times of sudden human population expansion (Stiner et al. 1999). Once societies adopted agriculture as a permanent, if not dominant mode of subsistence, then continued population pressure would stimulate further intensification to meet ever-increasing resource demands (Boserup 1965).

In all these explanations, environmental and demographic factors are closely intertwined. They also share a common emphasis on negative triggers preceding the change; their consensus is that human societies were pushed more than they were pulled into agriculture. If this consensus is correct then it is unfair to say that agriculture was humanity's worst *mistake*, even if the price was very high. A mistake entails a bad choice in the face of better alternatives, and it is unlikely that pre-agricultural circumstances presented many other options. Our first farmers probably arrived at their decisions with difficulty, choosing agriculture as a lesser of evils: a necessary rather than preferable solution to their subsistence problems.

That said, there are alternative explanations that emphasize positive rather than negative triggers. One of these explanations is derived from a biological theory of niche construction, in which organisms alter their environments to create niches for themselves, their descendants, and other species (Odling-Smee, Laland, and Feldman 2012). Viewed from this lens, adaptations are not simply one-way responses to surrounding conditions; they also interact with other adaptations to shape those same environments. Cultural Niche Construction Theory applies these dynamics to learned human practices, and in the case of agriculture, it proposes that the initial domestication of plants was neither an adaptive response to adverse environmental conditions or to unchecked human population growth. Instead, it was the result of deliberate human enhancements to their surrounding environments. Thus, Paleolithic foragers may have played an active role in selecting for particular species and favorable traits in the flora and fauna around them (Smith 2012). In particular circumstances, these gradually constructed environments presented increasing opportunities for cultivation up to a certain threshold,

after which the transition to agriculture became greatly accelerated.

These examples of cultural niche construction can also be framed in terms of Optimal Foraging Theory, which predicts that human subsistence practices will seek to achieve maximum nutritional returns with a minimum expenditure of time and energy. Accordingly, plant domestication became more energetically efficient than foraging in certain Late Pleistocene environments (Gremillion and Piperno 2009; Piperno et al., 2017). As some environments warmed at the end of the last Ice Age, changes would have occurred in certain regions that made them more conducive to plant domestication than to foraging, thus pulling rather than pushing some societies into agriculture. Such changes may have included the transformation of savanna-like areas to neotropical forests. At the same time, however, the depletion of resources in other regions might still have pushed people into agriculture because of the declining efficiency of foraging relative to primary food production. Thus the dominance of pull factors in some regions does not negate the dominance of push factors in other regions.

None of these explanations are necessarily exclusive of the others, and it is unlikely that any single theory can sufficiently address the many different contexts in which the transition to primary domestication occurred. Yet regardless of whether agriculture was a preferred choice or a necessary evil, its eventual worldwide dominance still presents a quandary: why did it persist and spread in so many different circumstances? At least some environments would have allowed foraging to persist, but subsequent changes in other environments would have allowed some agricultural societies to return to this original lifestyle. We know of societies that oscillated between foraging and farming, and we continue to see these oscillations in contemporary times (Kelly 1995). However, for the vast majority of human societies, the transition from primary foraging to primary agriculture was a one-way trajectory that, although a gradual process, occurred very rapidly in relation to the much longer time frame in which biologically modern humans have existed on this planet. Even among the few societies that oscillated, most wound up on the farming side of the "fence," literally as well as figuratively. The net result is what we see today: agriculture is the primary mode of subsistence for more than 99.99 percent of the human population.

The short answer is that agriculture was nearly always an irreversible decision. Agriculture transformed natural landscapes; it deforested wilderness through slash and burn practices and reshaped open areas by shovel and plow. Crop fields, grazing ranges, and human settlements displaced wild plants and animals, eventually reducing their numbers. Even when agricultural societies were surrounded by foraging-friendly environments, the per capita ranges for practical foraging would have been insufficient to feed their larger and denser populations. Additionally, while many agricultural societies often retained some of their earlier foraging abilities, much of the highly specialized foraging knowledge, skills, and experience would have been lost over generations. Finally, agricultural societies were unlikely to forego the military advantages of having a large and settled population with food reserves, especially when facing competition from similar societies along their borders. If anything, competition and conflict spurred the further growth of agricultural populations and their food supplies. In these ways, ironically, agriculture grew like a weed.

2.2 Examining the health of dead people

Having considered some of the hows and whys of the shift to primary agriculture, we can begin examining its impact on human health and disease. The bulk of this evidence comes from ancient skeletal individuals because even after thousands of years, ancient bones can display markers of disease from the past (Buikstra 2019; Ortner 2003). A variety of infectious and non-infectious diseases affect the skeleton, though these are mostly restricted to chronic conditions. For example, tuberculosis, Hansen's disease (a.k.a. leprosy), as well as treponemal infections such as syphilis and yaws, can result in permanent and detectable pathologies (lesions) on bones or teeth (Buikstra 2019; Ortner 2003). Some non-infectious diseases also leave their marks on the skeleton; these include certain forms of cancer, rheumatoid arthritis, osteoarthritis, and many of the nutrient deficiencies we examined in the previous chapter, amongst others (see Figure 2.2). Skeletons can also reveal permanent signs of trauma as well as periods of physiological and psychosocial stress that were experienced over the course of people's lives, especially during critical periods of growth and development in childhood. When skeletal signs of specific diseases are absent, biomolecular techniques for recovering ancient DNA and proteins from human tissues can help identify certain diseases such as TB, pneumonia, and plague (Arning and Wilson 2020; Austin et al. 2022; Donoghue 2019; Spyrou et al. 2016).

Even when a skeletal indicator does not point to the effects of a particular stressor, it can nevertheless point to the severity and duration of stress that an individual experienced over a lifetime (Goodman and Martin 2002). It is well established that prolonged exposure to stress-response hormones, such as cortisol, can inhibit human growth and suppress immune function (McDade 2005). For this reason, even non-specific indicators of stress and physiological disruption can be used as proxies for estimating overall health states of ancient populations (Reitsema and McIlvaine 2014).

It should be noted, however, that there are many diseases, infectious and otherwise, that are not detectable in ancient human bodies with our current scientific methods. Even when obvious skeletal pathologies are present, they often are not specific enough to diagnose a specific disease. Most acute conditions, including acute infectious diseases do not affect the body long enough to create changes in skeletal tissues, and ancient pathogen DNA or other diagnostic biomolecules may or may not be preserved in skeletal tissue (Buikstra 2019). In the face of these challenges, paleopathologists and bioarcheologists are usually more concerned with the broader health implications of skeletal pathologies, such as their impact on daily living or the relative burden of caregiving in a given community, rather than the frequencies of specific diseases (Ortner 2011; Tilley and Schrenk 2017). Such interpretations are made with the understanding that health is more than the absence of physical pathologies. Human health also encompasses social and psychological states that cannot be reconstructed from skeletal evidence alone (Reitsema and McIlvaine 2014; Temple and Goodman 2014).

(a)

(b)

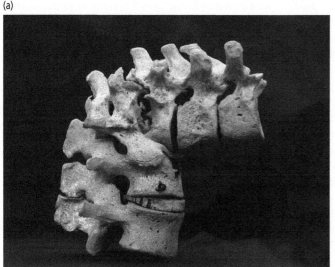
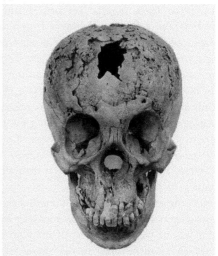

Figure 2.2 Bone pathologies due to specific infections. a. Thoracic spine showing collapsed vertebrae from a tuberculosis infection. Photo by Brian Spatola. CCA 2.0 generic. b. Skull of a World War I era individual with untreated tertiary syphilis at a very late stage. Missing bone around the nasal area and lesions on the cranial vault (caries sicca) are indicative of this disease. Otis Historical Archives National Museum of Health & Medicine. CCA 2.0 generic.

Sources: a. Brian Spatola. Otis Historical Archives Nat'l Museum of Health & Medicine. CCA 2.0 generic. https://commons.wikimedia.org/wiki/File:Spine_-_Kyphosis_from_Tuberculosis.jpg b. Otis Historical Archives Nat'l Museum of Health & Medicine. CCA 2.0 generic. https://commons.wikimedia.org/wiki/File:Syphilis_of_Skull_-_World_War_I_Era.jpg

When attempting to reconstruct the physical health of ancient societies, analysis can be complicated by the fact that most assemblages of skeletons, such as those found in cemeteries, are not statistically representative of their once living populations (DeWitte and Stojanowski 2015; Jackes 2011; Ortner 1991; 1992; Vaupel et al. 1979; Wissler 2021; Wood et al. 1992). One reason for this is that the skeletal individuals that emerge from the archaeological record may have been selectively preserved due to factors that had nothing to do with their prior health. These include post-mortem climate and soil conditions, age at death, and differences in mortuary practices. Another bias that is highly relevant to health assessments arises because individuals in the archeological record, when they were alive, varied in their vulnerability to harm, such as disease and death, from stressors. More specifically, bioarcheologists and paleopathologists often look to age-adjusted risk of death as a measure of what is operationally defined as frailty.

Just as in living populations today, some of these ancient people were more vulnerable to stressors than others, an issue known as heterogeneity in frailty. On average, the more resilient (i.e., less frail) survived, going on to die and enter the archaeological record at older ages. In contrast, those individuals in the skeletal assemblage—the ones we exhume—were by this measure of survivorship the frailest and most vulnerable at each age compared with their surviving peers, which is known as selective mortality.[6] It is challenging enough to determine these differences within and between living populations, but it is even more difficult to make these determinations for ancient individuals. This is due to the possibility of hidden sources of frailty, which can be difficult or impossible to detect through existing methods of analysis. Consequently, it is possible to overlook health issues by which the same stressor may have a greater impact on some populations than others.

Another complication arises from the possibility that older individuals with many pathologies and skeletal indicators of stress may represent those who were healthier and more resilient than their counterparts with relatively unmarked skeletons.

This is because they may have been better able to survive these insults, perhaps through some combination of genetics, better nutrition, or living conditions. A greater burden of disease could, in some circumstances, indicate resilience rather than frailty—the capacity to survive illness but accumulate their scars. For this latter reason especially, it is important to include a variety of contextual data, such as age at death, when assessing the health of ancient populations from skeletal assemblages. We will address these issues of heterogenous frailty, selective mortality, and resilience throughout the chapter.

Keeping in mind these limitations and challenges, there are many skeletal indicators of physiological stress, as well as markers of some specific diseases, that can be used to determine the impact of the agricultural transition on population health. Many of these indicators appear on the teeth, which because of their high mineral content are often the best-preserved parts of the skeleton in the bioarcheological record. Teeth can record periods of stress during growth and development because formation of dental enamel can be interrupted by stress.

In a growing body, dental enamel is secreted and deposited in sequential layers over time, much like the rings of a tree. A prolonged period of stress, caused by events such as disease, undernutrition, and psychosocial trauma, can cause a disruption in the enamel deposition, which appears as a layer or band of thinner enamel known as a linear enamel hypoplasia (Guatelli-Steinberg, 2015). Linear enamel hypoplasias (LEHs) are visible to the naked eye, and they can also be detected by running a fingernail over the surface of the tooth (see Figure 2.3). High frequencies of LEHs are often associated with poorer health and lower life expectancies in skeletal assemblages as well as in living populations (Boldsen 2007; Miszkiewicz 2015; Zhou and Corruccini 1998).

Diseases affecting the teeth, such as dental cavities or caries, are also very useful for determining stress and inferring health states. Dental caries are the most commonly examined markers of oral health due to their frequency in both present day and ancient societies (Marklein et al. 2019). They represent areas of demineralized enamel that develop in the presence of specific oral bacteria

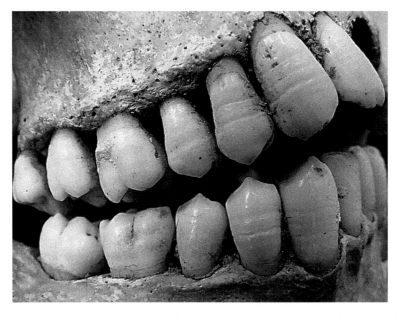

Figure 2.3 Linear enamel hypoplasias revealing periods of physiological stress, such as malnutrition or infectious diseases, during critical periods of growth and development. Photograph by Rebecca Watts.

Source: Rebecca Watts.

and particular diets rich in processed carbohydrates or simple sugars with sticky textures (Soames and Southam 2005).

Dental abscesses and loss of teeth before death are also common indicators of oral health. These develop when oral bacteria are introduced into the tooth root cavity through the tooth pulp or through an open wound on the gum (Robertson and Smith 2009). When unchecked by the immune system (or antibiotics in the present day), these bacteria ultimately form an abscess that can be evident in the bone of the jaw (Nair 2004). The loss of teeth before death, known as antemortem tooth loss (AMTL) occurs when the surrounding bone can no longer secure the tooth. This often occurs with chronic gum disease, and is often associated with caries, abscesses, and tooth pulp exposure from the extensive wear of the teeth. These pathologies are strong indicators of poor oral health in particular, but also of stress and poor overall health in general (Buikstra 2019).

Periosteal reactions are another common indicator of stress and disease as well as a proxy measure for certain health states (Weston 2008). These reactions entail the inflammation of periosteum, the fibrous outer membrane of the bone responsible for providing blood and feeling as well as growth and repair. The periosteum is the first tissue to respond to conditions affecting the bone such as trauma, tumors, and notably, infectious diseases. As the inflammation subsides, tissues heal with the regrowth of bone, resulting in a roughened appearance consisting of pits, bumps, and/or striations (see Figure 2.4). These reactions can be found in association with specific infections such as syphilis, tuberculosis, and leprosy, metabolic diseases like vitamin C deficiency, traumatic injuries, and other processes that can not be determined from skeletal evidence alone (Ortner 2003). In some cases, their specific location can suggest infection in neighboring areas, for example: oral infections with lesions on the lower jaw, and lower respiratory infections with lesions on the inner rib surfaces (Davies-Barrett et al. 2019; Liu et al. 2019). In any of these instances, the presence of periosteal reactions is often associated with higher mortality risk (DeWitte 2014).

There are also porous lesions on the skull which can serve to indicate poor health. These include cribra orbitalia (CO) and porotic hyperostosis (PH), which are among the most common disease indicators found in ancient human skeletons. These appear as porous, often coral-like lesions on the

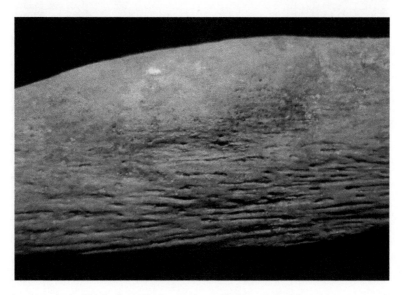

Figure 2.4 Periosteal reaction, clearly visible by the roughed appearance on this femur. Periosteal reactions are commonly associated with gram positive bacterial infections.

Source: Dennis Van Gerven

orbital roof (CO) and the cranial vault (PH), and are often caused by an expansion of the spongy bone inside of these flat areas of the skull as the outer and more dense layers reabsorbed in body (Rivera and Mirazón 2017) (see Figure 2.4). This process generally occurs during growth and development in infancy and childhood (Wapler, Crubezy, and Schultz 2004). Both CO and PH are lesions that were once considered to be caused by genetic or acquired anemias, like iron deficiency anemia[7] (Angel 1966; Smith-Guzmán 2015). However, deficiencies in other micronutrients, such as vitamin B12, folic acid, or vitamin C, have been more recently tied to these lesions, depending on the location where they occur (Walker et al. 2009). Several studies have found that CO and PH can have very different causes (Brickley 2018; Rivera and Mirazón 2017). However, both CO and PH are often found in association with individuals that have experienced some form of malnutrition and/or infectious disease (Hens, Godde, and Macak 2019). A deficiency in any one of the above micronutrients is often accompanied by deficiencies in others. As discussed in Chapter 1, any one of them results

in compromised immunity and increased risk for infection. Porotic lesions in living populations are closely associated with poor health and increased vulnerability to disease and death (Piperata et al. 2014).

Long bones, such as the femur and tibia in the leg, may also reveal periods of interrupted growth during childhood, indicating the presence of major stressors such as malnutrition and disease. Growth arrest and recovery produce linear changes in the density of endochondral growth plates, the ends of long bones that add layers as we grow before fusing at the end of growth (Steinbock 1976). These linear changes, known as Harris lines,[8] are clearly visible as opaque horizontal bands in X-rays and magnetic resonance imaging (MRI) images. It should be noted, however, that Harris lines are among the more debated forms of bioarcheological evidence owing to their many potential causes, including non-pathological processes, and sometimes unreliable correlations with other indicators of stress and disease (Mays 1985). But in instances when these latter correlations are more reliable, Harris lines can support other evidence

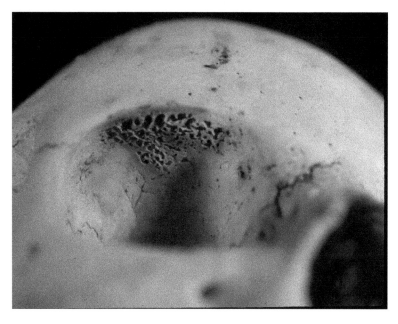

Figure 2.5 A special form of porotic hyperostosis known as cribra orbitalia, seen in flat bones of the inner eye orbit. Porotic hyperostoses are often caused by long-term anemia which, in turn, increases susceptibility to infectious diseases.

Source: Dennis Van Gerven

for health comparisons between different samples of ancient skeletons (Papageorgopoulou et al. 2011).

Long bones play a more important role in determining human stature, or adult height, which is often used as a proxy measure for the health of ancient as well as living populations. The lengths of long bones correlate with the stature of living people, allowing bioarcheologists and paleopathologists to use appropriate regression formulas to determine the height of ancient populations when they were alive (Ortner 2003). Stature is influenced by both genetic and environmental factors. The latter entail chronic stress, disease, and malnutrition especially (Roberts and Manchester 2005; Walker et al. 2007). Short stature, which is defined by a value that falls into the first quartile of the height distribution for a specific sex and population, strongly reflects conditions experienced early in life, and like the previous measures, it associated with poor health and an increased risk of premature death (Marklein et al. 2016; McEniry 2013; Steckel 1995).

It is important to note, however, that although bone length and stature are correlated, the specific differences between bone and body length can vary by the genetic distance between populations. Unfortunately, it is difficult to find living groups that are closely related to ancient groups for the purpose of making these comparisons. Yet as with the other non-specific indicators discussed, stature measurements can be highly relevant when comparing the health of two or more genetically related ancient populations that lived under changing social and environmental conditions at different points in time. Fortunately, the archaeological record provides us with these "natural experiments," opportunities to examine and compare the relative health of ancient societies before, during, and after the shift from primary foraging to primary agriculture. Moreover, these data have been uncovered in different geographic regions and historical eras, which allows us to identify some common variables despite particular differences in cultural trajectories and surrounding environments.

Even when specific diagnoses are possible, multiple lines of evidence are nevertheless required to verify particular observations and reconstruct ancient health and disease states. This integration is also needed to infer the events that we cannot observe, such as the presence of infections too acute to leave skeletal traces. Even the proverbial smoking gun of ancient pathogen DNA may not be detectable in the tissues of individuals affected by a particular infection. To infer such infections, and more importantly, the overall disease burden of a population, we must rely on a wide variety of additional evidence in the context of daily living in local environments.

The latter includes biomolecular evidence of diet and dietary composition. For example, lactose can be recovered from human dental calculus, indicating when emerging pastoralist and agricultural societies began consuming milk and dairy foods (Warinner et al. 2014). The evidence also includes geochemical analyses of human bones and teeth. Ratios of carbon and nitrogen isotopes in bones and teeth can be used to determine the proportions of meat from land or marine animals and the different types of plants consumed (Bickle 2018; Bird et al. 2021). And as we discussed in the last chapter, direct evidence of diet and disease can be recovered from coprolites as well as biomolecules recovered from bones (Reinhard et al. 2013). Finally, the analysis of genomic variations in present-day pathogens can help us determine when earlier pathogens emerged and evolved in ancient human populations (Harkins and Stone 2015).

2.3 Comparing societies in transition

Researchers have used the previously described methods to determine the health changes that accompanied the transition from primary foraging to primary agriculture in numerous regions throughout all the permanently inhabited continents (Clark, Tayles, and Halcrow, 2014; Cohen and Armelagos 2013 [1984]; Eshed et al., 2010). Each region comprises multiple ancient societies at different time periods within different specific environments. The scope of these studies covers a considerable range of cultural and environmental diversity so we should not be surprised to learn that the particular trajectories to primary agriculture are at least as diverse. Yet as with the Paleolithic, our aim is not to make sweeping generalizations about the

Neolithic. We are simply attempting to understand relevant patterns and trends amid the variation.

Early studies found that the transition from foraging to farming had a straightforwardly positive effect on human populations. The transition was initially thought to have produced reliable food sources, increased free time, decreased physiological stress, and extended human longevity (Boserup 1965; Childe 1936; Hayden et al. 1981). However, later research found the transition was fraught with negative health consequences, and that the relationships between agrarian modes of living and human wellbeing were much more complex than had been previously theorized (Cohen and Armelagos 2013 [1984]; Cohen and Crane-Kramer 2007; Marklein et al. 2019).

The first systematic analysis of the health impacts of agriculture, *Paleopathology at the Origins of Agriculture*, co-edited by one of us (Armelagos), synthesized more than 30 regional case studies of human skeletal samples from populations undergoing agricultural intensification. It examined skeletal and oral markers of stress as well as lesions from specific disease conditions (Cohen and Armelagos 2013 [1984]). Results from these studies indicated that most populations experienced overall declines in physiological health associated with the transition to intensive agriculture. By comparing skeletal individuals from the same ancient societies at different stages of transition, these studies found common trends of decreasing stature and increasing signs of under-nutrition, stress, and disease.

More recent large-scale studies have produced similar results. A systematic review of studies published since 1984 found evidence of stature decline as reliance on agriculture increased among transitioning societies (Mummert et al. 2011). This correlation was consistent across global regions and it occurred regardless of whether the transition took place in the Neolithic or thousands of years later. In all these cases, the intensification of agriculture was associated with nutritional deficiencies, dense populations, and increasing rates of infectious diseases that had a particularly negative impact on children.

These same health declines were corroborated by a systematic examination of 12,250 skeletal individuals, historic and prehistoric, from 65 composite locations in North and South America (Steckel and Rose 2002). A standardized health index was developed for these individuals based on the number and severity of nearly all the previously mentioned skeletal pathologies, as well as stature, lifespan, and the presence of degenerative joint diseases indicative of hard manual labor (Steckel et al. 2002). The authors then applied this index to data from hundreds of archaeological sites through the Western Hemisphere (Goodman and Martin 2002). Among the several dozen sites reflecting the transition to primary agriculture, the health indices were significantly lower in post-transition societies than in their earlier foraging periods. Average lifespans were also significantly reduced and average life expectancies at birth were inversely proportionate to the rates of pathological lesions (McCaa 2002). Together, these extensive samples reflect frailer and less healthy populations with agricultural intensification. And lastly, this study found that agricultural societies with reduced dietary breadth had much lower health index scores than did Paleolithic foraging societies, strongly suggesting the negative impact of nutritional deficiencies on immunological vulnerability to infectious diseases (Steckel et al. 2002).

Having examined the evidence at the global level, we turn to particular regions and sites to see these dynamics at higher resolution. Beginning with the earliest known sites of primary agriculture, skeletal samples from the Fertile Crescent reveal higher rates of child mortality from the Late Paleolithic to the Neolithic and Iron Ages (Rathbun 2013 [1984]). They also reveal increased evidence of growth disruptions, periods of nutritional inadequacy, and signs of gastrointestinal and parasitic infections during the transition. In the Levant region of the Middle East, such changes were not immediately apparent when agriculture first appeared, but later intensification, along with increases in population size and density, was associated with marked declines in nutrition, growth, and development (Eshed et al. 2010; Smith, Bar-Yosef, and Sillen, 2013 [1984]).

Population growth also played a key role in the impacts of agriculture in many of these local contexts. In the Eastern Mediterranean, for instance, agriculture appeared gradually and sporadically over many centuries but then intensified in a relatively short time frame concurrent with a 10- to 50-fold increase in population density (Angel 2013 [1984]). During this time, 20 percent of the land was converted for intensive farming and grazing. This was followed by soil depletion, as well as skeletal evidence of macro- and micronutrient deficiencies, namely protein, iron, and zinc. There was also increasing skeletal evidence of specific parasitic infections, including malaria. In South Asia, there is strong evidence that population expansion and pastoralism occurred prior to intensive agriculture (Kennedy 2013 [1984]). Here, seed crops brought food stability to growing numbers of people. However, this security came at the price of food quality, as indicated by declining stature and increasing growth interruptions, micronutrient deficiencies, periodontal disease, and pathologies indicative of vitamin C and D deficiencies.

Prior to the European invasions, North American societies experienced health declines with the widespread adoption of maize, though not to the catastrophic levels that would occur after the invasions. These declines were likely to have been due to steadily increasing populations and declining opportunities for foraging. The Lower Illinois Valley saw overall increases in developmental stress markers (i.e., LEH, CO, PH) as well as significant increases in treponemal infections, and the appearance of lesions attributable to tuberculosis (Buikstra 2013 [1984]; Cook 2013 [1984]). Similar associations were found in the Central Ohio Valley (Cassidy 2013 [1984]; Perzigian, Tench, and Braun, 2013 [1984]). In one of these village sites, one-third of all children died before five years of age and 30 percent of adult individuals displayed periosteal reactions. That said, the authors are careful to note that maize production was not a simple independent variable, but rather a key player in the positive feedback between subsistence, population, and available resources. In this context, declining health was a known cost in the face of other expenses, "the balance struck between dietary quantity and quality, and population size" (Cassidy 2013 [1984], p. 338).

In particularly dry regions, the natural (nonintentional) mummification of human bodies allows for direct analysis of soft tissues and sometimes pathogens as well. This is the case for Maitas Chirubaya and other ancient societies located in six

arid regions of Chile and Peru (Allison 2013 [1984]). The results of these analyses show very high rates of acute respiratory infections: 50–88 percent in children, 27–47 percent in adults. These infections are largely attributed to Group A streptococci and *M. tuberculosis*, many with extrapulmonary complications and comorbidity with non-specific gastrointestinal infections. Children were most impacted by these infections; 28–50 percent died before 15 years of age. These childhood mortality rates were much higher than when these societies primarily relied on hunting, gathering, and fishing.

Socio-economic differences can sometimes be inferred based on the relative quality and quantity of tombs and mortuary artifacts (Babić 2005; Rakita et al. 2005). For example, in the Lower Illinois Valley adult males buried in well-constructed tombs with valuable grave items were significantly taller than their contemporaries, though there is some debate as to whether stature or status came first (Buikstra, 2013 [1984]). Yet in one Maitas Chirubaya cemetery, the direction of causality is supported by dramatic differences in bone pathology (Allison 2013 [1984]). High-status male religious leaders were significantly taller than commoner males, the latter had more than three times the number of bone lesions, and commoner females had 62 percent more lesions than commoner males. Clearly the deficiencies and diseases of agriculture were experienced unequally in this society.

A much larger example with mummified remains is a population of Sudanese Nubians who were uncovered from 33 excavations over a period of 70 years (Martin et al., 2013 [1984]). These ancient communities spanned five major time periods, beginning with late Mesolithic foragers in 11,500 BCE and ending with highly agrarian Christians in 1350 CE (Martin et al. 2013 [1984]). As they increasingly adopted agriculture during the Neolithic, we see the first evidence of CO and PH and an 18-fold increase in dental caries. Around 350 BCE, Harris lines and LEHs appeared, most likely revealing severe physiological stress during growth and development. Additionally, adult females manifested signs of premature osteoporosis, a strong indication of malnutrition in which calcium was diverted from their bones to meet the additional demands of pregnancy and nursing.

Sex-based differences are also found in other archeological centers. Returning to the Levant, both male and female stature declined during the early stages of agricultural adoption, but then female stature declined further than among males during later agricultural intensification (Smith and Horowitz 2007). Across Europe, stature decreased significantly for males and females starting in the Late Paleolithic, but then further declined for males during the Mesolithic (Holt and Formicola 2008). Along the Georgian coast of North America, females had greater declines in stature than did males during agricultural intensification; they also exhibited more dental caries and more periosteal reactions (Larsen, 2013 [1984]). These stature differences likely reflect gender-based inequalities that have also been detected in other transitioning societies in the Middle East and Mesoamerica (Littleton 2007; Storey, Morfin, and Smith, 2002)

Lastly, one of the most complete records of agricultural transition comes from the excavations at the Dickson Mounds burial complex, located in the southern region of what is now the US state of Illinois (Goodman et al., 2013 [1984]). Here, the archaeological record reveals a geographically and culturally delineated society that experienced a relatively rapid transformation from foraging to intensive agriculture. This allows us to make comprehensive health measurements of a single population throughout the 250-year transition period, much like the analyses performed by Steckel and Rose (2002). Furthermore, analysis of inherited dental traits shows that this population was genetically well delineated, with very little in-migration from neighboring communities. Thus, we can generally exclude the possibility that health-related changes were due to population-level genetic changes.

The baseline data for Dickson Mounds starts around the Late Woodland Period (95–1100 CE), when this area hosted periodic campsites occupied by foragers: small groups of 75 to 125 people who were engaged in seasonal hunting and gathering (Goodman et al., 2013 [1984]). Over the next century, these foraging groups became increasingly influenced by their Mississippian neighbors, a large society of over 30,000 sedentary agriculturalists living 180 kilometers to the south. By the following century, known as the Middle Mississippian Period

(1200–1300 CE), these former foragers had settled into just over 200 hamlet structures with support camps and work structures for 600–1200 people (Harn 1978). This same period saw the intensification of maize agriculture as a primary means of subsistence, increased trade with neighboring communities, and a marked increase in population size and density.

Compared to their foraging ancestors a few centuries earlier, these settled farmers display many pathological markers of health decline as well as reduced life expectancies at every age interval (Goodman et al., 2013 [1984]). Findings include a fourfold increase in CO and PH and as much as a threefold increase in periosteal reactions as compared to their foraging ancestors. These early farmers also experienced an overall decrease in stature and cortical bone thickness, and significantly higher rates of traumatic injuries and degenerative spinal conditions, which may be associated with heavy manual labor demands.

As with other populations, the health consequences of intensive agriculture were unequally experienced at Dickson Mounds (Buikstra 2013 [1984]). Here we find that socio-economic status, inferred from mortuary data, is positively associated with better nutrition and growth, just as it is inversely associated with skeletal markers of infectious diseases and other adverse health conditions. Moreover, these differences are most pronounced when comparing groups of people who were buried with at least some decorative artifacts with people who were buried with nothing at all.

Finally, the children of Dickson Mounds bore the heaviest burden of these deficiencies and infections. Skeletons of children display the highest frequencies of PH during the years after weaning and before adolescence. Similarly, linear enamel hypoplasias indicate early growth interruptions and very early ages at the time of weaning. Both are major risk factors for childhood infections, and these are likely to be reflected in the presence of periosteal reactions. Furthermore, the evidence for under-nutrition and infection is not only highly correlated in this population but in many instances they co-occur in the same individuals. In these comorbid cases, both diseases were more severe than if they occurred separately. This is consistent with far too many observations of children living in severe poverty today. Under-nutrition and infection continue to be the most common determinants of mortality among children under five years of age around the world (Walson and Berkly 2018).

Children are the most vulnerable members of any population, and a society with too many sick children is a sick society, one that can no longer buffer itself from the diseases, deficiencies and other threats from the surrounding environment (Sandberg and Van Gerven 2016). Even for the more resilient individuals who survived childhood in these ancient societies, the risk for further infection would have remained higher because of developmental impairments in their immune systems. Much of this development, such as the maturation of the thymus and lymphatic system, occurs in early childhood (Bourke et al. 2016; Prentice 1999). This is the same period when we observe signs of growth impairment in the skeleton. These are only a few of the developmental processes that explain why, among present-day populations living in severe poverty, low birth weight and early childhood hardships often result in greater disease susceptibility throughout adulthood, a phenomenon addressed in the Barker Hypothesis (a.k.a. the developmental origins of health and disease (DOHaD) (Armelagos et al. 2009; Barker 2004; Kuzawa and Quinn 2009).[9] Thus, we should not be surprised that at Dickson Mounds, a 15-year-old agrarian adolescent might have expected to live 18 fewer years than his or her foraging ancestor of the same age (Cohen 1977).

We have reviewed these studies with the relatively modest aim of determining potential health changes with the Neolithic transition. Anything more ambitious would have to account for a tremendous variety of cultures, local environments, and historical details. Even at this lower resolution, we should note particular differences in the timing and manifestation of health changes. In some societies, the first indications of health decline appear in the early stages of agricultural adoption, while in other societies they appear in the later stages of agricultural intensification. In a few other instances, there are even signs of initial health improvement before an overall decline. Yet despite particular differences, all these studies support the same general conclusion: the transition from primary foraging to primary agriculture made overall health much worse, and it made dying from infection much more likely.

2.4 Exceptions to patterns and challenging interpretations

Given our scope of inquiry, we should expect to discover exceptions to the patterns in the previous studies: ancient societies that experienced no significant health changes or those that sustained improvements during their transition to agriculture. As we will see, the exceptions actually provide important clues regarding the more proximate determinants of health decline during the Neolithic, as well as precedents for the ways in which low- and middle-income countries experience infectious diseases today.

The archeological record includes several instances with evidence of unchanged or improved health with increasing populations and shifts toward agricultural activities. In the lower central valley of California, foraging populations increased in size and density around the time they began harvesting acorns in a quasi-agricultural manner (Dickel, Schultz, and McHenry, 2013 [1984]). Frequencies of skeletal stress indicators were mixed in these populations, and there is evidence of improved child survivorship, though overall life expectancy declined over time. In the pre-ceramic village of Paloma, Peru, successive experiments in cultivation were accompanied by declines in growth interruptions, increased stature, and reduced mortality among children and older people (Benfer 2013 [1984]). In northeast Thailand, the intensification of rice agriculture was also accompanied by decreased growth interruptions and increased stature, though these trends reversed in later centuries (Clark et al. 2014). In coastal Georgia and the Florida panhandle, the adoption of maize agriculture did not correspond to changes in stature, though there were increased frequencies of periosteal reactions, dental caries, and linear enamel hypoplasias (Larsen et al. 2007).

These four examples underscore the importance of dietary diversity in the context of a mixed subsistence strategy. The Californian communities continued to exploit a variety of wild food resources while taking advantage of acorns, a highly preservable staple crop, to buffer themselves from periodic shortages. Over time, the Paloma community increasingly relied on domesticated crops, but they also continued a variety of foraging activities, and they shifted their primary reliance to seafood during periods when agriculture was not sufficient. Similarly, the northeast Thai community was able to supplement their rice crops with robust fishing activities, a common pattern in other parts of ancient southeast Asia. And in Georgia and Florida, utilization of marine resources may have played a protective role in buffering populations from the under-nutrition typically associated with intensive maize farming. All of these societies maintained a fairly diversified subsistence portfolio, and many engaged in fishing, which helped to mitigate the health costs of agriculture (see also Ahedo et al. 2021).

That said, we should be careful not to overgeneralize the relative importance of dietary breadth in comparison with other factors associated with Neolithic health trajectories. For instance, most studies in the previous section also note the greatest health declines in communities with the highest population densities. Recall that Steckel and Rose (2002) found that plant domestication and settlement size had the greatest impact on declining health, although their conclusion is based on the combined effect of both variables. With respect to population characteristics alone, larger settlements scored much lower in the health index than smaller, more mobile groups (Steckel and Rose 2002).

It should also be noted that there is not a strictly linear relationship between overall subsistence strategies and some of the skeletal markers of stress and disease we discussed. This is particularly true for oral stress indicators like dental caries, abscesses, and antemortem tooth loss. A broad assessment of data from almost 200 archaeological sites found that, although Neolithic agricultural groups averaged more dental caries than Paleolithic foragers, there is a large overlap between them, and no significant difference in abscess and antemortem tooth loss frequencies (Marklein et al. 2019). More specifically, while maize agriculture is associated with increases in dental caries, this is not the case for rice agriculture (Cucina et al. 2011).

The latter may be attributed to differences in the specific carbohydrates within these plant species as well as differences in their modes of preparation. These findings remind us that foraging and farming are not generic activities but rather broad categories that encompass many subsistence traditions.

Earlier in this chapter we introduced some of the challenges and limitations of determining the health states of ancient populations based on skeletal data. Some of these major challenges include heterogeneous frailty, selective mortality, and both the presence and absence of stress and disease markers, all in relation to ages at death. These challenges are then compounded by biased representations of skeletal samples compared to their once-living populations (DeWitte and Stojanowksi 2015; Jackes 2011; Wissler 2021). Yet even when we account for these and other challenges, a very large body of evidence points to overall health declines with the intensification of agriculture.

There was certainly regional, temporal, and population-level variation in these studies, but there were also common themes revealed by the multiple measurements of many different populations, environments, and time periods (Cohen 2009). Some of these findings, such as declining stature and increasing LEHs, have well-established links to under-nutrition and immuno-susceptibility in contemporary populations, especially among those living in extreme poverty (Miszkiewicz 2015). Increased child mortality is probably the strongest indicator of declining health in early farming societies,[10] contributing to declines in life expectancy at birth in all cases where such estimates are possible (McCaa 2002). And with the intensification of agriculture, we see the rise of gender and status-based differences in nutritional status, disease risk, and mortality (Larsen 2013 [1984]; Smith and Horwitz 2007) (.All told, the evidence for health decline is overwhelming.

Finally, although we have seen that the intensification of agriculture is positively correlated with the growth and concentration of human populations, we must also remember that correlation is not the same as causation. Subsistence strategies and population dynamics are closely intertwined in cycles of mutual feedback. When both have shifted, it is neither productive nor feasible to attribute either as the greater determinant without accounting for covariates or further evidence. As with foraging in the Paleolithic, farming in the Neolithic was more than just a collection of methods for obtaining food. Both describe entire modes of living that shaped our social and natural environments, and for better and worse, they shaped our microbial environments as well.

2.5 Subsistence, settlement, and social organization

Thus far, we have only confirmed associations between the intensification of agriculture, overall health decline, and the increased burden of disease in ancient human populations. However, we have not sufficiently examined some of the specific ways that agrarian living might have led to these consequences. To make a better case for these causative processes, we must also examine direct evidence for those broader lifestyle changes that are known to impact human health and disease in living as well as ancient populations, especially with regards to the evolution of potential human pathogens and their spread as acute infectious diseases. For this, we revisit the same themes of subsistence, settlement, and social organization that we addressed for mobile foragers in Chapter 1.

With respect to dietary subsistence, ancient pollen and spore samples provide direct evidence of decreasing nutritional diversity with the intensification of agriculture. We find this in South Asia, for instance, where the intensification of agriculture stabilized the seasonal availability of food but did so with the restriction of edible plant resources (Kennedy 2013 [1984]). Similarly, the expansion of agriculture in the Mediterranean was accompanied by monocropping practices that led to the overuse and depletion of soil nutrients (Angel 2013 [1984]). As they began settling into permanent residences, the early farmers of ancient Nubia and Dickson Mounds became increasingly dependent on a single staple crop, maize, for their caloric intake (Martin et al., 2013 [1984]). Although maize is a great source of nutritional energy, it is deficient in zinc and the amino acid lysine, both of which are essential for healthy immune function. Depending on how it is processed, maize can also be deficient in vitamin

B3 (Niacin), which can lead to fatal nutritional deficiencies (Thompson et al. 2019). These crop data are an important link in the chain of causality between subsistence practices and susceptibility to infectious diseases.

Regarding settlement patterns, we not only see the population expansion with agriculture but perhaps more importantly, the concentration of these farming populations in permanent settlement clusters (i.e., sedentism). These population changes have led some anthropologists to argue that more than agriculture per se, sedentism was the primary trigger for the first emergence of acute human infections (Cohen and Armelagos, 2013 [1984]). We know that this settlement theory is supported by many of the studies that we have examined, but it is difficult to weigh settlement above other factors without first determining its precise location in the sequence of causality. For instance, there are many archaeological examples in which the size and density of human populations preceded the further intensification of agriculture. Yet as we stated earlier, we do not know if population pressure might be the result of earlier changes of subsistence. Subsistence and settlement changes were clearly linked to one another, but they are like chickens and eggs when it comes to determining which came first.

Less obvious is the impact of agriculture on the settlement of non-human animals. Whether for food or labor, the domestication of animals increased the size and densities of animal populations, just as it did for their human handlers. It also brought humans and animals into close proximity with one another, and it did so for longer periods of time than when Paleolithic foragers hunted for meat in the wild. Combining these factors could have created a "perfect storm" for the spread of zoonotic diseases from animal to human hosts. Thus it is with little surprise that we find many major human infections have their evolutionary origins as zoonotic diseases (Quammen 2012; Weiss 2001).

Here we find evidence tracing the origins of many common and deadly infections to domesticated ruminants. The smallpox virus is closely related to the cowpox virus, a variant of which is the *vaccinia* strain that had long been used to inoculate humans against the more virulent disease. Within the complex of mycobacterial strains associated with various kinds of tuberculosis (MTBC), those associated with human TB are closely related to those associated with bovine TB, and the latter can also infect humans as well as cattle and deer (Ver-Cauteren et al. 2018).[11] The measles virus originated with the rinderpest virus in cattle, which most likely made the leap to human populations in the eleventh to twelfth centuries (Furuse et al. 2010). Phylogenetic studies of influenza A viruses, human and otherwise, show they are essentially avian influenzas insofar as they can all thrive in the guts of waterfowl that have been variously domesticated by a number of human societies (Barrett 2010).

Lastly, we can consider the evidence for health-related changes in social organization associated with primary agriculture. Among the transitioning societies we examined earlier, we saw examples in which health declines were significantly greater among females and lower-status individuals than among their male and higher-status counterparts. These health inequalities are even more striking in instances of political centralization. In the Sudanese Nubian populations, for example, life expectancies were inversely correlated with the degree of centralization, and notably, these effects were more pronounced among women and other subgroups who were living on the periphery of major political centers (Van Gerven et al., 1990). Ironically, these health declines were most pronounced when the Nubian kingdoms of Meroë and Makuria were at their heights of wealth and power. We then see signs of improved health in the same subgroups during the declines of these kingdoms. These patterns are best explained by the kingdoms exerting greater control over their populations to extract additional labor and resources from peripheral subgroups—a common and recurring theme in human history.

In different forms, the same theme has persisted to the present day: people with more resources tend to be healthier than people with less resources. Societies having greater resource differences will tend to have greater health differences, and so on. But it is important to note that although these differences can be traced to prehistoric antiquity, they are not as old as humanity itself but rather hierarchy itself. The latter is largely a product of the Neolithic Transition. Combined with declining nutritional quality, increasing population density, and proximity to non-human animals, these social changes brought the first major rises of acute infectious diseases in the human species.

Notes

1. Although quite popular, it should be noted that *Guns, Germs and Steel* has received a great deal of scholarly criticism from anthropologists for its oversimplification, Eurocentrism, and for discounting the effects of colonialism and conquest in favor of environmental determinism to support its primary thesis (Blaut 1999; Wilcox 2010). We refer to the book and related article at the beginning of this chapter because for many readers, these may have previously been the sole source of information about this topic.

2. Henceforth, we generalize to 11,000 years ago.

3. Interestingly, nutritional status was not associated with levels of ecological knowledge in these three societies. The authors suggest that this may be due to food sharing practices, a subject we will examine later in this chapter.

4. Many mobile pastoral societies have also engaged in horticulture. Pastoralism is a subsistence strategy based on extensive, mobile livestock production. It should also be noted that pastoralism represents an ancient way of living that does not fit into the foraging, horticultural, or agricultural categories. Pastoralism is worthy of examination within the history of human economy relative to health, and notably, pastoralists have encountered some of the same barriers due to emerging infectious diseases that pastoralists have (Gifford-Gonzalez 2000). However, we are omitting such studies in this book for the sake of our focus on foraging and agricultural societies.

5. There are also Marxian and cultural materialist theories that emphasize changing modes of production in the rise of agriculture (see Cohen 2009). But these theories explain historical change rather than agriculture, which is itself a mode of production. It would be circular logic to propose that agriculture arose *because of* a changing mode of production.

6. Issues pertaining to heterogeneity in frailty (especially the hidden kind) and selective mortality—along with changes in the distribution of births, deaths, and migration—are often grouped together under an concept known as the osteological paradox.

7. Several lines of evidence suggest that the rapid loss and consequent overproduction of red blood cells seen in some kinds of anemias, like hemolytic and megaloblastic anemia, are the most likely causes of PH (Walker et al. 2009). Inherited, or genetic anemias, like sickle cell anemia, can point to evidence of infection with specific infectious diseases, specifically malaria. However, malaria is one of the few disease conditions that does leave distinctive lesions on the skeleton, specifically a distinctive pattern of lesions (Smith-Guzmán 2015).

8. Also known as growth arrest lines or radiopaque lines.

9. DOHaD emphasizes the role of exposure to environmental factors, such as undernutrition, early in life in determining the development of human diseases during adulthood. This includes epigenetic causes of adult chronic noninfectious diseases, like diabetes and type 1 diabetes, and the potential for such environmental causes to influence disease risk across generations (intergenerational risks) (Godfrey et al. 2007). In addition to numerous studies on living, present-day populations, bioarchaeologists have also found support for DOHaD in past populations (Armelagos et al. 2009).

10. It is worth noting that, in the Fertile Crescent, Nubian, and Dickson Mounds studies, linear enamel hypoplasias become more frequent in younger than in older skeletal individuals with the intensification of agriculture (Goodman et al. 2013 [1984]; Martin et al. 2013 [1984]; Rathbun 2013 [1984]). Because these lesions only occur in early ages, their diminished frequency in older individuals strongly suggests that higher proportions of juvenile skeletal individuals in post-agricultural samples are a function of increased child mortality rather than increased fertility. The latter possibility is one

of the confounding variables of nonstationary populations that have been discussed in relation to the osteological paradox (Gage and DeWitte 2009; Wood et al. 1992).

11. It should be noted that, although these strains are closely related, recent evidence shows that *M. tuberculosis* was probably ancestral to *M. bovis*, suggesting that domesticated cows originally contracted TB from their human handlers. As we will see in Chapter 5, the "spillover" of pathogens between human and animal populations can happen in both directions.

References

Ahedo, Virginia, Débora Zurro, Jorge Caro, and José Manuel Galán. 2021. "Let's go fishing: A quantitative analysis of subsistence choices with a special focus on mixed economies among small-scale societies." *PLoS One* 16 (8): e0254539. https://doi.org/10.1371/journal.pone.0254539

Allison, Marvin J. 2013. "Paleopathology in Peruvian and Andean Populations." In *Paleopathology at the Origins of Agriculture*, edited by Mark N. Cohen and George J. Armelagos, 515–530. Gainesville: University Press of Florida.

Angel, J. L. 1966. "Porotic Hyperostosis, Anemias, Malarias, and Marshes in the Prehistoric Eastern Mediterranean." *Science* 153 (3737): 760–763. http://www.jstor.org/stable/1719125

Angel, J. Lawrence. 2013. "Health as a Crucial Factor in the Changes from Hunting to Developed Farming in the Eastern Mediterranean." In *Paleopathology at the Origins of Agriculture*, edited by Mark N. Cohen and George J. Armelagos, 51–73. Gainesville: University Press of Florida.

Armelagos, George J., and Mark Nathan Cohen. 2013 [1984]. *Paleopathology at the Origins of Agriculture.* Orlando: Academic Press.

Armelagos, George J., Allen H. Goodman, and Kenneth H. Jacobs. 1991. "The origins of agriculture: Population growth during a period of declining health." *Population and the Environment* 13 (1): 9–22.

Armelagos, G.J., Goodman, A. H., Harper, K. N., and Blakey, M. L. 2009. "Enamel hypoplasia and early mortality: Bioarcheological support for the Barker hypothesis." *Evolutionary Anthropology* 18 (6): 261–271. https://doi.org/https://doi.org/10.1002/evan.20239

Arning, Nicolas, and Daniel J. Wilson. 2020. "The past, present and future of ancient bacterial DNA." *Microbial Genomics* 6 (7): 1–19.

Austin, Rita M., Molly Zuckerman, Tanvi P. Honap, Lee Hedwig, Geoff K. Ward, Christina Warinner, Krithivasan Sankaranarayanan et al. 2022. "Remembering St. Louis individual—Structural violence and acute bacterial infections in a historical anatomical collection." *Communications Biology* 5 (1): 1–10.

Babić, Stasa. 2005. "Status Identity and archaeology." *In The Archaeology of Identity. Approaches to Gender, Age, Status, Ethnicity and Religion,* edited by Margarita Díaz-Andreu, Sam Lucy, Stasa Babić, and David N. Edwards. New York: Routledge.

Bar-Yosef, Ofer. 2011. "Climatic fluctuations and early farming in West and East Asia." *Current Anthropology* 52 (4): 175–193.

Barker, David J.P. 2004. "The developmental origins of chronic adult disease." *Acta Paediatrica* 93: 26–33.

Barrett, Ronald. 2010. "Avian Influenza and the Third Epidemiological Transition." In *Plagues and Epidemics: Infected Spaces Past and Present,* edited by Ann Herring and Alan C. Swedlund, 81. New York: Bergin.

Barrett, Ronald, Christopher W. Kuzawa, Thomas McDade, and George J. Armelagos. 1998. "Emerging and re-emerging infectious diseases: The third epidemiologic transition." *Annual Review of Anthropology:* 247–271.

Benfer, Robert A. 2013[1984]. "The Challenges and Rewards of Sedentism: The Preceramic Village of Paloma, Peru." In *Paleopathology at the Origins of Agriculture,* edited by Mark N. Cohen and George J. Armelagos, 531–558. Gainesville: University Press of Florida.

Berkes, Fikret. 2008. *Sacred Ecology.* 1st ed. Abingdon: Routledge.

Bickle, Penny. 2018. "Stable isotopes and dynamic diets: The Mesolithic-Neolithic dietary transition in terrestrial central Europe." *Journal of Archaeological Science: Reports* 22: 444–451.

Binford, Louis. 1968. "Post Pleistocene Adaptations." In *New Perspectives in Archaeology,* edited by Sally R. Binford and Louis R. Binford, 313–341. New York: Routledge.

Bird, Michael I., Stefani A. Crabtree, Jordahna Haig, Sean Ulm, and Christopher M. Wurster. 2021. "A global carbon and nitrogen isotope perspective on modern and ancient human diet." *Proceedings of the National Academy of Sciences* 118 (19): e2024642118.

Blaut, James M. 1999. "Environmentalism and eurocentrism." *Geographical Review* 89(3): 391–408.

Boldsen, Jesper L. 2007. "Early childhood stress and adult age mortality—A study of dental enamel hypoplasia in the medieval Danish village of Tirup." *American Journal of Physical Anthropology* 132 (1): 59–66. https://doi.org/10.1002/ajpa.20467

Boserup, Ester. 1965. *The Conditions of Agricultural Growth: The Economics of Agrarian Change Under Conditions of Population Growth.* Chicago: Aldine.

Bourke, Claire D., James A. Berkley, and Andrew J. Prendergast. 2016. "Immune dysfunction as a cause and consequence of malnutrition." *Trends in Immunology* 37 (6): 386–398.

Braidwood, R.J. 1967. *Prehistoric Men.* Glenview: Scott Foresman.

Brickley, Megan B. 2018. "Cribra orbitalia and porotic hyperostosis: A biological approach to diagnosis." *American Journal of Physical Anthropology* 167 (4): 896–902. https://doi.org/10.1002/ajpa.23701

Brown, Terence A., Martin K. Jones, Wayne Powell, and Robin G. Allaby. 2009. "The complex origins of domesticated crops in the Fertile Crescent." *Trends in Ecology & Evolution* 24 (2): 103–109.

Buikstra, Jane. 2013[1984]. "The Lower Illinois River Valley Region: A Prehistoric Context for the Study of Ancient Diet and Health." In *Paleopathology at the Origins of Agriculture,* edited by Mark N. Cohen and George J. Armelagos, 215–234. Gainesville: University Press of Florida.

Buikstra, Jane, ed. 2019. *Ortner's Identification of Pathological Conditions in Human Skeletal Remains.* 3rd ed. New York: Academic Press.

Cassidy, Claire Monod. 2013 [1984]. "Skeletal Evidence for Prehistoric Subsistence Adaptation in the Central Ohio River Valley." In *Paleopathology at the Origins of Agriculture,* edited by Mark N. Cohen and George J. Armelagos, 307–345. Gainesville: University Press of Florida.

Childe, V. Gordon. 1936. *Man Makes Himself.* London: Watts.

Clark, A. L., N. Tayles, and S. E. Halcrow. 2014. "Aspects of health in prehistoric mainland Southeast Asia: Indicators of stress in response to the intensification of rice agriculture." *American Journal of Physical Anthropology* 153 (3): 484–495. https://doi.org/10.1002/ajpa.22449

Cohen, Mark Nathan. 1977. *The Food Crisis in Prehistory: Overpopulation and the Origins of Agriculture.* New Haven: Yale University Press.

Cohen, Mark Nathan. 2009. "Rethinking the origins of agriculture." *Current Anthropology* 50 (5): 591–595. https://doi.org/10.1086/603548

Cohen, Mark Nathan, and Gillian M. Mountford Crane-Kramer. 2007. *Ancient Health: Skeletal Indicators of Agricultural and Economic Intensification.* University Press of Florida.

Cook, Della Collins. 2013[1984]. "Subsistence and Health in the Lower Illinois Valley: Osteological Evidence." In *Paleopathology at the Origins of Agriculture,* edited by Mark N. Cohen and George J. Armelagos, 235–269. Gainesville: University Press of Florida.

Cucina, Andrea, Cristina Perera Cantillo, Thelma Sierra Sosa, and Vera Tiesler. 2011. "Carious lesions and maize consumption among the Prehispanic Maya: An analysis of a coastal community in northern Yucatan." *American Journal of Physical Anthropology* 145 (4): 560–567. https://doi.org/https://doi.org/10.1002/ajpa.21534

Davies-Barrett, Anna M., Daniel Antoine, and Charlotte A. Roberts. 2019. "Inflammatory periosteal reaction on ribs associated with lower respiratory tract disease: A method for recording prevalence from sites with differing preservation." *American Journal of Physical Anthropology* 168 (3): 530–542.

DeWitte, Sharon N. 2014. "Mortality risk and survival in the aftermath of the medieval Black Death." *PLoS One* 9 (5): e96513. https://doi.org/10.1371/journal.pone.0096513

DeWitte, Sharon N., and Christopher M. Stojanowski. 2015. "The osteological paradox 20 years later: Past perspectives, future directions." *Journal of Archaeological Research* 23 (4): 397–450. https://doi.org/10.1007/s10814-015-9084-1

Diamond, Jared. 1987. "The worst mistake in the history of the history of the human race." *Discover.*

Diamond, Jared. 1998. *Guns, Germs and Steel: A Short History of Everybody in the Last 13,000 Years.* New York: W.W. Norton.

Dickel, D.N., P.D., Schultz, and H.M., McHenry 2013 [1984]. "Central California: Prehistoric Subsistence Changes and Health." *In Paleopathology at the Origins of Agriculture*, 2nd ed., edited by M.N. Cohen and G.J. Armelagos, 439–462. University Press of Florida.

Donoghue, H.D. 2019. "Tuberculosis and leprosy associated with historical human population movements in Europe and beyond–an overview based on mycobacterial ancient DNA." *Ann Hum Biol* 46 (2): 120–128.

Eshed, V., A. Gopher, R. Pinhasi, and I. Hershkovitz. 2010. "Paleopathology and the origin of agriculture in the Levant." *American Journal of Physical Anthropology* 143 (1): 121–133. https://doi.org/10.1002/ajpa.21301

Flannery, Kent V. 1969. "Origins and Ecological Effects of Early Domestication in Iran and the Near East." In *The Domestication and Exploitation of Plants and Animals*, edited by P.J. Ucko and G.W. Dimbleby, 73–100. London: Duckworth.

Flannery, Kent V., and Joyce Marcus. 2012. *The Creation of Inequality: How Our Prehistoric Ancestors Set the Stage for Monarchy, Slavery, and Empire.* Cambridge, MA: Harvard University Press.

French, Jennifer C. 2016. "Demography and the Palaeolithic archaeological record" *Journal of Archaeological Method and Theory* 23 (1): 150–199. https://doi.org/10.1007/s10816-014-9237-4

Furuse, Yuki, Akira Suzuki, and Hitoshi Oshitani. 2010. "Origin of measles virus: Divergence from rinderpest virus between the 11th and 12th centuries." *Virology Journal* 7 (1): 52–55.

Gehlsen, Duane. 2009. *Social Complexity and the Origins of Agriculture: the Complex-systems Theory of Culture.* Saarbrücken: VDM Verlag.

Gifford-Gonzalez, Diane. 2000. "Animal disease challenges to the emergence of pastoralism in sub-Saharan Africa." *African Archaeological Review* 17 (3): 95–139.

Godfrey, Keith M., Karen A. Lillycrop, Graham C. Burdge, Peter D. Gluckman, and Mark A. Hanson. 2007. "Epigenetic mechanisms and the mismatch concept of the developmental origins of health and disease." *Pediatric Research* 61 (7): 5–10.

Goodman, A., and Martin, D. 2002. "Reconstructing Health Profiles from Skeletal Remains." In *The Backbone of History: Health and Nutrition in the Western Hemisphere* edited by R.H. Steckel and J.C. Rose, 11–60. Cambridge University Press.

Goodman, Alan H., John Lallo, George J. Armelagos, and Jerome C. Rose. 2013[1984]. "Health Changes at Dickson Mounds, Illinois (A.D. 950–1300)." *In Paleopathology at the Origins of Agriculture*, edited by Mark N. Cohen and George J. Armelagos, 271–306. Gainesville: University Press of Florida.

Gremillion, Kristen J., and Dolores R. Piperno. 2009. "Human behavioral ecology, phenotypic (developmental) plasticity, and agricultural origins: Insights from the emerging evolutionary synthesis." *Current Anthropology* 50 (5): 615–619. https://doi.org/10.1086/605360

Groman-Yaroslavski, Iris, Ehud Weiss, and Dani Nadel. 2016. "Composite sickles and cereal harvesting methods at 23,000-years-old Ohalo II, Israel." *PLoS One* 11 (11): e0167151. https://doi.org/10.1371/journal.pone.0167151

Guatelli-Steinberg, Debbie. 2015. "Dental stress indicators from micro- to macroscopic." *In A Companion to Dental Anthropology*, 450–464.

Harkins, Kelly M., and Anne C. Stone. 2015. "Ancient pathogen genomics: Insights into timing and adaptation." *Journal of Human Evolution* 79: 137–149.

Harn, Alan D. 1978. "Mississippian Settlement Patterns in the Central Illinois River Valley." *In Mississippian Settlement Patterns*, 233–268. Elsevier.

Hayden, Brian, Sandra Bowdler, Karl W. Butzer, Mark N. Cohen, Mark Druss, Robert C. Dunnell, Albert C. Goodyear et al. 1981. "Research and development in the Stone Age: Technological transitions among hunter-gatherers [and comments and reply]." *Current Anthropology* 22 (5): 519–548. http://www.jstor.org/stable/2742287

Hens, S. M., K. Godde, and K.M. Macak. 2019. Iron deficiency anemia, population health and frailty in a modern Portuguese skeletal sample. *Plos One* 14(3): e0213369. https://doi.org/10.1371/journal.pone.0213369

Holt, Brigitte M., and Vincenzo Formicola. 2008. "Hunters of the Ice Age: The biology of Upper Paleolithic people." *American Journal of Physical Anthropology* 137 (S47): 70–99.

Jackes, Mary. 2011. "Representativeness and Bias in Archaeological Skeletal Samples." In *Social Bioarchaeology*, edited by Anne L. Grauer, 107–146. Hoboken: Wiley Blackwell.

Jovanovic, J., R.C. Power, C. de Becdelievre, G. Goude, and S. Stefanovic. 2021. "Microbotanical evidence for the spread of cereal use during the Mesolithic-Neolithic transition in the Southeastern Europe (Danube Gorges): Data from dental calculus analysis." *Journal of Archaeological Science* 125 (105288). https://doi.org/10.1016/j.jas.2020.105288

Kelly, Robert L. 1995. *The Foraging Spectrum: Diversity in Hunter-Gatherer Lifeways*. Washington DC: Smithsonian Institution Press.

Kennedy, Kenneth A.R. 2013[1984]. "Growth, Nutrition, and Pathology in Changing Paleodemographic Settings in South Asia." In *Paleopathology at the Origins of Agriculture*, edited by Mark N. Cohen and George J. Armelagos, 170–192. Gainesville: University Press of Florida.

Kuijt, Ian, and Nigel Goring-Morris. 2002. "Foraging, farming, and social complexity in the pre-pottery neolithic of the southern Levant: A review and synthesis." *Journal of World Prehistory* 16 (4): 361–440. https://doi.org/10.1023/A:1022973114090

Kuzawa, Christopher W., and Elizabeth A. Quinn. 2009. "Developmental origins of adult function and health: evolutionary hypotheses." *Annual Review of Anthropology* 38: 131–147.

Larsen, Clark S., Dale L. Hutchinson, and Christopher M. Stojanowski. 2007. "Health and lifestyle in Georgia and Florida: Agricultural origins and intensification in regional perspective." In *Ancient Health: Skeletal Indicators of Economic and Political Intensification*, edited by M. N. Cohen and G.M.M. Crane-Kramer, 20–34. University Press of Florida.

Larson, Clark S. 2013[1984]. "Health and Disease in Prehistoric Georgia: The Transition to Agriculture." In *Paleopathology at the Origins of Agriculture*, edited by Mark N. Cohen and George J. Armelagos, 367–392. Gainesville: University Press of Florida.

Larson, Greger, Dolores R. Piperno, Robin G. Allaby, Michael D. Purugganan, Leif Andersson, Manuel Arroyo-Kalin, Loukas Barton et al. 2014. "Current perspectives and the future of domestication studies." *Proceedings of the National Academy of Sciences of the United States of America* 111 (17): 6139–6146.

Littleton, Judith. 2007. "The political ecology of health in Bahrain." In *Ancient Health: Skeletal Indicators of Agricultural and Economic Intensification*, edited by M.N. Cohen and G. Crane-Kramer, 1: 176–189. University Press of Florida.

Liu, D., J. Zhang, T. Li, C. Li, X. Liu, J. Zheng, Z. Su et al. 2019. "Chronic osteomyelitis with proliferative periostitis of the mandibular body: Report of a case and review of the literature." *The Annals of The Royal College of Surgeons of England* 101 (5): 328–332.

Marklein, Kathryn E., Rachael E. Leahy, and Douglas E. Crews. 2016. "In sickness and in death: Assessing frailty in human skeletal remains." *American Journal of Physical Anthropology* 161 (2): 208–225.

Marklein, Kathryn E., Christina Torres-Rouff, Laura M. King, and Mark Hubbe. 2019. "The precarious state of subsistence: reevaluating dental pathological lesions associated with agricultural and hunter-gatherer lifeways." *Current Anthropology* 60 (3): 341–368.

Martin, Debra L., George J. Armelagos, Alan Goodman, and Dennis P. Van Gurven. 2013[1984]. "The Effects of Socioeconomic Change in Prehistoric Africa: Sudanese Nubia as a Case Study." In *Paleopathology at the Origins of Agriculture*, edited by Mark N. Cohen and George J. Armelagos, 51–73. Gainesville: University Press of Florida.

Mays, Simon A. 1985. "The relationship between Harris line formation and bone growth and development." *Journal of Archaeological Science* 12 (3): 207–220.

McCaa, Robert. 2002. "Paleodemography of the Americas: From Ancient Times to Colonialism and Beyond." In *The Backbone of History: Health and Nutrition in the Western Hemisphere*, edited by Richard H. Steckel and Jerome C. Rose, 94–124. Cambridge, UK: Cambridge University Press.

McDade, Thomas W. 2005. "The ecologies of human immune function." *Annual Review of Anthropology* 34: 495–521.

McEniry, Mary. 2013. "Early-life conditions and older adult health in low- and middle-income countries: A review." *Journal of the Developmental Origins of Health and Disease* 4 (1): 10–29. https://doi.org/10.1017/s2040174412000499

Miszkiewicz, Justyna J. 2015. "Linear enamel hypoplasia and age-at-death at medieval (11th–16th centuries) St. Gregory's Priory and Cemetery, Canterbury, UK." *International Journal of Osteoarchaeology* 25 (1): 79–87.

Mummert, Amanda, Emily Esche, Joshua Robinson, and George J. Armelagos. 2011. "Stature and robusticity during the agricultural transition: evidence from the bioarchaeological record." *Economics & Human Biology* 9 (3): 284–301.

Nair, P.N. Ramanchandran. 2004. "Pathogenesis of apical periodontitis and the causes of endodontic failures." *Critical Reviews in Oral Biology & Medicine* 15 (6): 348–381.

Odling-Smee, John, Kevin N. Laland, and Marcus W. Feldman. 2012. *Niche Construction: The Neglected Process in Evolution*. Berkeley: University of California Press.

Ortner, Donald J. 1991. Theoretical and methodological issues in paleopathology. *Human paleopathology: Current syntheses and future options*: 5–11.

Ortner, Donald J. 1992. "Skeletal Paleopathology: Probabilities, Possibilities, and Impossibilities." In *Disease and Demography in the Americas*, edited by John W. Verano and Douglas H. Ubelaker, 5–13. Washington, DC: Smithsonian Institute Press.

Ortner, Donald J. 2003. *Identification of Pathological Conditions in Human Skeletal Remains*. New York: Academic Press.

Ortner, Donald J. 2011. "Human skeletal paleopathology." *International Journal of Paleopathology* 1 (1): 4–11. https://doi.org/10.1016/j.ijpp.2011.01.002

Papageorgopoulou, Christina, Susanne Suter, Frank Ruhli, and Frank Siegmund. 2011. "Harris lines revisited: Prevalence, comorbidities, and possible etiologies." *American Journal of Human Biology* 23 (3): 381–391.

Perzigian, Anthony J., Patricia A. Tench, and Donna J. Braun. 2013. "Prehistoric Health in the Ohio River Valley." In *Paleopathology at the Origins of Agriculture*, edited by Mark N. Cohen and George J. Armelagos, 347–366. Gainesville: University Press of Florida.

Piperata, Barbara A., Mark Hubbe, and Kammi K. Schmeer. 2014. "Intra-population variation in anemia status and its relationship to economic status and self-perceived health in the Mexican family life survey: Implications for bioarchaeology." *American Journal of Physical Anthropology* 155 (2): 210–220.

Piperno, Dolores R., Anthony J. Ranere, Ruth Dickau, and Francisco Aceituno. 2017. "Niche construction and optimal foraging theory in Neotropical agricultural origins: A re-evaluation in consideration of the empirical evidence." *Journal of Archaeological Science* 78: 214–220.

Prentice, Andrew M. 1999. "The thymus: A barometer of malnutrition." *British Journal of Nutrition* 81 (5): 345–347.

Quammen, David. 2012. *Spillover: Animal Infections and the Next Human Pandemic*. New York: Norton.

Rakita, Gordon, Jane E. Buikstra, Lane A. Bekc, and Sloane R. Williams, eds. 2005. *Interacting with the Dead: Perspectives on Mortuary Archaeology for the New Millennium*. Gainesville: University Press of Florida.

Rathbun, Ted A. 2013[1984]. "Skeletal Pathology from the Paleolithic Through the Metal Ages in Iran and Iraq." In *Paleopathology at the Origins of Agriculture*, edited by M.N. Cohen and G. Armelagos, 137–167. Cambridge, UK: Academic Press.

Reinhard, Karl J., Luis Fernando Ferreira, Françoise Bouchet, Luciana Sianto, Juliana M.F. Dutra, Alena Iniguez, Daniela Leles et al. 2013. "Food, parasites, and epidemiological transitions: A broad perspective." *International Journal of Paleopathology* 3 (3): 150–157.

Reitsema, Laurie J., and Britney K. McIlvaine. 2014. "Reconciling 'stress' and 'health' in physical anthropology: What can bioarchaeologists learn from the other subdisciplines?" *American Journal of Physical Anthropology* 155: 181–185.

Reyes-Garcia, Victoria, Maximilien Gueze, Isabel Diaz-Reviriego, Romain Duda, Alvaro Fernandez-Llamazares, Sandrine Gallois, Lucentezza Napitupulu et al. 2016. "The adaptive nature of culture: A cross-cultural analysis of the returns of local environmental knowledge in three indigenous societies." *Current Anthropology* 57 (6): 761–784. https://doi.org/10.1086/689307

Richerson, Peter J., Robert Boyd, and Robert L. Bettinger. 2001. "Was agriculture impossible during the Pleistocene but mandatory during the Holocene? A climate change hypothesis." *American Antiquity* 66(3): 387–411.

Rivera, Frances, and Marta Mirazón Lahr. 2017. "New evidence suggesting a dissociated etiology for cribra orbitalia and porotic hyperostosis." *American Journal of Physical Anthropology* 164 (1): 76–96.

Roberts, Charlotte, and Keith Manchester. 2005. *The Archaeology of Disease*. 3rd ed. Ithaca: Cornell University Press.

Robertson, Douglas, and A.J. Smith. 2009. "The microbiology of the acute dental abscess." *Journal of Medical Microbiology* 58 (2): 155–162.

Salamini, F., H. Ozkan, A. Brandolini, R. Schafer-Pregl, and W. Martin. 2002. "Genetics and geography of wild cereal domestication in the Near East." *Nature Reviews Genetics* 3 (6): 429–441. https://doi.org/10.1038/nrg817

Sandberg, Paul A., and Dennis P. Van Gerven. 2016. "Canaries in the Mineshaft: The Children of Kulubnarti." In *New Directions in Biocultural Anthropology*, edited by M.K. Zuckerman and D.L. Martin, 159–176. Hoboken: Wiley-Blackwell.

Smith, Bruce D. 2012. "A cultural niche construction theory of initial domestication." *Biological Theory* 6: 260–271.

Smith-Guzmán, N.E. 2015. *The skeletal manifestation of malaria: An epidemiological approach using documented skeletal collections*. https://doi.org/10.1002/ajpa.22819

Smith, P., and L.K. Horwitz, 2007. "Ancestors and inheritors: A bioanthropological perspective on the transition to agropastoralism in the Southern Levant." In *Ancient Health: Skeletal Indicators of Agricultural and Economic Intensification*, Vol. 1, edited by M.N. Cohen and G. Crane-Kramer, 207–222. University Press of Florida.

Smith, Patricia, Ofer Bar-Yosef, and Andrew Sillen. 2013[1984]. "Archaeological and Skeletal Evidence for Dietary Change during the Late Pleistocene/Early Holocene in the Levant." In *Paleopathology at the Origins of Agriculture*, edited by Mark N. Cohen and George J. Armelagos, 101–136. Gainesville: University Press of Florida.

Soames, James Victor, and John Chambers Southam. 2005. *Oral pathology*. Oxford University Press.

Spyrou, Maria A., Rezeda I. Tukhbatova, Michal Feldman, Joanna Drath, Sacha Kacki, Julia Beltrán de Heredia, Susanne Arnold et al. 2016. "Historical Y. pestis genomes reveal the European Black Death as the source of ancient and modern plague pandemics." *Cell Host & Microbe* 19(6): 874–881.

Steckel, Richard H. 1995. "Stature and the standard of living." *Journal of Economic Literature* 33(4): 1903–1940. http://www.jstor.org/stable/2729317

Steckel, Richard H., and Jerome C. Rose. 2002. "Patterns of Health in the Western Hemisphere." In *The Backbone of History: Health and Nutrition in the Western Hemisphere*, edited by Richard H. Steckel and Jerome C. Rose, 563–582. Cambridge, UK: Cambridge University Press.

Steckel, Richard H., Paul W. Sciulli, and Jerome C. Rose. 2002. "A Health Index from Skeletal Remains." In *The Backbone of History: Health and Nutrition in the Western Hemisphere*, edited by Richard H. Steckel and Jerome C. Rose, 61–93. Cambridge, UK: Cambridge University Press.

Steinbock, R. 1976. *Paleopathological Diagnosis and Interpretation: Bone Disease in Ancient Human Populations*. Springfield, IL: Charles Thomas Publisher.

Stiner, Mary C., Natalie D. Munro, Todd A. Surovell, Eitan Tchernov, and Ofer Bar-Yosef. 1999. "Paleolithic population growth pulses evidenced by small animal exploitation." *Science* 283 (5399): 190–194. https://doi.org/10.1126/science.283.5399.190

Storey, Rebecca, Lourdes Marquez Morfin, and Vernon Smith. 2002. "Social Disruption and the Maya civilization of Mesoamerica." In *The Backbone of History: Health and Nutrition in the Western Hemisphere*, edited by R.H. Steckel and J.C. Rose, 283–306. Cambridge, UK: Cambridge University Press.

Temple, Daniel H., and Alan H. Goodman. 2014. "Bioarcheology has a 'health' problem: Conceptualizing 'stress' and 'health' in bioarchaeological research." *American Journal of Physical Anthropology*

155 (2): 186–191. https://doi.org/https://doi.org/10.1002/ajpa.22602

Tilley, Lorna, and Alecia A. Schrenk. 2017. *New Developments in the Bioarchaeology of Care: Further Case Studies and Expanded Theory*. New York: Springer International Publishing.

UN FAO. 2020. "Sustainable Food and Agriculture." Food and Agriculture Organization of the United Nations. https://www.fao.org/sustainability/news/detail/en/c/1274219/

Van Gerven, Dennis P., J. Hummert, K. Pendergast Moore, and M.K. Sanford. 1990. "Nutrition, disease and the human life cycle: A bioethnography of a medieval Nubian community." *Primate Life History and Evolution* 1: 297–324.

VanDerwarker, Amber M., Dana N. Bardolph, Kristin M. Hoppa, Heather B. Thakar, Lana S. Martin, Allison L. Jaqua, Matthew E. Biwer et al. 2016. "New World paleoethnobotany in the New Millennium (2000–2013)." *Journal of Archaeological Research* 24 (2): 125–177. https://doi.org/10.1007/s10814-015-9089-9

Vaupel, James W., Kenneth G. Manton, and Eric Stallard. 1979. "The impact of heterogeneity in individual frailty on the dynamics of mortality." *Demography* 16 (3): 439–454.

VerCauteren, Kurt C., Michael J. Lavelle, and Henry Campa III. 2018. "Persistent spillback of bovine tuberculosis from white-tailed deer to cattle in Michigan, USA: Status, strategies, and needs." *Frontiers in Veterinary Science* 5: 301.

Walker, Phillip L., Rhonda R. Bathurst, Rebecca Richman, Thor Gjerdrum, and Valerie A. Andrushko. 2009. "The causes of porotic hyperostosis and cribra orbitalia: A reappraisal of the iron-deficiency-anemia hypothesis." *American Journal of Physical Anthropology* 139 (2): 109–125.

Walker, Susan P., Theodore D. Wachs, Julie Meeks Gardner, Betsy Lozoff, Gail A. Wasserman, Ernesto Pollitt, Julie A. Carter et al. 2007. "Child development: Risk factors for adverse outcomes in developing countries." *The Lancet* 369 (9556): 145–157. https://doi.org/10.1016/s0140-6736(07)60076-2

Walson, Judd L., and James A. Berkley. 2018. "The impact of malnutrition on childhood infections." *Current Opinion in Infectious Diseases* 31 (3): 231.

Wapler, Ulrike, Eric Crubezy, and Michael Schultz. 2004. "Is cribra orbitalia synonymous with anemia? Analysis and interpretation of cranial pathology in Sudan." *American Journal of Physical Anthropology* 123 (4): 333–339.

Warinner, Christina, Jessica Hendy, Camilla Speller, Enrico Cappellini, Roman Fischer, Christian Trachsel, Jette Arneborg et al. 2014. "Direct evidence of milk consumption from ancient human dental calculus." *Scientific Reports* 4 (1): 1–6.

Weiss, Robin A. 2001. "The Leeuwenhoek Lecture 2001. Animal origins of human infectious disease." *Philosophical Transactions of the Royal Society of London Series B: Biological Sciences* 356 (1410): 957–977.

Weston, Darlene A. 2008. "Investigating the specificity of periosteal reactions in pathology museum specimens." *American Journal of Physical Anthropology* 137 (1): 48–59. https://doi.org/10.1002/ajpa.20839

Wilcox, Michael. 2010. "Marketing conquest and the vanishing Indian: An indigenous response to Jared Diamond's Guns, germs, and steel and Collapse." *Journal of Social Archaeology* 10(1): 92–117.

Wissler, A. 2021. *Engaging the osteological paradox: A study of frailty and survivorship in the 1918 influenza pandemic.* Unpublished PhD Dissertation. Arizona State University.

Wood, James W., George R. Milner, Henry C. Harpending, and Kenneth M. Weiss. 1992. "The osteological paradox: Problems with inferring prehistoric health from skeletal samples." *Current Anthropology* 33 (4): 343–370. https://doi.org/10.1086/204084

Zhou, Liming, and Robert S. Corruccini. 1998. "Enamel hypoplasias related to famine stress in living Chinese." *American Journal of Human Biology* 10 (6): 723–733. https://doi.org/10.1002/(sici)1520-6300(1998)10:6<723:aid-ajhb4>3.0.co;2-q

PART 2

The Second Epidemiological Transition

CHAPTER 3

When Germ Theory Didn't Matter

There is an Hour when I must die,
Nor do I know how soon 'twill come;
A thousand Children young as I
Are call'd by Death to hear their Doom.
Isaac Watts (1715). *Divine Songs*

Parents should never have to bury their children. Yet tragically, childhood death was all too common from the Neolithic to the early twentieth century, when it remained prevalent even among the wealthier societies of Europe and North America (Volk and Atkinson 2013). This was the case in Victorian England, when child elegies were a popular form of verse and comfort books were written to help surviving mothers and fathers deal with their grief (Jalland 1996). Some spoke with platitudes of heroism, early salvation, and playmates in heaven, while others wrestled with the unjust tragedy of premature death. Emily Dickinson took both approaches in her poem, *On such a night, or such a night*, likening a cemetery to a playground filled with the ghosts of deceased children, while also lamenting that, for all their dreams in life, "feet so precious charged should reach so small a goal" (Dickinson 1896: I, 146).

The scale of these tragedies is reflected in the mortality statistics of the time. In the years just prior to 1840, three out of 10 English children died before the age of 15, and in London, only 44 percent survived to their mid-20s (Wrigley et al. 1997). With an average of five children, English parents were likely to lose at least one son or daughter before the child reached adulthood. At the population level, high childhood mortality restricted life expectancies to little more than 40 years of age (Omran 1971). These were averages of course; many people lived well into their 60s and beyond. However, they first had to reach adulthood before old age was a realistic possibility. This meant surviving a gauntlet of childhood infections.

The situation in England was similar to most societies following the First Epidemiological Transition: an ongoing pattern of high mortality offset with a slightly higher fertility resulting in a net increase in total population. It was a global trend that had persisted since the prehistoric origins of intensive agriculture. Then, in the early years of the Industrial Revolution, England and several other European and American countries began to see modest epidemiological changes. Successive waves of major infectious disease epidemics became less frequent; this had a leveling effect on episodic (a.k.a. "crisis") mortality peaks (Omran 1971). Despite these improvements, however, overall mortality remained high due to the endemic persistence of these same infections.

Industrialization also brought additional health problems with the expansion of urban centers that were ill-equipped to handle increasing concentrations of poor and working-class populations. By the early nineteenth century, British sanitary reformers had brought government attention to these problems. Within the jurisdiction that comprised England and Wales,[1] the government had already developed a registry to adjudicate property claims using standardized life tables. By the late 1830s, a General Registry Office (GRO) was established and the registry itself expanded to include known

Emerging Infections. Second Edition. Ron Barrett, Molly K. Zuckerman, Matthew R. Dudgeon, with George J. Armelagos, Oxford University Press.
© Ron Barrett, Molly K. Zuckerman, Matthew R. Dudgeon (2024). DOI: 10.1093/oso/9780192843135.003.0004

causes of death as well as socio-economic and environmental measures that might prove to be disease risk factors (Eyler 1979; Rosen 1993). In this way, England and Wales were able to amass the world's most comprehensive public health statistics from 1841 to 1911. Despite having a number of shortcomings, these data are generally considered to be the most reliable quantitative measurements of state-level health and socio-demographic changes during this time period.

Not long after the English and Welsh began collecting these statistics, their mortality figures declined substantially, falling even more sharply in the early twentieth century. Other wealthy countries showed similar declines around the same time period (Eyler 1979; Omran 1971). These improvements primarily reflected a reduction in deaths from infectious diseases, especially those contracted in childhood. These declines were so dramatic that they drove an exponential rise in total human populations, despite the fact that fertility rates had been declining during the same period. Eventually chronic, non-infectious diseases replaced acute infections as the major causes of death in these populations.

These disease-related population changes constitute the "Classic Model" of Abdel Omran's Epidemiological Transition Theory (Omran 1971). However, as we noted in the Introduction, Omran's theory was initially applied only to changes that occurred over the last few centuries. (see Figure 0.2 on pg. 6). Lacking the viewpoint of a much deeper time frame, the model did not consider whether the initial proximate conditions—highly prevalent acute infectious diseases—were actually a 10,000-year-old consequence of a much earlier epidemiological transition. Given our knowledge of the Neolithic, we understand that these later historical changes are best described as the Second Epidemiological Transition.

On several levels, the Second Transition is the reverse of the First Transition. Declining mortality rates stand in obvious contrast to the ancient increases we examined in Chapter 2. The Second Transition also presents reverse examples of the ways that human modes of subsistence, settlement, and social organization shape the evolution of microorganisms and determine our risk for infectious diseases. The Second Transition would

eventually spread to more than 95 percent of the world. However, as we will see in Chapter 4, there were problematic differences in the ways that the later versions of this transition played out in low- and middle-income countries. To improve our understanding of these later problems, we must first examine the earliest instances of infectious disease decline in the wealthier nations of Europe and North America. We need to know what went right in these places so that we can understand what went wrong in other places.

This chapter critically examines the ideas and events surrounding the first instances of the Second Epidemiological Transition. Because it is the best documented example of these early transitions, we will focus much of our attention on the case of England and Wales during the nineteenth and early twentieth centuries. We will also clarify some major myths about these events. Chief among them is that Germ Theory was largely responsible for the mortality and infectious disease declines via its revolutionary transformations in biomedicine. Belying this myth, the largest declines in infectious diseases occurred before many of its subsequent medical discoveries were fully realized. Until then, Germ Theory did not contribute as much to the decline in infectious disease as other factors, such as nutrition, sanitation, and housing reforms, especially among working-class communities. These factors harken back to the same themes of subsistence, settlement, and social organization that drove the first emerging infections of the Neolithic.

3.1 Miasma and more

There is little doubt that Germ Theory transformed the fields of biology and biomedicine. It revealed entire worlds of microorganisms, the knowledge of which would eventually lead to life-saving medicines and immunizations against all manner of diseases. Germ Theory also revolutionized surgical practices and food safety procedures. These later changes had a major impact on human health and wellbeing in the later decades of the nineteenth century. That said, more than 50 years had passed between the first clinically relevant microbial discoveries and the development of effective antibiotics and most of the major vaccines we use today. Given this half-century delay, it is worth examining the dominant biomedical theories that preceded Germ Theory. Although some of these ideas were eventually disproven, they nevertheless informed a set of health policies that greatly reduced infectious disease mortality. They also worked in tandem with other ideas that laid the foundation for epidemiological science.

Cursory studies of biomedical history often reveal two generalizations about the biomedical predecessors to Germ Theory in the late nineteenth century. The first is that *miasma*, an ancient Greek term referring to the poisonous gases emitted by decayed organic matter, was the singularly dominant explanation for febrile and epidemic diseases leading up to this period. The second is that miasmic beliefs stood in opposition to contagionist beliefs until they were eventually overwhelmed by the empirical evidence of microscopic observations.

Closer studies, however, reveal a more complex story. Prior to the widespread adoption of Germ Theory, miasmic theories certainly prevailed when it came to explaining febrile and epidemic diseases. However, these theories did not operate alone, nor were they used to explain all instances and aspects of what we now consider to be infectious diseases. There were multiple and overlapping explanations that were variously applied to specific diseases (Baldwin 1999; Hamlin 1992). These explanations typically fell into at least one of three etiological categories:

(1) Environmentalist explanations regarding the role of local conditions such as air quality, water quality, and overall climate in producing or preventing certain diseases. Miasma-like factors were often included in these explanations, sometimes prominently, but they were often listed among other factors whose relative emphasis depended upon the particular diagnosis.

(2) Constitutionalist explanations regarding the susceptibility or resistance of certain people and populations to specific diseases. Some of these explanations were based on racist ideas of inherited dispositions; others blamed certain groups for the chronic effects of bad habits. Yet still other theories took a more syndemic approach, emphasizing the longer-term consequences of poverty and under-nutrition on the susceptibility of populations to clusters of different diseases.

(3) Contagionist explanations regarding the transmission of certain diseases from person to person, though with different ideas as to the nature of the agents being transmitted, such as whether they were gaseous or particulate, inanimate poisons or, in a few instances, living seeds.

All three etiological categories were rooted in the ideas of Classical Greek or Roman medicine. These ideas were further developed in later centuries by physicians and schools in the eastern Mediterranean, North Africa, the Middle East, and eventually, the post-Enlightenment healing traditions that are often referred to as "Western" medicine (Pickstone 1992). These historical trajectories saw many changes in medical theory and practice, but historians would be hard pressed to find a single tradition in which any one of these three explanatory categories was entirely absent. As we will see, there were many instances in which all three explanations were combined to address a particular infection.

Environmental conditions played a central role in the Classical Greek medical treatises attributed to Hippocrates (Jouanna 2012). In this Hippocratic corpus, it was the bodily humors whose balance determined the various states of health and disease. These humors could also be characterized according to different combinations of temperature and moisture, which were in turn associated with different seasons. Informed by this theory, several treatises explain how febrile and epidemic diseases result from the inhalation of putrified air from swamps, marshes, and the decomposed bodies of humans and animals. In the treatise entitled *Breaths*, Hippocrates states:

"Common fever is common because everyone breathes the same air; the same air is mixed with the body in the same way, and so the fevers are identical." And furthermore, "[w]hen the air is infected by miasmas (μιασμασιν), which are harmful to human nature, then men are sick."

(Breaths: Chapter 6. 98.2f. L.
cited in Jouanna 2012: c4 59).

This quotation is exceptional, however, because miasma rarely appears in the Hippocratic corpus[2] (Jouanna 2012). The same is true for the writings of Galen six centuries later, when he famously updated and expanded these Hippocratic theories. The term was also absent from 281 plague tractates written in the years during and after the Black Death, though many of these texts refer to the dangers of putrid and pestilential air. It was not until the seventeenth century that "miasma" was revived by an Italian physician to describe the poisonous effluvia responsible for malaria—apropos, given that the Italian *mal'aria* refers to "bad air" (Sterner 1948).

Miasma resurfaced again in the eighteenth century with a variety of explanations for the causal role of toxic corpuscles in contagious diseases (Wilson 1995). Even then, the proposed agents were of an inanimate nature, and the term "miasma" was not evoked as often as the ancient theory it described: that poisonous gases emitted by decomposing plants and animals were the proximate cause of most febrile diseases, regardless of whether they appeared to be contagious.

Word and theory came together in nineteenth-century England, and miasma became the primary focus of attention for prominent sanitary reformers such as Edwin Chadwick, Thomas Southwood Smith, William Farr, and Florence Nightingale. Chadwick probably had the most influence on mid-century domestic health policies. Trained in the law and inspired by the liberal utilitarianism of Jeremy Bentham, his friend and benefactor, Chadwick eventually rose through the civil ranks to become chief member of the commission to reform and oversee the Poor Law (Halliday 2001). From this position, Chadwick and Smith formed a team to investigate the health of England's poorer populations, publishing a much-read *Report on the Sanitary Conditions of the Labouring Population of Great Britain*. This report led the British government to pass a series of acts aimed at improving urban infrastructure, primarily through water, drainage, and sewage projects designed to eliminate miasma from the most common places where its stench arose. In the words of Chadwick:

"All smell is, if it be intense, immediate acute disease; and eventually we may say that, by depressing the system and rendering it susceptible to the action of other causes, all smell is disease."

(Chadwick 1846 cited in Halliday 2001).

Yet despite Chadwick's significant influence, many English sanitarians did not share his myopia for miasma, nor did they share his nearly singular emphasis on the most proximate environmental causes of disease. Many were also influenced by constitutionalist theories that explained why some populations were predisposed to disease more than others. Once again, these views had ancient roots and a longstanding history. Hippocrates described a variety of constitutional factors to explain the comparative observations he made of different people during his Mediterranean travels, and Galen made similar claims to explain why plague affected some communities more than others (Jouanna 2012). Centuries later, these ideas informed a sanitarian concern with deprivation, particularly with respect to nutritional states, and their role in the greater susceptibility of impoverished communities to many diseases. Florence Nightingale was one of these sanitarians. She was a strong supporter of Chadwick and his miasmic ideas; these informed her hospital reforms, which emphasized the importance of cleanliness and ventilation. Yet additionally, Nightingale strongly advocated for good nutrition, which she thought essential for building the physical constitution of patients (Gill and Gill 2005).

William Farr had similar concerns about the effects of nutrition on the human constitution. As the first statistician of the General Registrar's Office (GRO), Farr effectively crafted and oversaw a new system for measuring the health of the country's population in a series of annual government reports on births, deaths, and marriages. He owed his career to Chadwick, and the two worked closely together on the reports (Halliday 2000). Nevertheless, tensions arose between them during the drafting of their first report in 1839, when Farr classified starvation as an official cause of 63 deaths among a total of 148,000 deaths that year (Hamlin 1995). He wrote to Chadwick that the numbers may even be higher:

"Hunger destroys a much higher proportion than is indicated by the registers in this and in every other country, but its effects, like the effects of excess, are generally manifested indirectly, in the production of diseases of various kinds."

(cited in Hamlin 1995: 857).

In making the constitutional case for deprivation, Farr was effectively arguing for a syndemic of malnutrition and many diseases that were disproportionately impacting the poor populations of Britain. But although Chadwick recognized the problem, he argued forcefully against the inclusion of starvation as a nosological category in the annual reports (Hamlin 1995; Pickstone 1992). Chadwick claimed that the category did not account for breastfeeding difficulties among infant deaths, and that it was ambiguous with respect to the many deprivations, such as cold weather, that often accompany hunger. Chadwick also stated that, as an etiological category, starvation was too broad and remote in comparison to all the other more "exciting" (i.e., proximate) physiologically based causes in the Registry. Chadwick prevailed. Although miasma would be disproven by Germ Theory a few decades later, Chadwick's central focus on proximate, singular, and physiological causes became—for better and worse—an enduring theme in biomedicine and public health (Hamlin 1992).

Politics may have also played a role in the Chadwick–Farr exchange. In his analysis of the controversy, Christopher Hamlin discusses Chadwick's conflict of interest as Chief Administrator for the implementation of the New Poor Law (1995). As a proxy for public relief, the New Poor Law offered workhouses and workhouse diets (based on prison diet experiments) that were designed to provide the barest sustenance to poor families, who were also required to be separated while they were receiving assistance. These austerities were meant to deter lazy and irresponsible behavior while still providing for basic survival. Yet the workhouses proved so unpopular that many preferred to live in abject poverty and some even opted for prison. The New Poor Law became known as the "Starvation Law" by working-class and poor communities, who fervently opposed the policy and its institutions.[3] Notwithstanding his stated concerns about medical nosology, it was not in Chadwick's political interest to have starvation enumerated in official public health records.

Contagion was far less controversial than starvation in the annual reports. Contagious diseases were listed first among the five major classes under which the causes of death were organized (Farr

2000 [1856]). These Class I, *zymotic* (cf. fermenting) diseases included smallpox, plague, influenza, cholera, syphilis, and several other acute fevers. The transmissibility of these diseases had been recognized since the time of Hippocrates. However, the nature of the contagion was another matter, and there was no suggestion at that time of invisible organisms. Instead, the zymotic diseases were attributed to (i) miasmas that could be transmitted from person to person; (ii) poisons that could be transmitted by direct contact or puncture; (iii) transmission between food and blood; and (iv) direct transmission by visible parasites.

Physicians and scholars may have debated these causes with respect to particular diseases, but with the exception of the parasites, the annual reports reflected a medical consensus that did not allow for organismic causes. This is famously illustrated in John Snow's investigations of the London cholera epidemics that occurred during the first decade of this classification (Figure 3.1). Snow's investigation of the Broad Street neighborhood during the 1848 cholera epidemic, and his petition to have the pump handle removed from the neighborhood's contaminated well is an oft-cited legend in the public health community (Figure 3.2). But it was Snow's London-wide comparison of changes between the 1848 and 1854 epidemics, the so-called Grand Experiment, that provided the strongest evidence for the water-borne transmission of cholera (Johnson 2006).

Working with data provided by William Farr, Snow analyzed the geographic distribution of London cholera deaths for the two epidemics, paying particular attention to water supply (Snow 1855). During the 1848 epidemic, 10 major water companies had exclusive rights to and infrastructure in different areas of the city. Most had intake pipes within the tidal basin of the Thames River, which was highly contaminated with sewage. These included the Lambeth and Southwark & Vauxhall (S&V) companies, and in 1848, cholera mortality was comparable in their respective neighborhoods. But in 1852, Lambeth shifted its intake above the tidal reach of the river, and during the 1855 epidemic, cholera mortality in its recipient neighborhoods was almost five times less than those supplied by the S&V company. Unintended circumstances had

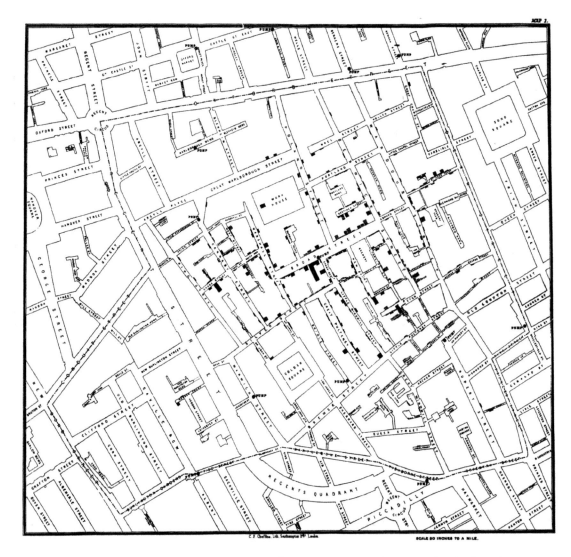

Figure 3.1 John Snow's original map depicting a geographic cluster of cholera cases in the Broad Street area of London during the 1854 epidemic. This was part of a much larger statistical comparison of two cholera epidemics that demonstrated the waterborne contagion of the disease.

Source: John Snow (1855). On the Mode of Communication of Cholera, 2nd Ed, John Churchill: London, England.

resulted in a crossover experiment with case and control groups totaling more than 300,000 people. It certainly was a grand experiment, albeit a naturalistic one, that required only thoughtful observation of unfolding events (Frerichs 2000; Johnson 2006).

This mortality difference between the London neighborhoods eventually convinced Farr to change his mind about cholera transmission. That said,

Farr did not publicly acknowledge the water-borne theory until 1866, after Snow's death, the Great Stink of London, another cholera epidemic, and perhaps most relevantly, Chadwick's retirement (Halliday 2001). Even then, the water-borne theory did not necessitate the existence of a living microscopic pathogen. Water could simply be another medium for the transmission of a non-living agent. Along these lines, it is interesting to note that Snow ambiguously referred to the agent as the "cholera poison" in his publication (1855).

The evidence for microbial agents was quickly accumulating by the time that Snow's theory was publicly recognized. But as we will see, Germ Theory was more than just another explanation. It challenged an existing social order as well as a major scientific consensus. Consequently, it would take more than pure evidence to change people's minds.

3.2 Shifting paradigms

In *The Structure of Scientific Revolutions*, Thomas Kuhn disputes the generalization that scientific developments inevitably proceed in an incremental and linear fashion, such that theories rise and fall in response to the steady, stepwise accumulation of new evidence (1996). Instead, he proposes a dialectical scenario in which the steady stream of scientific development, if given enough time, is punctuated by revolutionary discoveries that result in profound disciplinary changes.

Kuhn refers to the steady discoveries as a typical activity of "normal science," the process by which discoveries build upon and challenge existing theories, but not to the degree that they overturn fundamental ideas that are considered axiomatic by the scientific consensus. According to Kuhn, these fundamental ideas are the *paradigms* of scientific disciplines. They are the "norms" of normal science.

Unlike the theories of normal science, revolutionary theories occasionally arise to challenge an existing paradigm. They often do so by explaining a major puzzle in a better way than had previously been attempted or solving a previously intractable problem. If the challenge is successful, then a paradigm shift occurs, thus changing one or more scientific disciplines. In many cases, paradigm shifts also change the ways that societies view the world around them (Kuhn 1996; Bird 2012).

In the early half of nineteenth-century Europe and North America, *inanimate cause* was the dominant paradigm to explain the various etiologies of febrile and epidemic diseases. Provided that this paradigm went unchallenged, scientists were encouraged to debate and develop new theories, regardless of whether they leaned toward environmental, constitutional, or contagious causes. Scientists could freely consider whether the miasma of plague could be exhaled by a patient, or a cholera substance moved through the water instead of the air. They could even debate whether external causes or internal health states had a greater impact on disease-affected populations. None of these competing ideas caused a great stir, provided that they continued to assume that the external agent of disease was an inanimate poison instead of a living pathogen.

Germ Theory, however, constituted a whole new paradigm of *contagium vivum*. If accepted, it would do more than supplant old theories. It would also bring about profound changes in multiple scientific disciplines, altering their language and methods of inquiry, and revising curricula for the teaching of biology, chemistry, and medicine. It would also threaten the reputations of senior scholars and health officials. For the latter group especially, the shift would be even more than a matter of personal politics because it also entailed changes to trade and migration policies. Given these stakes, it is not surprising that Germ Theory faced considerable resistance from certain people with power.

To be fair, some of the resistance was based on scientific concerns about the evidence at the time. Even with the development of the microscope, the evidence was literally obscured by a series of technical challenges. In the 1670s, Antoni van Leeuwonhoek, a Dutch draper and amateur scientist, designed a single lens microscope that allowed him to see free-swimming microorganisms in natural media such as pondwater and human saliva (Fassin 1934). Based on these observations, he described the shapes and motions of numerous microorganisms which he called "animalcules" (Figure 3.2).

After sending numerous letters, and even giving away many of his microscopes with instructions on their use, van Leeuwenhoek captured the attention of the Royal Society as well as that of several reputable scholars. More than three centuries later, follow-up studies of van Leeuwenhoek's instruments and notes determined that he probably made the first observations of individual bacteria (van Zuylen 1981). But the instruments he donated were of variable quality, and van Leeuwenhoek's observations were difficult to

(a)

(b)

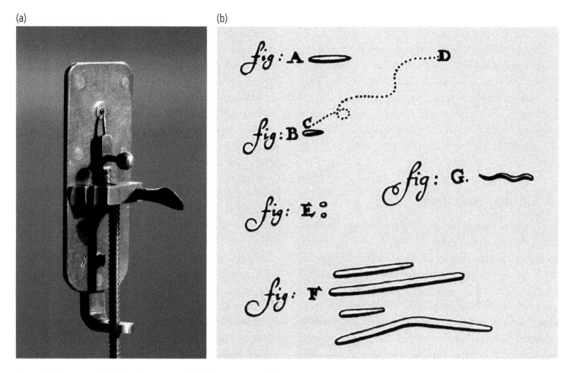

Figure 3.2 van Leeuwhoek's microscope and sketches. a. Replica of the single lens microscope used to make his observations. b. Sketches sent to the Royal Society depicting the shapes and movements of bacteria obtained from the human mouth.

Sources: a: Jerome Rowkema. cca-sa 3.0 unported. b: van Leeuwonhoek letter 39. 17 September, 1683.

replicate. Consequently, the proposed animalcules were eventually met with considerable skepticism (Lane 2015).

That van Leeuwenhoek received any consideration at all was at least partly due to the work of a highly regarded contemporary. A decade earlier, Robert Hooke, the English polymath and Royal Society member who had already contributed to a variety of fields, published a book about his observations with a compound microscope (1665). *Micrographia* presented exquisitely detailed illustrations of plant and animal microstructures, as well as those of other natural and manufactured objects. These included the honeycomb-like structures of cork, for which Hooke first coined the term "cells." They also included microfungi in mold samples, with stalk-like structures that suggested some kind of reproductive function (Gest 2004). Nevertheless, Hook's microscope did not approach the magnification of van Leewenhoek's simpler instrument, and the bacterial "animalcules" were too small to catch his eye.

Despite its potential, the compound microscope encountered chromatic and spherical aberrations at higher magnification. The first problem was solved by John Dolland, who patented an achromatic lens in 1759 (Araki 2017). The second problem was solved in 1830 by Joseph Jackson Lister (father of the famous surgeon, Joseph Lister), when he discovered a way to combine the effects of lower magnification lenses. From that point forward, the compound microscope was capable of resolving bacteria-level images (Figure 3.3).

Yet even with these developments, microscopy needed more than good lenses for its observations to be clinically relevant. Challenges remained with the staining of transparent specimens and fixing any of them in order to characterize and distinguish microbial species. Even today, these challenges are well known to anyone who has worked with a microscope. Then as now, microscopy was as much a craft as it was a science. Without a mastery of both, it was difficult to ascertain the visual evidence for living germs.

(a)　　　　　　　　　　　　　　　(b)

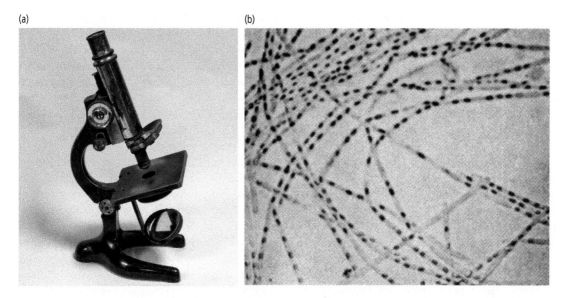

Figure 3.3 Improved microscopy in the late 19th Century. a. Siebert compound microscope of the same model used by Robert Koch in the early stages of his work. b. Photomicrograph of Bacillis anthracis using a different instrument published by Koch in 1877.
Sources: a. Hans Grobe/AWI. CCA-SA 3.0 unported. b. Koch (1877). "Verfahren zur Untersuchung, zum Konservieren und Photographieren der Bakterien." Ders: 27-50.

Neither was the skepticism that greeted Germ Theory a simple matter of conservative resistance to a new idea. On the contrary, *contagium vivum* had an ancient and prolific history, with many accounts of inferences drawn from observable processes such as the spread of decay, the growth of molds, and the leavening of bread (Wilson 1995). In Pre-Classical Greece, Anaxagoras inferred from seed growth the infinitesimal origins of all living things (Vlastos 1950). This doctrine of *panspermia* was popular among Greek and Roman thinkers over the following centuries. Among them was Marcus Torentius Varro (1783) who, in the first century BCE, warned that "in swampy places minute creatures live that cannot be discerned with the eye and they enter the body through the mouth and nostrils and cause serious disease" ([1783] 1934: L.1,12,2).

Tracing these ideas from Imperial Rome to the Renaissance, Vivian Nutton (1983) draws particular attention to the work of Galen, who proposed that the "seeds" of plague could be transmitted from affected to healthy people, thus making them sick. From this proposition, Nutton extrapolates "that the object posited is a living entity; that is in origin very small; and that it contains within itself the potentiality for growth" (1983: 3). These ideas arose many times until the early sixteenth century, when

Girolamo Fracastoro famously (though perhaps not independently) proposed that some diseases are caused by invisible "semenaria" that could be transmitted by direct contact, via surfaces (fomites), or at a distance (Nutton 1983).[4]

Thus the seeds of Germ Theory were at least as old as the inanimate theories of Britain's nineteenth-century medical establishment. Unlike its counterparts, however, *contagium vivum* had darker associations. In what is perhaps the best-known analysis of the controversy, William Ackerknecht (1948) describes its association with the Medieval quarantine practices that were considered archaic in Post-Enlightenment times. Derived from the Venetian *quaranta giorni* (40 days), quarantine applied the Old Testament practice of forced isolation, not only to persons in transit but also to entire communities and anyone under suspicion during the Black Death. By the beginning of the fifteenth century, quarantines were widely adopted by European nations, becoming emblems of collusion between the Universal Church and authoritarian states. Sanitarians wanted nothing to do with them.

Quarantines also presented an empirical problem for Germ Theory when they were used to control indirectly transmitted diseases. Speaking against contagionism in 1834, J.A. Rouchoux cited the failure of quarantines to contain the yellow fever and typhus epidemics during the Napoleonic Wars (1834). Both are vector-borne diseases: typhus being transmitted by lice, and yellow fever by the mosquito *Aedes egypticus*. No quarantine could contain such tiny creatures, and even the contagionists of the time did not suspect the role of insects in the transmission of pathogens across human boundaries (Ackerknecht 1948). The same could be said for water and food-borne diseases such as typhoid and cholera, which could freely move through plumbing, infecting thousands of healthy people who had not previously been in contact with the sick.

Faced with ambiguous evidence, the sordid histories of quarantine, and what appeared to be counterexamples of microbial contagion, we can understand why many nineteenth-century European scientists were critical of Germ Theory. From this perspective, Ackerknecht claims that their criticism was viewed as "a fight for science, against outdated authorities and medieval mysticism; for observation and research against systems and speculation" (1948: 9).

The controversy was also informed by economic and political agendas. Citing the Sanitarian consensus, the English, French, and Dutch empires had relaxed their international quarantine restrictions, regarding goods and people, between the 1820s and 1840s (Ackerknecht 1948). This had the effect of increasing the flow of goods between commercial ports and land borders, while incentivizing and enabling colonial expansion. At the same time, Germ Theory entailed a different set of effects: immigration restrictions, quarantine taxes, and exclusive trade corridors that were variously implemented by the German states, Eastern Europe, and the Ottoman Empire (Baldwin 1999; Hamed-Troyansky 2021). Powerful interests could be found on both sides of the paradigm debates. Here, we could draw analogies with the political and economic dynamics surrounding some of the debates about COVID-19 responses today.

Considering the stakes, practical outcomes may have outweighed theoretical explanations. If so, the successes of sanitarian reform provided the best defense of their causal theories. These successes were systematically documented and statistically measured via the new discipline of epidemiology. In England, the leading epidemiologist was William Farr, the effective (though not official) head of the General Registry Office. From this office, his outcome measurements were the nineteenth-century equivalent of today's big data science. Combined with Chadwick's bureaucratic power and ideological zeal, miasmic sanitation was a major reckoning force in England.

Despite mistaken ideas about the etiology of infectious diseases, Chadwick's model of sanitation reduced many infectious diseases through infrastructural improvements in water quality, sewage, drainage, and waste disposal. It also promoted individual cleanliness not only through personal hygiene but also by the curtailing of perceived vices such as indolence, immoderate drinking, and illicit sexual relations (Baldwin 1999; Eyler 1979). Yet when it came to managing the health of the British military, and the many nations of its empire, Chadwick did not hold a candle to the "Lady with the Lamp."

Florence Nightingale was probably the most influential sanitary health reformer and epidemiologist of her day. Despite pressure from her high-status family, she eschewed marriage and instead chose to become a nurse, which at the time was considered to be a socially low profession. In addition to nursing, Nightingale was personally tutored by Adolph Quetelet, France's pioneering statistician (Diamond and Stone 1981). After gaining clinical experience in London's Soho district (walking distance from John Snow's infamous pump), she used her family connections to obtain the support of the War Minister for an experimental intervention that involved bringing a team of personally selected nurses to the Scutari Barracks Hospital at the height of the Crimean War (Kopf 1916).

At the time, the British military was losing more soldiers to fever diseases than they could replace. In Scutari, Nightingale's team cleaned up the hospital wards, regularly bathed the patients, and changed their linens daily. Nightingale also improved patient nutrition by hiring new cooks, creating better menus, and forming a separate supply chain to guard against corruption. As a committed miasmist, she also ensured that all hospital windows remained open for ventilation (McDonald 2001).

Reporters from the *Times of London* documented all these activities, including Nightingale's famous night rounds with the lamp. The stories had a very positive impact on public morale back home. Yet for the military commanders, Nightingale made her best case with "coxcomb" charts and the latest statistics of the time. They clearly demonstrated a 20-fold decline in patient deaths within six months of instituting her sanitary reforms (see Figure 3.4).

After her success at Scutari, Nightingale's reforms became a standard for military hospitals throughout the British Empire (Attewell 2010). She published extensively, and designed curricula for her own schools of nursing and midwifery (*Notes on Nursing*). The latter became models for training a new class of "professional" nurses in England and abroad, generations of healer-educators who promoted her model of sanitation.

Additionally, Nightingale's social capital sometimes outweighed that of other physicians on matters of clinical practice. A notable example concerned the prevention of puerperal fever, a major cause of maternal mortality (Chamberlain 2006). Her investigations led to the same conclusion as Oliver Wendell Holmes and Ignaz Semmelweis, that birth attendants (especially physicians) were the primary vectors of contagion between patients (Lane et al. 2021; Noakes 2008). However, Nightingale's published recommendations received greater attention and acceptance than those of her physician predecessors (Nightingale 1871).

It is possible that the more positive reception to Nightingale's recommendations was informed by the greater acceptance of Germ Theory at the time of publication, even though the author herself had not yet come around to the idea.[5] Regarding

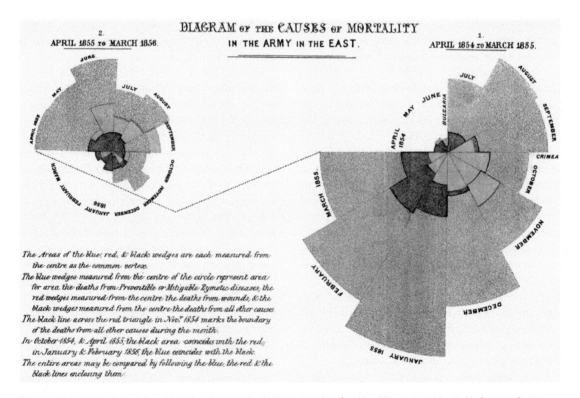

Figure 3.4 Florence Nightingale's coxcomb chart depicting the decline in mortality of British soldiers at Scutari hospital before and after her reforms from April, 1855 to March, 1856. The light grey portion (blue on the original) represents "preventable deaths" that were likely due to infectious diseases.

Source: Nightingale, F. (1858). Notes on Matters Affecting the Health, Efficiency, and Hospital Administration of the British Army. London: Harrison & Sons.

matters of hygiene, germ theorists were unlikely to have had philosophical quarrels with even the most ardent miasmists. The recognition of microbial pathogens only served to underscore the importance of clean practices and clean environments for preventing the growth and transmission of infectious diseases. If anything, germ theorists were likely to go even further with their advocacy for cleanliness.

This was the case with Joseph Lister's famous methods of antiseptic surgical practice, which he began publishing in the years between Semmelweiss' and Nightingale's puerperal fever studies (Lister 1867; 1870). Lister was strongly influenced by Louis Pasteur's research, though he must have been exposed to microbial concepts at an early age via his father's interest in the compound microscope. Lister applied Pasteur's findings to clinical research on the problem of gangrene and postoperative sepsis (Worboys 2013). Although initially based on a selective sample of patient observations, Lister's data accumulated over the years while he continued to revise and improve his methods. It should also be noted that Lister worked in close partnership with his wife, Agnes Lister, a botanist and meticulous researcher who is thought to have co-authored many of his publications (Richardson 2013).

Lister continued to make evidence-based revisions to his specific methods, but the overall system always included the same basic elements: rigorous handwashing, the wearing of gloves, and the use of carbolic acid (a.k.a. phenol) dilutions for bandages, sutures, and wounds. All of these elements were direct applications of Germ Theory. The phenol was used as an *anti-septic*, a chemical that destroyed the microbes acquired through open trauma and surgical procedures. The washing and gloves were *a-septic* measures intended to prevent any additional microbes from being introduced to the patient. Lister's aseptic methods entailed a level of cleanliness that exceeded even Nightingale's standards.

The Listerian system proved challenging to many surgeons, and the new methods were often reluctantly and partially adopted over the years. But Lister was persistent in his mission of surgical reform, which included practical arguments for those who remained skeptical of germs:

"If anyone chooses to assume that the septic material is not of the nature of the living organisms, but a so-called chemical ferment destitute of vitality, yet endowed with a power of self-multiplication equal to that of the organism associated with it, such a notion, unwarranted though I believe it to be by any scientific evidence, will in a practical point of view be equivalent to a germ theory, since it will inculcate precisely the same methods of antiseptic management."

(footnote to Lister (1870), cited by Worboys 2013: 204).

This statement reflected a greater interest in improving patient outcomes than in winning a theoretical argument. The etiological beliefs of Lister's colleagues did not matter so long as they followed his recommended surgical practices. As a fellow clinician, Lister knew that could appeal to the pragmatism of his profession by demonstrating the efficacy of these practices. Ironically, this pragmatic approach was very similar to that of the sanitary reformers in previous years. Indeed, Lister adopted some of their epidemiological methods to make his case (Worboys 2013).

By the last decades of the nineteenth century, the paradigm had shifted in favor of Germ Theory. Improved microscopes and staining techniques revealed previously invisible microbes, and an emerging guild of microbiologists was systematically determining its role in human diseases and other natural processes. Louis Pasteur discovered the bacterial origins of fermentation and food spoilage, and he led a team of scientists to establish the field of immunology (Zaman 2020). Robert Koch and his team developed a set of postulates for linking particular bacterial species to particular diseases (Blevins and Bronze 2010; Brock 1988). These included the bacilli responsible for anthrax, cholera, and tuberculosis. Others followed suit: Alexandre Yersin identified the plague bacillus, Armauer Hansen the leprosy bacillus, and so forth (Butler 2014; Hansen 1875).

These were important and exciting discoveries. Yet even with surgical reform, some new vaccines, and food safety improvements, the practical contributions of Germ Theory to overall mortality decline were relatively modest for at least fifty years. In the interim, the same sanitary reform model (regardless of explanation) dominated the practical domains of human health. Even with germs in mind, biomedical physicians continued to prescribe good nutrition, healthy behavior, and a clean environment for disease prevention. Such prescriptions were well-founded, for they were largely responsible for the decline of infectious diseases more than a hundred years prior to the end of the Second World War. Germ Theory gained favor in the 1870s, but the paradigm shift was not fully realized until well into the twentieth century.

3.3 The McKeown thesis

Despite ground-breaking discoveries in microbiology and immunology, medical technologies made little contribution to the decline of infectious diseases in England and Wales in the nineteenth and early twentieth centuries. In his classic work on the topic, Thomas McKeown (1976, 1988) convincingly illustrates this point with graphs that relate the decline of specific infectious diseases to the development of their respective vaccines and effective antimicrobial medicines. Tuberculosis was an emblematic example. Popularly

known as "consumption" or "phthisis," tuberculosis probably killed more people than any other infectious disease at the end of the nineteenth century, having been attributed to one in seven deaths worldwide. Even so, TB mortality was already well in decline by then, with 57 percent reduction in totals deaths between 1838 and 1971 (see Figure 3.5).

Effective biomedical treatments for TB were not available until the mid-twentieth century. The first antibiotic cure for TB, streptomycin, was not prescribed until 1947, and the BCG vaccination against the bacillus was not made available until 1954. While these and subsequent medicines have played a tremendous role in the prevention and treatment of tuberculosis, they contributed relatively little to the total decline since the previous century was surprisingly small.[6] Assuming that TB would have continued its decline without antibiotics and vaccinations at the same rate as its decline just before their appearance (1921–1946), and generously assuming that antibiotics and immunization have reduced TB mortality by 50 percent, then the contribution of these medicines to the decline

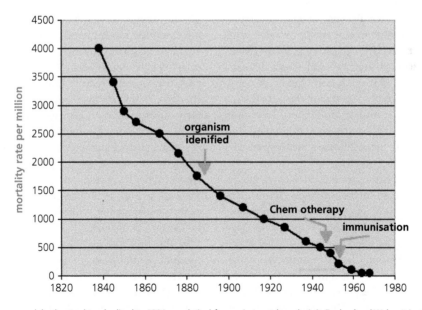

Figure 3.5 Mean annual death rates (standardized to 1901 population) for respiratory tuberculosis in England and Wales. It is striking to see that most of this decline occurred before the availability of effective anti-TB medications.

Source: Thomas McKeown (1979). The Role of Medicine: Dream, Mirage, or Nemesis. Oxford: Basil Blackwell. p. 92. Reproduced with the permission of John Wiley & Sons.

between 1838 and 1971 would be about 3.2 percent (Mckeown 1976).

To be fair, McKeown acknowledges the role of new medicines in some diseases (1978). The small-pox vaccine had been made available throughout the British Empire since the early 1800s, and it is likely to have played a major role in the early stages of the decline a century before the government began collecting of cause-of-death statistics. Immunizations for typhus and tetanus, and antitoxin for diphtheria, also played important roles. Nevertheless, the combined mortality for these four diseases comprised only a minority of the total infection-related deaths. To be sure, these new pharmaceuticals saved many lives, but non-pharmaceutical factors must have played a greater role. This conclusion is well established among medical historians and epidemiologists, including Omran, who reasonably extends it to other relatively affluent nations in his Classic Transition Model (Omran 1971).

Perhaps more controversially, McKeown is also skeptical of the primary role played by sanitation on the health of the national population (1976). As with the newer medicines, sanitary reform made substantial contributions to the British population, especially in the cities. Because of the movement, the British government embarked on ambitious infrastructure projects for improving urban drinking water as well as drainage and waste disposal systems (Rosen 1993). However, many of these projects were not fully realized until the last decades of the nineteenth century. Until then, sanitation went from poor to worse in expanding cities with increasingly dense populations. Once again, this assertion is well-documented.

At this point in his argument, McKeown cites a popular quotation from the Sherlock Holmes stories: "When we have eliminated the impossible, whatever remains, no matter how improbable, must be the truth." Having ruled out the two other major possibilities, McKeown identifies improved nutrition as the most prominent remaining factor, and thus, the primary determinant in the decline of infection-related mortality. This hypothesis is often referred to as the McKeown Thesis.

In addition to the argument by elimination, the McKeown Thesis rests on two additional lines of empirical evidence. The first concerns the baseline prior to the decline, for which McKeown cites the established relationship between undernutrition and infection. In Chapter 1, we reviewed some of the ways that different nutritional deficiencies impair certain mechanisms and structures of immune function. Tragically, there is no shortage of contemporary examples to demonstrate these relationships in the twenty-first century as McKeown does for the nineteenth century.

The Food and Agriculture Organization (FAO) of the United Nations estimates that by the end of 2020, there were between 720 and 811 million people facing hunger and food in the world, include 22 percent of all children under five years of age (UN FAO 2021). Under-nutrition is associated with at least half of all child deaths each year, and more than half of all deaths due to infectious pneumonias and diarrheal diseases (Walson and Berkly 2018). Combining these data with well-known physiological mechanisms, it stands to reason that overall dietary improvements would have led to substantial declines in infectious diseases.

The second line of empirical data addresses demographic changes that occurred during the decline, namely an acceleration of population growth that would have been unlikely without increased food output and availability. Here, McKeown points to improved agricultural methods and transportation networks (1988). Although historians debate the exact timing of the agricultural changes, there is broad agreement that improvements in crop rotation increased soil nitrogen levels while diversifying produce by the second half of the eighteenth century (Allen 2008 Overton 1996). Along with major irrigation projects, these changes substantially increased crop yields, almost twofold for some staples, by the second half of the eighteenth century—coinciding with the earliest indicators of the Second Transition.

In the first half of the nineteenth century, the products of these improved crop yields were distributed to populations better than ever before, through faster, cheaper, and more extensive transportation networks. Railways accelerated transport by 10-fold at less than half the cost, and a combination of industrial interests and turnpike trusts supported the construction and maintenance of extensive road networks (Bogart 2013). The result was a major increase in the availability, variety, and affordability of food. Thus, improved nutrition may have been the best medicine for England and other industrialized nations during that time, even as their cities faced problems of poverty, crowding, and lagging infrastructure.

Evidence that these circumstances led to actual nutritional improvements is further suggested from generational changes in body height and the timing of first menstruation. James Tanner, the pediatrician who developed the world's most widely used scales for childhood growth and development, maintains that such measures are "a mirror of the conditions of society" (Tanner 1987: 96). This is certainly the case for human stature, which has a well-established link with the nutritional status of populations just as it does for individuals (Tanner 1992). With this link in mind, it is notable that the European populations (inclusive of England and Wales) that experienced major mortality declines in the second half of the nineteenth century also experienced average stature increases of 1 to 3 centimeters during that same time period (Cole 2000).

From the Paleolithic to the present, stature has always been closely associated with mortality and disease states. A major contemporary study of 31 population cohorts in 10 European countries, as well as in England and the United States, shows a significant negative correlation between the stature and mortality of young children, especially infants between 28 days and one year of age (Bozzoli et al. 2009). Most of these deaths are attributed to respiratory and gastrointestinal infections. In low-income societies, maternal stature is closely associated with gestational growth and birth weights (Kramer 1998; Kramer et al. 1992). Birth weights, in turn, are closely associated with later growth as well as adult susceptibility to infectious and non-infectious diseases, even when environments improve in the interim (Barker 2004; Kuzawa et al. 2020). From fetus to child, child to adult, and then again to fetal offspring, the physical effects of deprivation and disease can become persistent cycles across multiple generations.

The age of menarche (i.e., first menstruation) is also a sensitive indicator of nutritional status, though as with overall growth, it can also be influenced by other physical and psychological stressors (Bogin 2020; Worthman et al. 2019). Along with generational increases in stature, the European and North American countries that experienced mortality declines around the same time as England and Wales also saw a decrease in their ages of menarche when they began recording these data in the late nineteenth and early twentieth centuries (Euling et al. 2008). This trend was especially evident in Scandinavian countries when the mean age of menarche fell 12 months per decade until the Second World War (Cole 2000).

These trends also correlate with declining variability in the age of menarche. In Belgium, for instance, the age of the oldest 10 percent declined the fastest while the youngest 10 percent hardly changed at all (Hauspie et al. 1997). These latter observations suggest that well-nourished populations may be reaching the lower age limits for menarche in our species. Indeed, the mean age of menarche appears to have stabilized in recent decades among the world's affluent societies. But more importantly, these observations also suggest that the reduction of inequalities can improve the health of entire populations, not just the least privileged within them. This is further supported by the reduction of variation in mortality rates between European countries during the same periods of mortality decline (Vallin 1991). The lesson here is that everyone can benefit from an equitable distribution of resources for health and wellbeing.

That said, we should be cautious about attributing growth and pubertal data to improved nutrition when they could simply be markers of overall stress (i.e., allostatic load). As we learned from the osteological evidence presented in Chapter 2, physiological outcomes are often ambiguous with respect to their specific proximal inputs such as undernutrition vs. disease burden. In the same way we approached the health of ancient populations, we must take care to consider data from multiple methods and different contexts, as well as alternative explanations, when considering the first instances of declining infections during the Industrial Revolution.

There is little debate about the relatively minor role played by biomedical discoveries in the mortality declines of high-income nations during the nineteenth and early twentieth centuries. Beyond this broad agreement, however, there are criticisms about some of the evidence used to support the McKeown Thesis, and some researchers propose alternative explanations to its claim about the primary role of nutrition (Colgrove 2002; Harris 2004).

One criticism is that most of the evidence for declining infections in England and Wales is based on outdated diagnostic criteria and a system of disease classification (nosology) from an earlier century. Counting people and the number of deaths is relatively straightforward, so we can reasonably conclude that mortality declined overall. But attributing portions of this decline to infectious diseases requires an accurate determination of the causes of death. From the 1840s to the 1910s, the standards for these determinations were established by William Farr, who was not a germ theorist (Eyler 1979). Even among the physicians who were germ theorists, and whose individual diagnoses directly contributed to the primary data, no individual clinician had the practical means to identify specific pathogens for many years. Considering the standards and their inputs, how could a medical historian distinguish between infectious and non-infectious diseases?

The answer depends on the level of precision needed to distinguish the two categories. The diagnostic criteria for determining a specific infectious disease by nineteenth-century standards might not distinguish the most common differential diagnoses based on twenty-first-century standards. But if the large majority of the twenty-first-century diagnoses are also infectious diseases, then the precision of the nineteenth-century diagnoses is sufficient to make the distinction from non-infectious diseases.

We can test this proposition with another source that uses the same criteria and data as McKeown: Arthur Newsholm's (1889) oft-cited synopsis of English health over the previous 50 years. Following Farr, Newsholm identifies the most common causes of death in the General Registry. The "zymotic" causes are diarrhea diseases, enteric fevers, scarlet fever, whooping cough, measles, smallpox, and diphtheria. All these either have distinctive clinical presentations or, in the case of diarrheal diseases, they are usually attributable to water and food-borne pathogens. Respiratory diseases, including

phthisis (TB) make up the largest category, but even if they were poorly distinguished, the majority of non-infectious causes would probably be related to tobacco. Unless there was a major decline in the use of tobacco during this time period, these respiratory deaths were most likely caused by microbial pathogens.

Even with the advantages of recent biomedical science, physicians continue to face challenges attributing specific diseases to specific causes of death. Some of these challenges are matters of clinical error. Studies comparing officially recorded diagnoses on death certificates with follow-up diagnoses from autopsies find a wide range of discrepancies. Eighteen of these comparison studies were conducted between 1972 and 2000, finding discrepancies in 9 per cent to 80 percent of cases, the highest of which were among surgical and geriatric patients (Roulson et al. 2005). Focusing specifically on elderly deaths in long-term care facilities, one of these studies attributed the largest percentage of discrepancies to overlooked respiratory infections (Gross et al. 1988).

Other challenges stem from legal requirements to determine a primary cause of death when multiple and interacting diseases are involved. This is the case for HIV-related deaths, when the proximate causes are a suite of other infections due to immunosuppression. It is also common among influenza-related deaths, for which the proximal cause may not be a physiological reaction to the virus itself but rather a secondary bacterial pneumonia (Kalil and Thomas 2019). Indeed, influenza was long thought to be a bacterial infection, and the namesake of one of these secondary pathogens, *Hemophilis influenzae* (formerly, "Pfeiffer's bacillus"), turned out to be a misattribution (Crosby 2003).

Non-infectious diseases present an even greater challenge. Adult-onset diabetes is the chief determinant of chronic renal failure, and cardiovascular disease is the chief determinant of stroke. Separately, each of these four diseases are ranked among the 10 leading causes of death in high-income countries, but which among them should be put on a death certificate? With these dilemmas in mind, we might be suspicious of some of the heart conditions that are often entered into cause of death entries for long-term care patients in the United States (Gross et al. 1988). After all, the heart usually stops working by the time of the postmortem examination.

Another criticism is that the McKeown Thesis underestimates the role of smallpox inoculation in the early years of mortality decline between the late 1700s and early 1800s (Mercer 1985). Until the mid-eighteenth century, *the pox*[7] was endemic to British populations, as it was in many societies around the world. Well before the annual reports, the telltale signs of smallpox were easy to identify, and their alternative causes were unlikely (see Fenner et al. 1988). That said, data for inoculation rates are incomplete or absent for many English rural communities, just as they are for many other societies at the time

Inoculation may indeed have played a role in protecting certain subpopulations against smallpox, but it is likely that patient isolation played an even greater role. There is a strong precedent for this in the final years of smallpox eradication, when epidemiologists from the Centers for Disease Control (CDC) found themselves short of vaccines in West and Central Africa. Combining isolation measures with selective vaccination, the CDC team was able to control the spread of smallpox below the threshold needed to achieve herd immunity in these populations (Foege et al. 1975). Yet although these specific measures proved effective, we should be cautious in extending them to COVID-19. These were not only stopgap interventions but they were based on surveillance data from active detection efforts—sample-based surveys of general populations in the field rather than those who walk into clinics and testing centers. In the first years of the pandemic, active detection has not been a major component of most state-level COVID-19 responses.

Better lessons in the efficacy of isolation for the current pandemic can be drawn from early interventions for TB and influenza. Informed by miasmist principles, many TB patients were effectively isolated in remote sanitariums that were built for fresh air and rest (Dubos and Dubos 1987). And based on microbial principles during the 1918 influenza pandemic, municipal isolation measures, such as the closing of public facilities, explained some of the

variation in the disease curves of US cities (Markel et al. 2007). The latter are especially relevant to today's COVID-19 policies.

McKeown may have also discounted the educational contributions of professional health providers, especially with regard to teaching basic health practices to the general public. Miasma notwithstanding, North American and European countries adopted practices of nutrition, hygiene, and ventilation within increasingly standardized medical curricula. These practices, in turn, were further propagated with the expansion of home health and visiting nurse services in the early twentieth century, reaching out to communities while helping family members to care for each other in their homes (Kunitz 1991). Yet unlike Nightingale's hospital reforms, these community efforts did not enjoy the same level of statistical scrutiny.

Finally, although McKeown has fair reason to cite problems with urban housing and infrastructure in the early decades of the decline, he does little to acknowledge the potential contributions of their reforms in later decades. Motivated by concerns about fire as well as disease, later regulations set minimum room sizes and large industrial cities such as Manchester placed outright bans on their notorious cellar dwellings (Burnett 1991). By 1885, the country had established 28 Model Housing Trusts for working-class families. By the time of the housing reforms, many English cities made significant improvements in waste disposal and drainage, progress that was in an 1896 survey of sanitary conditions in London and five other European capitals (Woods 1991). It took time to implement Chadwick's ambitious plans, but many of them were realized by the turn of the twentieth century.

Considering these issues, perhaps the best criticism of the McKeown Thesis also comes with a qualified defense (Harris 2004). For England and Wales, the author makes a strong case for the role of nutrition in the decline of infectious diseases from the mid-nineteenth to the early twentieth centuries. The link between nutrition and immunity is clear, and the case is compelling for food availability, affordability, and diversity. But in the absence of quantitative comparisons, the strongest thesis is that nutrition was one of several important determinants. As with the Neolithic era increase in infectious diseases, nutrition, settlement, and social organization are strongly implicated in this English example of industrial-era decrease. Yet although this pattern was similar in several wealthy nations during the same time period, the majority of low- and middle-income nations had a very different experience of the Second Epidemiological Transition.

Notes

1. Although they are two of the four separate (and non-sovereign) countries that comprise the United Kingdom of Great Britain and Northern Ireland, England and Wales represented a single jurisdiction under English law and constitutional successor to the Kingdom of England. It is with this authority that the Government Registry Office gathered its population data.

2. Originally referring to "pollution" or "stain," Jacques Jouanna (2012: c7) argues that "miasma" was more commonly used in the context of ritual pollution in religious healing rather than the physical properties of air in secular healing practices. Ironically, the miasma of ritual pollution was often regarded as contagious through person-to-person contact (Jouanna 2012: c7).

3. Fredrick Engels wrote an extensive critique of the New Poor Law and workhouse conditions in *Condition of the Working Class in England in 1844* (1943 [1892]). Although the text did not cite Chadwick by name, it frequently describes the New Poor Law commissioners as major leaders in the Malthusian war of the bourgeoisie against the working classes in England during this period.

4. Fracastoro is also credited with giving syphilis its name, based on his widely read poem about the disease (Waugh 1982).

5. As with most of her medical colleagues, Florence Nightingale eventually accepted Germ Theory. This probably occurred by 1875, when she hired John Croft to teach Listerian methods

of antisepsis to her nursing students (Jones et al. 2017).

6. There is considerable debate about the current efficacy of the BCG vaccine against tuberculosis, though about 100 million children a year continue to be vaccinated. The median estimate is 18 percent protection against all forms of tuberculosis, with significantly higher efficacy in infants and young children (Martinez et al. 2022).

7. Syphilis has also historically been referred to as "the pox" in English-speaking societies.

References

Ackerknecht, E.H. 2009 [1948]. "Anticontagionism between 1821 and 1867." *International Journal of Epidemiology* 38 (1): 7–21.

Allen, Robert C. 2008. "The nitrogen hypothesis and the English agricultural revolution: A biological analysis." *Journal of Economic History* 68 (1): 182–210.

Araki, Tsutomu. 2017. "The history of the optical microscope." *Mechanical Engineering Reviews* 4 (1): 1–8. https://doi.org/10.1299/mer.16-00242

Attewell, Alex. 2010. "Florence Nightingale's relevance to nursing." *Journal of Holistic Nursing* 28 (1): 101–106.

Baldwin, Peter. 1999. *Contagion and the State in Europe: 1830–1930.* Cambridge, UK: Cambridge University Press.

Barker, D.J.P. 2004. "The developmental origins of chronic adult disease." *Acta Paediatrica* 93: 26–33. https://doi.org/10.1080/08035320410022730

Bird, Alexander. 2012. "The structure of scientific revolutions and its significance: An essay review of the fiftieth anniversary edition." *British Journal for the Philosophy of Science* 63: 859–883.

Blevins, Steve M., and Michael S. Bronze. 2010. "Robert Koch and the 'golden age' of bacteriology." *International Journal of Infectious Diseases* 14 (9): e744–e751.

Bogart, Dan. 2013. "The Transportation Revolution in Industrializing Britain." University of California-Irvine Department of Economics Working Papers.

Bogin, Barry. 2020. *Patterns of Human Growth.* Cambridge, UK: Cambridge University Press.

Bozzoli, Carlos, Angus Deaton, and Climent Quintana-Domeque. 2009. "Adult height and childhood disease." *Demography* 46 (4): 647–669.

Brock, Thomas D. 1988. *Robert Koch: A Life in Medicine and Bacteriology.* Washington, DC: American Society for Microbiology.

Burnett, J. 1991. "Housing and the Decline in Mortality." In *The Decline of Mortality in Europe*, edited by Roger Schofield, David Reher, and Alain Bideau, 158–176. Oxford: Oxford University Press.

Butler, Thomas. 2014. "Plague history: Yersin's discovery of the causative bacterium in 1894 enabled, in the subsequent century, scientific progress in understanding the disease and the development of treatments and vaccines." *Clinical Microbiology and Infection* 20 (3): 202–209.

Chamberlain, Geoffrey. 2006. "British maternal mortality in the 19th and early 20th centuries." *Journal of the Royal Society of Medicine* 99: 559–563.

Cole, T.J. 2000. "Secular trends in growth." *Proceedings of the Nutrition Society* 59: 317–324.

Colgrove, James. 2002. "The McKeown thesis: A historical controversy and its enduring influence. American journal of public health." *American Journal of Public Health* 92 (5): 725–729.

Crosby, Alfred W. 2003. *America's forgotten pandemic: The influenza of 1918*. Cambridge, UK: Cambridge University Press.

Diamond, Marion, and Mervyn Stone. 1981. "Nightgale on Quetelet." *Journal of the Royal Statistical Society* 144 (3): 332–351.

Dickinson, Emily. 1896. *Time and Eternity, Poem 24, Going in Poems of Emily Dickinson*. Boston: Robert Brother.

Dubos, René Jules, and Jean Dubos. 1987. *The white plague: Tuberculosis, man, and society*. New Brunswick, NJ: Rutgers University Press.

Engels, Fredrick. 1943 [1892]. *Condition of the Working Class in England in 1844* https://www.almendron. com/tribuna/wp-content/uploads/2016/03/The-Condition-of-the-Working-Class-in-England-in-1844.pdf

Euling, Susan Y., Sherry G. Selevan, Ora Hirsch Pescovitz, and Niels E. Skakkabaek. 2008. "Role of Environmental Factors in the Timing of Puberty." *Pediatrics* 121: S167–S171.

Eyler, John M. 1979. *Victorian Social Medicine: The Ideas and Methods of William Farr*. Baltimore: Johns Hopkins University Press.

FAO. 2021. *The State of Food Security and Nutrition in the World 2021: Transforming Food Systems for Food Security, Improved Nutrition and Affordable Healthy Diets 40or All*. Food and Agriculture Organization of the United Nations (Rome).

Farr, William. 2000 [1885]. "Vital statistics: memorial volume of selections from the reports and writings." *Bulletin of the World Health Organization* 78 (1): 88–96.

Fassin, Giustav. 1934. "Something about the early history of the microscope." *The Scientific Monthly* 38 (5): 452–459.

Fenner, F., D.A. Henderson, I. Arita, Z. Jezek, and I.D. Ladnyi. 1988. *Smallpox and its Eradication*. Geneva: World Health Organization.

Foege, William H., J.D. Millar, and D.A. Henderson. 1975. "Smallpox eradication in West and Central Africa." *Bulletin of the World Health Organization* 52 (2): 209–222.

Frerichs, Ralph R. 2000. "UCLA's John Snow Site." Department of Epidemiology, Jonathan and Karin Fielding School of Public Health, University of California Los Angeles. https://www.ph.ucla.edu/epi/snow. html Last accessed 08/16/2023.

Gest, Howard. 2004. "The discovery of microorganisms by Robert Hooke and Antoni van Leeuwenhoak, Fellows of the Royal Society." *Notes and Records of the Royal Society of London* 58 (2): 187–201.

Gill, Christopher J., and Gillian C. Gill. 2005. "Nightingale in Scutari: Her legacy reexamined." *Clinical Infectious Diseases* 40 (12): 1799–1805.

Gross, Joel S., Richard R. Neufeld, Leslie S. Libow, Isadore Gerber, and Manuel Rodstein 1988. "Autopsy study of the elderly institutionalized patient: review of 234 autopsies." *Archives of Internal Medicine* 148 (1): 173–178.

Halliday, Stephen. 2000. "William Farr: Campaigning statistician." *Journal of Medical Biography* 8: 220–227.

Halliday, Stephen. 2001. "Death and miasma in Victorian London: An obstinate belief." *British Medical Journal* 323: 22–29.

Hamed-Troyansky, Vladimir. 2021. "Ottoman and Egyptian quarantines and European debates on plague in the 1830s–1840s." *Past and Present* 253 (1): 235–270.

Hamlin, Christopher. 1992. "Predisposing causes and public health in early Nineteenth-Century medical thought." *Social History of Medicine* 5 (1): 43–70.

Hamlin, Christopher. 1995. "Could you starve to death in England in 1839? The Chadwick–Farr controversy and the loss of the 'social' in public health." *American Journal of Public Health* 85 (6): 856–866.

Hansen, Armauer. 1875. "On the etiology of leprosy." *The British and Foreign Medico-Chirurgical Review* 55 (110): 459–489.

Harris, Bernard. 2004. "Public health, nutrition and the decline of mortality: The McKeown thesis revisited." *Social History of Medicine* 17 (3): 379–407.

Hauspie, Ronald C., Martine Vercauteren, and Charles Susanne. 1997. "Secular changes in growth and maturation: An update." *Acta Paediatrica* 86 (S423): 20–27.

Hooke, Robert. 1665. *Micrographia: Or Some Physiological Descriptions of Minute Bodies Made by Magnifying Glasses with Observations and Inquiries Thereupon*. London: Royal Society.

Jalland, Patricia. 1996. *Death in the Victorian Family*. Oxford: Oxford University Press.

Johnson, Steven. 2006. *The Ghost Map: The Story of London's Most Terrifying Epidemic—And How it Changed Science, Cities, and the Modern World*. New York: Riverhead Books.

Jones, Claire L., Marguerite Dupree, Susan Gardner, and Anne Marie Rafferty. 2017. "Personalities, preferences and practicalities: Educating nurses in wound sepsis in the British hospital, 1870–1920." *Social History of Medicine* 31 (3): 577–604.

Jouanna, Jacques. 2012. *Greek Medicine from Hippocrates to Galen: Selected Papers*. Leiden: Brill.

Kalil, Andre C., and Paul G. Thomas. "Influenza virus-related critical illness: Pathophysiology and epidemiology." *Critical Care* 23 (2019): 1–7.

Kopf, Edwin W. 1916. "Nightingale as statistician." *Publications of the American Statistical Association* 15 (116): 388–404.

Kramer, Michael S. 1998. "Maternal nutrition, pregnancy outcome and public health policy." *Canadian Medical Association Journal* 159: 663–665.

Kramer, M.S., F.H. McLean, E.L. Eason, and R.H. Usher. 1992. "Maternal nutrition and spontaneous preterm birth." *American Journal of Epidemiology* 136 (5): 574–583.

Kuhn, Thomas. 1996. *The Structure of Scientific Revolutions*. 3rd ed. Chicago: University of Chicago Press.

Kunitz, Stephen J. 1991. "The Personal Physician and the Decline of Mortality." In *The Decline of Mortality in Europe*, edited by Roger Schofield, David Reher and Alain Bideau, 248–262. Oxford University Press.

Kuzawa, Christopher W. 2020. "Evolutionary life history theory as an organising framework for cohort studies: insights from the Cebu Longitudinal Health and Nutrition Survey." *Annals of Human Biology* 47 (2): 94–105.

Lane, Nick. 2015 [1677]. "The unseen world: Reflections on Leeuwenhoek (1677) 'Concerning little animals'." *Philosophical Transactions of the Royal Society B: Biological Sciences* 370 (1666): 20140344.

Lane, Hillary J., Nava Blum, and Elizabeth Fee. 2021. "Oliver Wendell Holmes (1809–1894) and Ignaz Philipp Semmelweis (1818–1865): Preventing the transmission of puerperal fever." *American Journal of Public Health* 100 (6): 1008–1009.

Lister, Joseph. 1867. "On the antiseptic principle in the practice of surgery." *British Medical Journal* 2 (351): 246–248.

Lister, Joseph. 1870. "A method of antiseptic treatment applicable to wounded soldiers in the present war." *British Medical Journal* 2 (505): 243–244.

Markel, Howard, Harvey B. Lipman, J. Alexander Navarro, Alexandra Sloan, Joseph R. Michalsen, Alexandra Minna Stern, and Martin S. Cetron. 2007. "Nonpharmacological interventions implemented by U.S. cities during the 1918–1919 influenza pandemic." *Journal of the American Medical Association* 298: 644–654.

Martinez, Leonardo, Olivia Cords, Qiao Liu, Carlos Acuna-Villaorduna, Maryline Bonnet, Greg J. Fox, Anna Cristina, C. Carvalho et al. 2022. "Infant BCG vaccination and risk of pulmonary and extrapulmonary tuberculosis throughout the life course: A systematic review and individual participant data meta-analysis." *Lancet Global Health* 10 (9): e1307–1316.

McDonald, Lynn. 2001. "Florence Nightingale and the early origins of evidence-based nursing." *Evidence Based Nursing* 4 (3): 68–69.

McKeown, Thomas. 1976. "Determinants of health." *Human Nature* 1: 57–62.

McKeown, Thomas. 1978. "Fertility, mortality and causes of death: An examination of issues related to the modern rise of population." *Population Studies* 32 (3): 535–542.

McKeown, Thomas. 1988. *The Origins of Human Disease*. Oxford: Basil Blackwell.

Mercer, Alex J. 1985. "Smallpox and epidemiological-demographic change in Europe: The role of vaccination." *Population Studies* 39 (2): 287–307.

Newsholme, Arthur. 1889. *The Elements of Vital Statistics*. 2nd ed. London: Swan Sonnnshein & Co.

Nightingale, Florence. 1871. *Introductory Notes on Lying-In Institutions: Together with a Proposal for Organising an Institution for Training Midwives and Midwifery Nurses*. Green: Longmans.

Noakes, Timothy D., J. Borresen, T. Hew-Butler, M.I. Lambert, and E Jordaan. 2008. "Semmelweis and the aetiology of puerperal sepsis 160 years on: An historical review." *Epidemiology & Infection* 136 (1): 1–9.

Nutton, Vivian. 1983. "The seeds of disease: An explanation of contagion and infection from the Greeks to the Renaissance." *Medical History* 27 (1–34).

Omran, Abdel R. 1971. "The epidemiologic transition: A theory of the epidemiology of population change." *Millbank Memorial Fund Quarterly* 49 (4): 509–538.

Overton, Mark. 1996. "Re-establishing the English agricultural revolution." *The Agricultural History Review* 44 (1): 1–20.

Pickstone, John V. 1992. "Dearth, Dirt and Fever Epidemics: Rewriting the History of British 'Public Health,' 1780–1950." In *Essays on the Historical Perception of Pestilence*, edited by Terrence Ranger and Paul Slack, 125–148. Cambridge, UK: Cambridge University Press.

Richardson, Ruth. 2013. "Joseph Lister's domestic science." *The Lancet* 82 (9898): E8–E9.

Rosen, G. 1993. *A History of Public Health*. Baltimore: Johns Hopkins University Press.

Rouchoux, Jean-André. 1834. *Dictionnaire de médecine, Vol, VIII*. Paris.

Roulson, Jo-an, E. W. Benbow, and Philip S. Hasleton. 2005. "Discrepancies between clinical and autopsy diagnosis and the value of post mortem histology; a meta-analysis and review." *Histopathology* 47 (6): 551–559.

Snow, John. 1855. *On the Mode of Communication of Cholera*. 2nd ed. London: John Churchill.

Sterner, Carl S. 1948. "A brief history of miasmic theory." *Bulletin of the History of Medicine* 22: 747.

Tanner, James M. 1987. "Growth as a mirror of the condition of society: Secular trends and class distinctions." *Acta Paediatrica Japonica* 29 (96–103).

Tanner, James M. 1992. "Growth as a measure of the nutritional and hygienic status of a population." *Hormone Research* 38 (Suppl. 1): 108–115.

Vallin, Jacques. 1991. "Mortality in Europe from 1720 to 1914: Long-Term Trends and Changes in Patterns by Age and Sex." In *The Decline of Mortality in Europe*, edited by Roger Schofield, David Reher, and Alain Bideau, 38–67. Oxford: Oxford University Press.

van Zuylen, J. 1981. "The microscopes of Antoni van Leeuwenhoek." *Journal of Microscopy* 121 (3): 309–328.

Varro, Marcus Trentius. 1934 [1783]. "On Agriculture, Book 1." In *Cato and Varro on Agriculture*, edited by W.D. Hooper and H.B. Ash, 160–305. Cambridge: Harvard University Press.

Vlastos, Gregory. 1950. "The physical theory of anaxagoras." *Philosophical Review* 59 (1): 31–57.

Volk, Anthony A., and Jeremy A. Atkinson. 2013. "Infant and child death in the human environment of evolutionary adaptation." *Evolution and Human Behavior* 34: 182–192.

Walson, Judd L., and James A. Berkley. 2018. "The impact of malnutrition on childhood infections." *Current Opinion on Infectious Diseases* 31 (3): 231–236.

Watts, Isaac. 1715. *Divine Songs: Attempted in Easy Language for the Use of Children: Facsimile Reproductions of the First Edition of 1715 and an Illustrated Edition of Circa 1840*. Oxford University Press.

Waugh, M.A. 1982. "Role played by Italy in the history of syphilis." *British Journal of Venereal Diseases* 58 (2): 92–95.

Wilson, Catherine. 1995. "Animalcula and the Theory of Animate Contagion." In *The Invisible World: Early Modern Philosophy and the Invention of the Microscope*, edited by Catherine Wilson, 140–175. Princeton: Princeton University Press.

Woods, Robert. 1991. "Public Health and Public Hygiene: The Urban Environment in the Late Nineteenth and Early Twentieth Centuries." In *The Decline of Mortality in Europe*, edited by Roger Schofield, David Reher, and Alain Bideau, 233–247. Oxford: Oxford University Press.

Worboys, Michael. 2013. "Joseph Lister and the performance of antiseptic surgery." *Notes and Records of the Royal Society* 67: 199–209.

Worthman, Carol M., Samantha Dockray, and Kristine Marceau. 2019. "Puberty and the evolution of developmental science." *Journal of Research on Adolescence* 29 (1): 9–31.

Wrigley, E.A., R.S. Davies, J.A. Oeppen, and R.S. Scofield. 1997. *English Population History from Family Reconstitution, 1580–1837*. Cambridge, UK: Cambridge University Press.

Yersin, Alexandre. 1894. "La peste bubonique à Hong Kong." *Annales de lInstitut Pasteur* 8: 662–667.

Zaman, Muhammad H. 2020. *Biography of Resistance: The Epic Battle Between People and Pathogens*. New York: HarperCollins.

CHAPTER 4

The Worst of Both Worlds

We live in a world where infections pass easily across borders—social and geographic—while resources, including cumulative scientific knowledge, are blocked at customs.

Paul Farmer (1996)

In the previous chapter, we examined the earliest examples of the Second Epidemiological Transition in England and Wales as well as a handful of European and North American nations from the late eighteenth to the early twentieth century. These nations represented the ideal, or Classic Model of the epidemiological transition as defined by Abdel Omran and described by the work of Thomas McKeown (McKeown 1976; Omran 1971). Although the Classic Model entailed a tradeoff between the declining infectious diseases and rising non-infectious diseases, the net result was extremely positive. These affluent societies experienced the largest recorded mortality declines since the Neolithic.

Encouraged by these outcomes, many health authorities in the 1970s hoped that the world's poorer nations would achieve similar levels of improvement once they became sufficiently "developed" (read "industrialized"). Likewise, they hoped that the latest vaccines, antibiotics, and other advanced medical technologies would spread among these throughout the world, thereby eradicating most infectious diseases by the end of the twentieth century. Adding credence to this optimistic projection, several poorer societies made rapid gains in the initial years of their second transitions (Soares 2007). These gains suggested a bright future for global health.

Sadly, this future was not fully realized. Despite initial positive gains in many lower income nations, the global spread of the Second Transition turned out to be slower and its health gains more modest

than expected. Many of these nations did not begin their shifts until after the end of the Second World War, and infectious disease declines began to taper after several years. Meanwhile, non-infectious diseases rose at similar if not greater rates than in wealthier nations. Rapid urbanization and declining fertility also resulted in larger proportions of elderly in societies that did not have the resources to support them (Kinsella and Velkoff 2001). Additionally, it is important to note that the mortality declines that began in the twentieth century must have depended more on the availability of antimicrobial medicines than the mortality declines that began in the nineteenth century. For late-transitioning societies, these medicines have buffered at least some such as the health consequences of ongoing problems of undernutrition and poverty. Given the rise of antimicrobial resistance, it is alarming to think of what will happen if and when these medicinal buffers become obsolete.

Because of these trends, poorer societies experienced a worst-of-both-worlds situation with regards to the Second Epidemiological Transition: modest-level health gains with respect to infectious diseases combined with the major-level health challenges of non-infectious diseases and aging populations comparable to those of affluent societies. This has resulted in a large overlap between infectious and non-infectious diseases in populations that are least equipped to deal with them, creating further opportunities for major syndemics such as HIV–tuberculosis (TB), cancer–influenza, and diabetes–COVID-19.

Emerging Infections. Second Edition. Ron Barrett, Molly K. Zuckerman, Matthew R. Dudgeon, with George J. Armelagos, Oxford University Press.
© Ron Barrett, Molly K. Zuckerman, Matthew R. Dudgeon (2024). DOI: 10.1093/oso/9780192843135.003.0005

Furthermore, by shouldering the greatest burden of these syndemics, the chronically ill and frail elderly of lower-income societies have become a growing reservoir for new and drug-resistant infections.

These problems, of course, are not restricted to poor societies. Given the porous nature of international borders, they are easily spread to nearly every nation in the world. Accelerated globalization has brought our species into a single disease ecology in which every syndemic can affect the wealthy as well as the poor, though with varying degrees of impact and very different means for prevention and control. To address these global problems effectively, it is necessary to understand the recent history of the Second Transition in poorer societies and the ways it has led us to the Third Transition that we are all experiencing today.

4.1 Delayed and incomplete transitions

There are sufficient data to identify starting points for the Second Epidemiological Transition in 119 countries (Riley 2005). Among these, only seven nations began their transition before 1850, and another 17 before 1900. In these nations, the Second Transition was roughly correlated with industrialization. Except for the inclusion of Mexico and Japan, this group represented the wealthiest nations of Western Europe and North America. The next major cluster of transitions occurred in the interwar period of the 1920s and 1930s among industrializing middle-income countries of Latin America, Eastern and Southern Europe, and a few countries within Asia and Africa. Almost all the remaining transitions occurred after the Second World War (see Figure 4.1).

These later transitions comprised most of the Second Epidemiological Transition, affecting the majority of the total human population. To provide some perspective, by 1875 only 10.5 percent of the human population was undergoing the Second Transition; by 1960, this figure increased to 96.4 percent. It was largely because of this expansion that the Second Transition has had a profoundly positive impact of human survival around the world. The estimated global life expectancy at birth has increased 20 years in four decades: from 52 years of age in 1963 to 72 years of age in 2019 (Bloom and Canning 2007; UN Population Division 2019).

Despite these impressive gains, the delayed transitions have masked important differences within and between societies. Second Transition continued to group into at least two different clusters. These clusters are often referred to as "convergence clubs" of low and high mortality (Liou et al. 2020). The Low Mortality Club consists of wealthy societies whose life expectancies reached the high 70s and low 80s by the early twenty-first century (World Bank 2022). In contrast, the High Mortality Club comprises the majority of poorer societies whose life expectancies at birth have leveled off to the low 60s by the turn of this century, a disparity of about 15 years. Despite its overall benefits, the Second Transition has had different trajectories in wealthier and poorer societies. In the remaining chapters, we will see how the continuing problems of the High Mortality Club is having a major impact on the health of the Low Mortality Club.

Even with this disparity, some may still argue that the High Mortality Club will eventually catch up with the Low Mortality Club. After all, the wealthy societies had more time to reach low mortality levels by virtue of the fact that they started the transition much earlier than their poorer counterparts. It could be further noted that many late transition countries made rapid gains in the initial years of their Second Transition, largely due to substantial improvements in child survival related to the global availability of affordable antimicrobials (Aksan and Chakraborty 2023; Liou et al. 2020). At the same time, the better trajectories have been tapering down: life expectancy at birth has recently leveled off in many high-income countries, a situation we will discuss in later chapters (Ho and Hendi 2018). As the health gains of wealthy countries slow down, it might be possible for the poor countries to catch up, though it would certainly be better if all countries gained at more rapid rates.

Contributing to health improvements thus far, many basic twentieth-century medicines have became available in lower income countries. These medicines have helped address endemic respiratory, gastrointestinal, and vector-borne infections, resulting in up to 50 percent of the mortality declines in LMICs up through the late 1970s

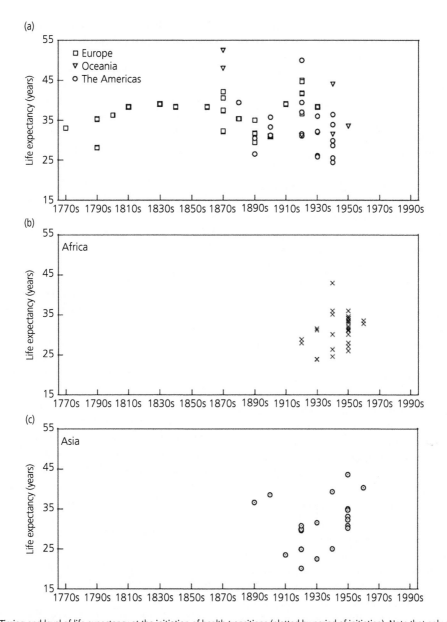

Figure 4.1 Timing and level of life expectancy at the initiation of health transitions (plotted by period of initiation). Note that only seven countries began the Second Transition before the early 1800s. The lowest income countries began the transition after WWII.

Source: Riley, John C. (2005). The Timing and Pace of Health Transitions around the World. Population and Development Review. 31(4): 744. Reproduced with the permission of John Wiley & Sons.

(Preston 1980). In the case of malaria, the combined availability of medicines, bed-nets, and vector control measures contributed to significant, though limited mortality declines in Sub-Saharan African societies, especially among pregnant women and children (Murray et al. 2012; Wang et al. 2016). From the mid-twentieth century onwards, these basic medicines have buffered the poorest societies against the health effects of inadequate living conditions.

Unfortunately, even these medical buffers may only provide short-term benefits. The anti-malarial campaigns of the twentieth century were insufficient to match the pace of rising drug resistance, and it was not long before clinical measures proved inadequate for the deadliest form of the disease (Cohen et al. 2012). Drug resistance also arose with basic antibiotics for respiratory and gastrointestinal infections, which continue to be the leading causes of mortality for children under five years of age in the world's poorest societies (Jasovský et al. 2016; Winskill et al. 2021). With the increasing obsolescence of these pharmacological buffers, the impoverished majority of the world's population has faced resurging infections related to fundamental issues that were never adequately addressed: food insecurity, crowding, limited access to clean water, and related problems of drainage and sanitation.

Health improvement is closely tied to economic improvement at both individual and societal levels. Life expectancy measurements are positively correlated with economic indicators such as per capita income level and gross domestic product (GDP). In some cases, lower-income societies have achieved health improvements despite little gains in GDP, and they have even occurred in the face of declining economic conditions (Soares 2007). But these examples, such as Costa Rica, and the Indian state of Kerala, are exceptions to the rule (Pesec et al. 2017; Thankappan and Valiathan 1998). As we shall see, health improvements in most of the world's perpetually impoverished societies have proven to be temporary and unsustainable precisely because of the importance of having adequate material resources for human wellbeing. Additionally, many low-income countries face challenges of political turmoil, widespread corruption, and armed conflicts that have impacted life expectancies at adult ages (Edwards 2011). Consequently, life expectancies remain especially low in many nations of Sub-Saharan Africa, Oceana, South and Central Asia (Aksan and Chakraborty 2023; Liou et al. 2020). Despite the so-called miracles of medical technology, ongoing problems with the living conditions that brought about the First Transition have limited the health benefits of the Second Transition in the world's poorest societies.

4.2 The nutrition transition and non-communicable diseases

Even with the persistence of long-standing infectious diseases, deaths from non-communicable diseases surpassed infectious disease mortality in all continents except Africa by the end of the twentieth century (Kanavos, 2006; Wang et al. 2016). These included several types of cancer, heart disease, and diseases associated with diabetes and other metabolic conditions. These non-communicable diseases have been nearly as prevalent in lower-income countries as they have in higher-income countries, reflecting a global shift toward a Western dietary pattern known as the Nutrition Transition (Caballero and Popkin 2002).

The Nutrition Transition began in the mid-twentieth century with the industrialization of food production in wealthier societies, followed by well-intended but often misguided attempts to alleviate global hunger by exporting these so-called reforms to poorer and less industrialized societies, efforts sometimes referred to as the "Green Revolution" (Jain 2010). Reminiscent of the Neolithic, these efforts emphasized high yields of starchy foods, as well as meat and dairy products, often at the expense of dietary diversity (Popkin 2015). The former products were also more lucrative such that many farmers shifted their production strategies from localized subsistence to larger-scale cash crops for international export. Consequently, the global price of food relative to real wages fell dramatically over the last 50 years. As a result, processed and packaged foods became more affordable, and more accessible, to lower-income and increasingly urbanized populations around the world (Armelagos et al. 2005).

These industrially produced foods have contributed to what is known as the "Western dietary pattern"[1] (Azzam 2021). This pattern is characterized by higher percentages of red meat (when available), the generous addition of saturated oils and fats, sodium, and sucrose, as well as a very high reliance on refined carbohydrates such as corn-based foods. It is also characterized by a relative paucity of high-fiber foods like fruits and vegetables, whole grains, nuts, and seeds. These foods are energy dense, with calories provided by the refined carbohydrates and saturated fats, and higher ratios of animal to vegetable protein. Yet at the same time, this mode of food production has come at the expense of dietary diversity, and many of its products are deficient in micronutrients and essential minerals (Popkin and Ng 2022). This situation is reminiscent of the dietary changes in the Neolithic; the chief difference is that the Nutrition Transition occurred much more rapidly.

The Nutrition Transition has been further accelerated and perpetuated by a phenomenon known as dietary delocalization. This occurs when local communities increasingly consume foods produced outside their region that do not fall within their traditional patterns of food consumption. Dietary delocalization has occurred for many centuries, driven by international trade, colonization, and migration across regions. But in the last century it has greatly expanded to large-scale international food production within multinational commodities markets, with the trades often occurring at the expense of primary food-producing communities (Leatherman et al. 2016; Pelto and Pelto 1983). At the consumer end, the non-local Westernized foods have exhibited a "trickle down" effect insofar as they were initially introduced to wealthier communities, then adopted by poorer communities as high-status items, finally becoming staples with the progressive displacement of local food sources (Fine et al. 2002).

Following these trends, obesity, heart disease, and metabolic disorders have also trickled down from wealthier to poorer communities. Consequently, health conditions that were once considered "diseases of affluence," in many of the poorer and middle-income communities of Latin America and Asia (Popkin and Ng 2021). A key example of this can be found in China, a middle-income country that rapidly shifted from subsistence agriculture to industrial agriculture while becoming deeply involved in international trade. Along with these economic changes, Chinese populations underwent a major shift toward the consumption of mass-produced foods (Wang et al. 2016). This shift was also accompanied by a proliferation of Western fast-food restaurants. Once seen as status symbols among the cosmopolitan elite, the appeal of these restaurants and their associated foods has broadened across socio-economic strata. The same can be

said for the prevalence of obesity and diabetes in China, where the disease burden is especially felt among poorer communities.

This trickle-down effect has also occurred in India. In rapidly expanding urban areas such as New Delhi, Western fast-food restaurants are often staffed with hosts bedecked with dress uniforms and stores sell the fattiest of traditional foods in pre-cooked packages for easy preparation (Barrett 2008). Throughout urban India, economic mobility has splintered extended families that once shared domestic cooking tasks, thereby increasing the need for convenient foods outside the home (Bailey et al. 2018). Although sugary and fatty foods have often been a part of many traditional diets, their proportions have greatly increased under these conditions, thereby increasing the prevalence of obesity and adult-onset diabetes (Weaver and Narayan 2008). Initial ethnographic research also indicates that this pattern is affecting at least some rural Indian communities as well (Nichols 2017). Together, China and India represent 38 percent of the world's population, yet the health challenges of the Nutrition Transition extend to many more LIMCs (Li et al. 2020). The same holds true for its impact on non-communicable diseases.

4.3 Non-communicable diseases and new syndemics

A common theme in the history and prehistory of human health is that diseases rarely occur in isolation, and they often interact with one another in synergistic ways. This has been the case for non-communicable as well as communicable diseases. Throughout this book, we have used the term *syndemic* to describe these synergistic interactions, and within a broader anthropological framework we recognize that this definition also includes root causes such as poverty and violence as health conditions themselves. As we will see in subsequent chapters, syndemics are a signature challenge in the Third Epidemiological Transition, even though they have been an ancient feature of our epidemiological past. Syndemics are also key to understanding the conditions that led to our present global situation. With this in mind, we must examine the syndemic interactions within the worst-of-both-worlds situation faced by societies for whom the health benefits of Second Epidemiological Transition were delayed and diminished.

One of the most notable associations between communicable and non-communicable diseases was first identified in the 1930s with the comorbidity of diabetes and tuberculosis (Root 1934). Epidemiologically, this association persists today, and the prevalence of these combined diseases is especially high in poorer populations (Stubbs et al. 2021). Although the physiological interactions between diabetes and TB are still being investigated, it has been observed that TB-related immunosuppression can increase the risk of diabetes as well as respiratory and cardiovascular diseases and several forms of cancer (Marais et al. 2013, Peltzer 2018).

The causal factors between these diseases may also be bidirectional; diabetes and the chronic obstructive pulmonary diseases have also been shown to greatly increase the risk of tuberculosis (Stubbs et al. 2021). In one southern Mexican population, a diagnosis of adult-onset diabetes presents a sevenfold increase in the risk for tuberculosis infection (Ponce-de-Leon et al. 2004). This higher risk is comparable to people diagnosed with HIV in the same population, which is striking, given that TB disease is the world's most common AIDS-defining medical condition. Furthermore, alterations to the microbiome, especially the gut microbiome, may also play a role in these dynamics. A growing body of research suggests that altered microbiomes related to diet, stress, and use of antimicrobials is a risk factor for development of these and other non-communicable diseases (Ahn and Hayes 2021; West et al. 2015).

Cancer presents further examples of synergistic interaction between noncommunicable and communicable diseases. Like diabetes and obesity, cancer was once thought to be a disease of affluence, but it is now the second leading cause of death in low and middle income countries (LIMCs), contributing to 56 percent of cases and 64 percent of deaths globally (Jemal 2011; Remais et al. 2013). Case mortality for cancer is significantly higher in poorer societies than in wealthier ones, and overall mortality in poorer societies is projected to rise 75 percent by 2030 (Beaulieu et al. 2009; Bray et al. 2021). The rising burden of cancer in lower income societies is mediated by multiple factors, including longer life expectancies, changes in diet and physical activity, smoking, and exposure to environmental toxins.

As with other non-communicable diseases, the specific relationships between cancers and infectious diseases are complex, but two categorical factors are prominent. First, cancers and their treatment regimens often result in immunosuppression. Leukemias and lymphomas target immune cells, cancers can break down protective barriers, and other varieties of cancer can overwhelm the immune system and reduce metabolic energy needed to prevent and fight off opportunistic infections (Naran et al. 2018). Chemotherapy and targeted immunotherapies can also cause substantial immunosuppression, which leaves patients vulnerable to new and dormant infections (Morrison 2014).

Second, at least seven viruses, one bacterium, and three parasites can directly induce cancers in the absence of other causal factors (Yasunaga and Matsuoka 2018). These include pathogens that are endemic to affluent communities, such as human papilloma virus and *Heliobacter pylori*. However, the global prevalence of infectious diseases produced by these and most other carcinogenic pathogens is inversely proportional to socio-economic status, especially with regard to HIV-1, Hepatitis B virus, and *Schistosomiasis haematobium* (Azevedo et al. 2020). Infectious diseases are responsible for 13 percent of cancer cases worldwide, but we should take care to note that the large majority of these cases occur in LIMCs (de Martel et al. 2017).

Although the net benefits of the Second Epidemiological Transition have spread across most human populations, the combined burden of non-communicable and communicable diseases continues to be substantially greater in LIMCs than their wealthier counterparts. The synergistic interactions between these diseases further compounds the problem. As we will see in Chapter 6, synergies have proven to be especially relevant to the emergence and spread of the coronavirus epidemics in recent decades: severe acute respiratory syndrome (SARS), Middle East respiratory syndrome (MERS), and, most recently, COVID-19. Along with the global trend of aging populations, these dynamics have set the epidemiological stage for our twenty-first century pandemics.

4.4 Aging and poverty

Since the 1980s more than half the world's people over 65 years of age live in LIMCs, and the elderly poor are projected to increase from 460 million people in 1990 to 1.4 billion in 2030 based on a relative growth rate that is almost three times faster than in wealthy societies (Chatterji et al. 2015; Kinsella and Velkoff 2001). By 2050, it is expected that these countries will be home to more than 80 percent of the world's elderly. Part of this increase represents the success of the Second Epidemiological Transition in lower-income societies, where increased survival to adulthood has improved the odds that their members will survive to older years. But the increased proportion of elderly in these populations is also driven by the fertility declines that have accompanied a global trend toward urbanization, largely driven by major shifts from small-scale agrarian production to city-based employment. These fertility declines resulted in "baby busts" (as opposed to baby booms) that have eventually lead to larger ratios of older to younger people as they grow and age throughout their lifespans.

These changes are best illustrated by population pyramids, which demonstrate the relative proportions of people at different ages, also known as population age structures. Figure 4.2 shows three population pyramids representing different age structures for the world population at three periods of time. Each pyramid consists of two bar graphs (a.k.a. histograms) that have been turned on their sides and placed beside each other to depict the relative numbers of males and females in five-year age increments over a human lifespan: from birth to five years of age at the bottom to 80+ years of age at the top. In this particular figure, each pyramid is essentially two pyramids: a darker interior pyramid representing the combined age structures of lower-income nations, and a lighter exterior pyramid representing those of higher-income nations.

The 1950 pyramid is fairly triangular, thus similar, for the lower- and higher-income nations alike.

Two factors are responsible for this triangular shape. The first is a relatively large number of births compared to previous years (not shown), a phenomenon known as the "baby boom" of the twentieth century that greatly broadened the base of the pyramid. The second is an increasing risk of death at older age that narrows the pyramid toward the top. It should be noted that the narrowing of this pyramid, compared with subsequent pyramids, reflects a lower level of survival at older ages, especially in the lower income countries. It should also be noted that the abrupt contraction at five to nine years of age reflects early child mortality levels, which were also more pronounced in lower-income nations than higher-income countries. But because of high fertility during this time period, the overall shape of the pyramid is triangular, reflecting many more newborns to elderly individuals. Once again, however, the triangularity is especially pronounced in the lower-income countries owing to their greater mortality levels across the lifespan (Ritchie and Roser 2019).

In the 1990 pyramid, higher income countries begin to bulge in the middle as the baby boomers survived to middle adult ages with greater levels of survivability to adulthood and later years than in the lower-income countries. The base and lower bars are much larger in the lower-income countries, reflecting higher fertility than their wealthier counterparts. The slight bulge in the lower-income countries reflects decreased mortality from childhood to young adult years, the key health benefit experienced by late transitioning societies.

The 2030 pyramid is projected to change from a triangular to a columnar or "beehive" appearance in both the dark and light portions. These two bulges represent the aging populations of lower- and higher-income nations. Although these aging trends appear somewhat similar, these statistical graphs mask an important difference. The base of the pyramid for lower-income countries is deceptively similar to that of the 1990 pyramid, but with the expansion of the total human population, this apparent stasis reveals that more people are having fewer children. As mentioned earlier, the aging of lower-income societies has been largely driven by baby busts accompanied rapid urbanization and rural-to-urban migration, which has led to steep fertility declines as large families became more costly, economic mobility became more important, and children were no longer needed for agricultural labor. This global trend has resulted in a major shift in kinship structures with contraction of traditional

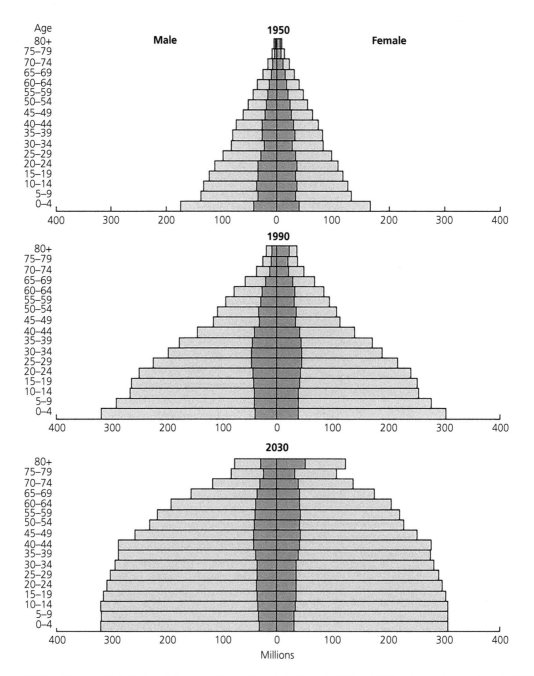

Figure 4.2 Population pyramids indicating relative ages of the world population by sex in 1950 and 1990, and a population estimate for 2030. The darker colors indicate developed nations. The lighter colors represent developing nations. Most societies, both rich and poor, are trending toward bulging pyramids with aging populations.

Source: Kinsella, K. and Velkoff, V.A. (2001). An Aging World: 2001. Washington D.C.: U.S. Census Bureau.

extended families, their fragmentation into nuclear subunits, and finally, their geographic dispersion, either due to the "push factors" of economic hardship, or the "pull factors" of economic opportunity.

This aging trend presents major challenges to both wealthy and poor societies. Among demographers and economists, these challenges are often framed in terms of dependency ratios, the average number of economically dependent people in relation to the economically productive people in a population. As anthropologists, we would also include domestically productive people in the latter group because family caregiving and household maintenance are as essential to the health and wellbeing of families as is the generation of income and other material resources. Taking into account this broader definition, dependency ratios with larger proportions of working age individuals are essential for the economic and social functioning of human societies (Choudry et al. 2016; Ritchie and Roser 2019). When these proportions are skewed toward higher dependency, the societal and health consequences can range from difficult to disastrous.

In wealthier societies, increasingly higher dependency ratios present difficult challenges. At the collective level, these include the challenges of funding pension programs and social security as a larger proportion of people leave the workforce. Public and private medical systems and health insurance plans must shoulder an increasing burden of chronic health conditions among a greater percentage of elderly. At the family level, older members can be an important asset for child-rearing and decision-making as well as household income generation and other domestic tasks. But with the increasing frailty of individuals at much older ages, these contributions can diminish, and second-generation working adults increasingly face the dual challenge of caring for their parents as well as their children. While there have been many names for the generations that followed the baby boomers, perhaps the best name for the generation facing this dual challenge is the Sandwich Generation (Parker and Patten 2013).

In poorer societies, higher dependency ratios are especially challenging. Lower-income countries have historically lacked the public resources to address the needs of their older members, much less the greater need of expanding older populations. Many of these societies have traditionally relied on the support of extended family members, but the recent trends of urbanization and economic migration have fragmented large families, thereby reducing household resources for caregiving and support. Consequently, the Sandwich Generations of poorer societies face a triple bind of not having the public, financial, or social resources to meet the needs of their youngest and oldest family members.

This challenge can reach crisis levels when older members become sick or disabled. Under these circumstances, impoverished families face difficult decisions about the allocation of resources: whether to pay for medicines instead of food, a clinic visit instead of a pair of shoes, or another hospitalization instead of another year of school fees. Compounding these dilemmas, the indirect costs of an illness are often higher than the direct costs. This is especially the case when working family members must forgo wage-earning labor to accompany a sick parent on long journeys to health providers or long waits in overcrowded clinics. Many hospitals in poor countries expect accompanying family member to provide meals and provide basic care such as bathing, laundry, and even routine administration of medications (cf. Barrett 2008). All of this can add up to days of missed wages for families surviving on narrow economic margins.

Faced with these expenses, it is not uncommon for impoverished families to forego, delay, or otherwise compromise the medical treatment of their elderly members. Such decisions may be reinforced by historical expectations about when and how elderly people are supposed to die. For instance, North Americans once referred to pneumonia as the "old man's friend," with the idea that was a relatively quick and painless way to die for people who did not usually live much beyond 65 years of age. But respiratory infections, such as influenza and TB, most often affect both the very young and the very old in U-shaped curves of infection by age. Consequently, higher rates of infection among the elderly can greatly increase the risk of infection among young children. In this manner, the "old man's friend" can quickly become the poor child's enemy.

As with the increase of chronic degenerative diseases, the aging of poor societies has created unwilling reservoirs for the evolution of virulent and drug resistant infections. A very good example of this can be found in the relationship between seasonal and pandemic influenzas. In wealthier societies, seasonal influenzas (the so-called "nonpathogenic" varieties) are often considered common and manageable conditions for which people may only have to miss a few days of work or school. However, few know that these common flus are responsible for between 290,000 and 645,000 worldwide deaths per year and that 41 percent of this mortality occurs among people over 75 years of age, mostly in low-income countries (Luliano et al. 2018). Furthermore, seasonal influenza epidemics contribute to the yearly antigenic variation of the virus, and the number and severity of cases increases the probability of emerging pathogenic strains, such as the H1N1 strain associated with the pandemic of 2009 (Boni et al. 2004; Roos 2011). In this way, the disproportionate impact of seasonal influenza among increasing populations of elderly people furthers the risk of a pathogenic influenza pandemic that could affect people of all ages.

Recall that influenza-related deaths are frequently caused by secondary bacterial pneumonias. There is experimental evidence that patients with pre-existing respiratory infections can become super-spreaders for additional infections, the so-called "cloud babies" and "cloud adults" capable of transmitting pathogens methicillin-resistant *Staphylococcus aureus* (MRSA) and SARS by sneezing airborne droplets of pathogens from the outer nasal area that are otherwise commonly transmitted via close contact or fomites (Chan et al. 2003; Sherertz 1996) (see Figure 4.3). More recent experiments indicate that sneezing could expel COVID-19-laden particles much further than their otherwise limited ballistic trajectories (Pöhlker et al. 2021). As with influenza, bacterial pneumonias, MRSA, and SARS have all disproportionally affected the elderly. And thus far in the COVID-19 pandemic, the elderly comprise more than 80 percent of deaths attributed to the disease (Booth et al. 2021; Sasson 2021).

Finally, elderly populations often serve as reservoirs for drug-resistant pathogens such as *Staphylococcus aureus*, *Pseudomonas auregenosa*, and *Klebsiella pneumoniae*, which became endemic to nursing homes and residential long-term care

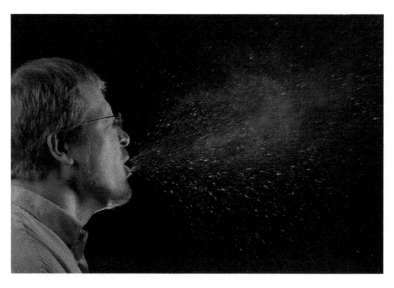

Figure 4.3 Sneeze in progress, depicting a cone-shaped plume of respiratory droplets being expelled from the nose and mouth. People with additional respiratory conditions can sometimes transmit a pathogen more effectively than if they were infected by one disease alone.
Source: Brian Judd (2009). CDC Public Health Image Library #11162.

facilities in the later decades of the twentieth century from which they spread to broader communities (Smith et al. 2000). Although these institutions have long been prevalent in wealthier societies, they are becoming an increasing feature of LIMCs where the socio-economic trends we previously discussed, such as urbanization, declining fertility, and economic mobility, have reduced and fragmented extended families, leaving them ill-equipped to address the chronic medical needs of their older members (Loyd-Sherlock 2014).

That said, a more common determinant of antimicrobial infections among the elderly in poorer societies is the inappropriate and incomplete use of antibiotics. Low-cost generic antimicrobials are widely available throughout the world, and they can be readily obtained without prescriptions in even the poorest communities. Such medicines present cheap alternatives to professional medical care when older people become sick and health services are either unaffordable or unavailable. As we will see in the next chapter, such practices have greatly contributed to the evolution of antimicrobial resistance.

4.5 When worlds collide

For better and worse, the Second Epidemiological Transition has effected the health of more than 95 percent of the human population. Despite the persistent poverty of late transitioning societies, no country in the world today has a life expectancy as low as that of the richest countries in 1800. Overall, the global life expectancy is now higher than it was for any country in the middle of the twentieth century (UN Population Division 2019; Zijdeman and Ribeira da Silva 2015). For the first time since the late Neolithic, infectious diseases are no longer the major cause of human mortality in most countries, and even with the rise of non-communicable diseases, the total world population continues to increase, despite declining fertility—a stark demonstration of improved human survival.

These improvements are undeniable, but global population statistics mask profound differences in the trajectories and outcomes of the Second Transition in rich vs. poor societies. More than 150 years

passed between the initial decline of infectious diseases in a handful of high-income countries and the declines that occurred in a larger and more populous set of low-income countries, a delay representing almost a billion foreshortened lives. In the high-income countries, infectious diseases had declined to the point that some medical authorities predicted near-total eradication by the end of the twentieth century. Yet around the same time as these optimistic predictions, various levels of economic underdevelopment produced a dose-related effect on the slope of infection declines in LIMCs. For 70 percent of the human population, the characteristic health benefit of the Second Epidemiological Transition turned out to be a case of too little, too late.

Short of true eradication, it was merely a matter of time before the persistent pathogens of poorer societies returned to infect the wealthier societies, even when some infections were merely endemic to smaller corners of the world. This is well illustrated in the recent histories of smallpox and polio. By the mid-twentieth century, smallpox had been all but eliminated in affluent Western societies. But the virus persisted in other parts of the world, especially in the poorer societies of Asia and Sub-Saharan Africa. Because of this, Europe and North America experienced no less than 53 so-called re-importation epidemics from the end of the Second World War to the final eradication of the disease in 1980 (Barrett 2006). Until then, even the wealthiest societies had to ensure that their populations were vaccinated to prevent what we would now call "re-emerging" infections.

The same could not be said for polio prevention, for which the United States alone has spent USD 35 billion on vaccinations from 1955 to 2005 (Thompson et al. 2021). As with smallpox prevention, all this money could be saved with the worldwide eradication of polio. We expect that most people do not think about health matters in purely fiscal terms, yet with the permeability of international borders to infectious diseases, the economic and ethical arguments are not exclusive of one another. On the contrary, they both make the same powerful and pragmatic case against medical isolationism.

The same arguments could be made for non-communicable diseases, given their synergistic relationships with major infectious disease threats, such as the highly pathogenic influenzas and coronaviruses with demonstrated their pandemic potentials. These synergies are also driving the evolution of antimicrobial resistance in the pathogens responsible for TB, malaria, and many historically deadly diseases that until recently we had come to regard as everyday infections. While the decline of infectious diseases has tapered in many poorer societies, becoming temporarily submerged rather than permanently eliminated, their increases in the burden of non-communicable diseases have been relatively rapid, especially among growing proportions of older people.

This is indeed a worst-of-both-worlds situation, but with accelerated globalization, the challenges faced by people living in the worst conditions were bound to spread to those living in the best conditions. Thus, over the last several decades, the pathogens and pathologies of nearly every human society have been converging into a single, global disease ecology. This convergence has been setting the stage for today's Third Epidemiological Transition.

Notes

1. Also known as the Standard American Diet, or SAD.

References

Ahn, Jiyoung, and Richard B Hayes. 2021. "Environmental Influences on the Human Microbiome and Implications for Noncommunicable Disease." *Annual review of public health* 42: 277.

Aksan, Anna-Maria, and Shankha Chakraborty. 2023. "Life expectancy across countries: Convergence, divergence and fluctuations." *World Development* 168: 106263.

Armelagos, George. J., Peter. J. Brown, and Bethany Turner. 2005. "Evolutionary, historical and political economic perspectives on health and disease." *Social Science & Medicine* 61 (4): 755–765. https://doi.org/10.1016/j.socscimed.2004.08.066.

Azevedo, Maria Manuel, Cidália Pina-Vaz, and Fátima Baltazar. 2020. "Microbes and cancer: friends or faux?" *International Journal of Molecular Sciences* 21 (9): 3115.

Azzam, Azzeddine. 2021. "Is the world converging to a 'Western diet'?" *Public health nutrition* 24 (2): 309–317.

Bailey, Claire, Vandana Garg, Deksha Kapoor, Heather Wasser, Dorairaj Prabhakaran, and Lindsay M Jaacks. 2018. "Food choice drivers in the context of the nutrition transition in Delhi, India." *Journal of nutrition education and behavior* 50 (7): 675–686.

Barrett, Ron. 2006. "Dark winter and the spring of 1972: Deflecting the social lessons of smallpox." *Medical Anthropology* 25 (2): 171–191.

Barrett, Ron. 2008. *Aghor Medicine: Pollution, Death, and Healing in Northern India*. Berkeley: University of California Press.

Beaulieu, Nancy, D Bloom, R Bloom, and R Stein. 2009. "Breakaway: The global burden of cancer—challenges and opportunities." *The Economist Intelligence Unit*.

Bloom, David E., and David Canning. 2007. "Mortality traps and the dynamics of health transitions." *Proceedings of the National Academy of Sciences* 104 (41): 16044–16049. https://doi.org/doi:10.1073/pnas.0702012104. https://www.pnas.org/doi/abs/10.1073/pnas.0702012104.

Boni, Maciej F, Julia R Gog, Viggo Andreasen, and Freddy B Christiansen. 2004. "Influenza drift and epidemic size: the race between generating and escaping immunity." *Theoretical population biology* 65 (2): 179–191.

Booth, Adam, Angus Bruno Reed, Sonia Ponzo, Arrash Yassaee, Mert Aral, David Plans, Alain Labrique, and Diwakar Mohan. 2021. "Population risk factors for severe disease and mortality in COVID-19: A global systematic review and meta-analysis." *PloS one* 16 (3): e0247461.

Bray, Freddie, Mathieu Laversanne, Elisabete Weiderpass, and Isabelle Soerjomataram. 2021. "The ever-increasing importance of cancer as a leading cause of premature death worldwide." *Cancer* 127 (16): 3029–3030.

Caballero, Benjamin, and Barry M. Popkin. 2002. *The nutrition transition: diet and disease in the developing world*. London: Academic Press.

Chan, JWM, CK Ng, YH Chan, TYW Mok, S Lee, SYY Chu, WL Law, MP Lee, and PCK Li. 2003. "Short term outcome and risk factors for adverse clinical outcomes in adults with severe acute respiratory syndrome (SARS)." *Thorax* 58 (8): 686–689.

Chatterji, Somnath, Julie Byles, David Cutler, Teresa Seeman, and Emese Verdes. 2015. "Health, functioning, and disability in older adults—present status and future implications." *The lancet* 385 (9967): 563–575.

Choudhry, Misbah Tanveer, Enrico Marelli, and Marcello Signorelli. 2016. "Age dependency and labour productivity divergence." *Applied Economics* 48 (50): 4823–4845. https://doi.org/10.1080/00036846.2016.1167823.

de Martel, Catherine, Martyn Plummer, Jerome Vignat, and Silvia Franceschi. 2017. "Worldwide burden of cancer attributable to HPV by site, country and HPV type." *International journal of cancer* 141 (4): 664–670. https://doi.org/10.1002/ijc.30716. https://pubmed.ncbi.nlm.nih.gov/28369882. https://www.ncbi.nlm.nih.gov/pmc/articles/PMC5520228/.

Edwards, Ryan D. 2011. "Changes in world inequality in length of life: 1970–2000." *Population and Development Review* 37 (3): 499–528.

Farmer, Paul. 1996. "Social Inequalities and Emerging Infectious Diseases." *Emerging Infectious Diseases.* 2(4): 259–269.

Fine, Ben, Michael Heasman, and Judith Wright. 2002. *Consumption in the age of affluence: the world of food.* Routledge.

Ho, Jessica Y, and Arun S Hendi. 2018. "Recent trends in life expectancy across high income countries: retrospective observational study." *Bmj* 362.

Jain, Hari Krishan. 2010. *Green revolution: history, impact and future.* The Green Revolution: Histor.

Jasovský, Dušan, Jasper Littmann, Anna Zorzet, and Otto Cars. 2016. "Antimicrobial resistance—a threat to the world's sustainable development." *Upsala journal of medical sciences* 121 (3): 159–164.

Jemal, Ahmedin, Melissa M Center, Carol DeSantis, and Elizabeth M Ward. 2010. "Global Patterns of Cancer Incidence and Mortality Rates and Trends." *Cancer epidemiology, biomarkers & prevention* 19 (8): 1893–1907.

Kanavos, Panos. 2006. "The rising burden of cancer in the developing world." *Annals of oncology* 17: viii15-viii23.

Kinsella, Kevin, and Victoria A. Velkoff. 2001. *An Aging World: 2001.* Washington D.C.: U.S. Census Bureau.

Leatherman, Thomas L., Morgan K. Hoke, and Alan H. Goodman. 2016. "Local nutrition in global contexts: critical biocultural perspectives on the nutrition transition in Mexico." In *New Directions in Biocultural Anthropology*: 49–45.

Li, Lian, Ning Sun, Lina Zhang, Guodong Xu, Jingjing Liu, Jingcen Hu, Zhiying Zhang, Jianjun Lou, Hongxia Deng, and Zhisen Shen. 2020. "Fast food consumption among young adolescents aged 12–15 years in 54 low- and middle-income countries." *Global health action* 13 (1): 1795438.

Liou, Lathan, William Joe, Abhishek Kumar, and SV Subramanian. 2020. "Inequalities in life expectancy: An analysis of 201 countries, 1950–2015." *Social Science & Medicine* 253: 112964.

Lloyd-Sherlock, Peter. 2014. "Beyond neglect: long-term care research in low and middle income countries." *International Journal of Gerontology* 8 (2): 66–69.

Iuliano, A Danielle, Katherine M Roguski, Howard H Chang, David J Muscatello, Rakhee Palekar, Stefano Tempia, Cheryl Cohen, Jon Michael Gran, Dena Schanzer, and Benjamin J Cowling. 2018. "Estimates of global seasonal influenza-associated respiratory mortality: a modelling study." *The Lancet* 391 (10127): 1285–1300.

Marais, Ben J, Knut Lönnroth, Stephen D Lawn, Giovanni Battista Migliori, Peter Mwaba, Philippe Glaziou, Matthew Bates, Ruth Colagiuri, Lynn Zijenah, and Soumya Swaminathan. 2013. "Tuberculosis comorbidity with communicable and non-communicable diseases: integrating health services and control efforts." *The Lancet infectious diseases* 13 (5): 436–448.

Morrison, Vicki A. 2014. "Immunosuppression Associated With Novel Chemotherapy Agents and Monoclonal Antibodies." *Clinical Infectious Diseases* 59 (suppl_5): S360-S364. https://doi.org/10.1093/cid/ciu592.

Murray, Christopher J. L., Lisa C. Rosenfeld, Stephen S. Lim, Kathryn G. Andrews, Kyle J. Foreman, Diana Haring, Nancy Fullman, Mohsen Naghavi, Rafael Lozano, and Alan D. Lopez. 2012. "Global malaria mortality between 1980 and 2010: A systematic analysis." *The Lancet* 379 (9814): 413–431. https://doi.org/10.1016/S0140-6736(12)60034-8.

Naran, Krupa, Trishana Nundalall, Shivan Chetty, and Stefan Barth. 2018. "Principles of Immunotherapy: Implications for Treatment Strategies in Cancer and Infectious Diseases." *Frontiers in microbiology* 9: 3158. https://doi.org/10.3389/fmicb.2018.03158. https://pubmed.ncbi.nlm.nih.gov/30622524. https://www.ncbi.nlm.nih.gov/pmc/articles/PMC6308495/

Nichols, Carly. 2017. "Millets, milk and maggi: Contested processes of the nutrition transition in rural India." *Agriculture and human values* 34: 871–885.

Parker, Kim, and Eileen Patten. 2013. *The Sandwich Generation: Rising Financial Burdens for Middle-Aged Americans.* (Pew Research Center). https://www.pewresearch.org/social-trends/2013/01/30/the-sandwich-generation/

Pelto, Gretel H., and Pertti J. Pelto. 1983. "Diet and Delocalization: Dietary Changes since 1750." *The Journal of Interdisciplinary History* 14 (2): 507–528. https://doi.org/10.2307/203719. http://www.jstor.org/stable/203719.

Peltzer, K. 2018. "Tuberculosis non-communicable disease comorbidity and multimorbidity in public primary care patients in South Africa." *African journal of primary health care & family medicine* 10 (1): e1–e6. https://doi.org/10.4102/phcfm.v10i1.1651.

Pesec, Madeline, Hannah L Ratcliffe, Ami Karlage, Lisa R Hirschhorn, Atul Gawande, and Asaf Bitton. 2017. "Primary health care that works: the Costa Rican experience." *Health Affairs* 36 (3): 531–538.

Pöhlker, Mira L, Ovid O Krüger, Jan-David Förster, Thomas Berkemeier, Wolfgang Elbert, Janine Fröhlich-Nowoisky, Ulrich Pöschl, Christopher Pöhlker, Gholamhossein Bagheri, and Eberhard Bodenschatz. 2021. "Respiratory aerosols and droplets in the transmission of infectious diseases." *arXiv preprint arXiv:2103.01188.*

Ponce-de-Leon, Alfredo, Ma de Lourdes Garcia-Garcia, Ma Cecilia Garcia-Sancho, Francisco J Gomez-Perez, Jose Luis Valdespino-Gomez, Gustavo Olaiz-Fernandez, Rosalba Rojas, Leticia Ferreyra-Reyes, Bulmaro Cano-Arellano, and Miriam Bobadilla. 2004. "Tuberculosis and diabetes in southern Mexico." *Diabetes care* 27 (7): 1584–1590.

Popkin, Barry M. 2015. "Nutrition transition and the global diabetes epidemic." *Current diabetes reports* 15: 1–8.

Popkin, Barry M., and Shu Wen Ng. 2022. "The nutrition transition to a stage of high obesity and noncommunicable disease prevalence dominated by ultra-processed foods is not inevitable." *Obes Rev* 23 (1): e13366. https://doi.org/10.1111/obr.13366.

Preston, Samuel H. 1980. "Causes and Consequences of Mortality Declines in Less Developed Countries during the Twentieth Century." In *Population and Econimic Change in Developing Countries*, edited by Richard A. Easterlin, 289–360. Chicago: University of Chicago Press.

Remais, Justin V, Guang Zeng, Guangwei Li, Lulu Tian, and Michael M Engelgau. 2013. "Convergence of non-communicable and infectious diseases in low-and middle-income countries." *International journal of epidemiology* 42 (1): 221–227.

Riley, James C. 2005. "Estimates of Regional and Global Life Expectancy, 1800–2001." *Population and Development Review* 31 (3): 537–543. https://doi.org/10.1111/j.1728-4457.2005.00083.x. https://onlinelibrary.wiley.com/doi/abs/10.1111/j.1728-4457.2005.00083.x

Ritchie, Hannah, and Max Roser. 2019. "Urbanization." Our World in Data. Accessed June 17, 2021. https://ourworldindata.org/urbanization

Roos, Robert. 2011. "Study puts global 2009 H1N1 infection rate at 11% to 21%," https://www.cidrap.umn.edu/h1n1-2009-pandemic-influenza/study-puts-global-2009-h1n1-infection-rate-11-21

Root, Howard F. 1934. "The Association of Diabetes and Tuberculosis." *New England Journal of Medicine* 210 (1): 1–13. https://doi.org/10.1056/nejm193401042100101. https://www.nejm.org/doi/full/10.1056/NEJM193401042100101

Sasson, Isaac. 2021. "Age and COVID-19 mortality." *Demographic Research* 44: 379–396.

Sherertz, Robert J, David R Reagan, Kenneth D Hampton, Kim L Robertson, Stephen A Streed, Helena M Hoen, Robert Thomas, and Gwaltney Jack M. Jr. MD. 1996. "A cloud adult: the Staphylococcus aureus-virus interaction revisited." *Annals of internal medicine* 124 (6): 539–547.

Smith, Philip W, Cindy W Seip, Stephen C Schaefer, and Connie Bell-Dixon. 2000. "Microbiologic survey of long-term care facilities." *American journal of infection control* 28 (1): 8–13.

Soares, Rodrigo R. 2007. "On the Determinants of Mortality Reductions in the Developing World." *Population and Development Review* 33 (2): 247–287.

Stubbs, B., K. Siddiqi, H. Elsey, N. Siddiqi, R. Ma, E. Romano, S. Siddiqi, and A. Koyanagi. 2021. "Tuberculosis and Non-Communicable Disease Multimorbidity: An Analysis of the World Health Survey in 48 Low- and Middle-Income Countries." *Int J Environ Res Public Health* 18 (5). https://doi.org/10.3390/ijerph18052439.

Thankappan, KR, and MS Valiathan. 1998. "Health at low cost: the Kerala model." *Lancet* 351: 1274–1275.

Thompson, Kimberly M, Dominika A Kalkowska, and Kamran Badizadegan. 2021. "A health economic analysis for oral poliovirus vaccine to prevent COVID-19 in the United States." *Risk Analysis* 41 (2): 376–386.

UN Population Division. 2019. *World Population Prospects 2019: Highlights.* Population Division United Nations Department of Economic and Social Affairs. https://www.un.org/development/desa/publications/world-population-prospects-2019-highlights.html.

Wang, Haidong, Mohsen Naghavi, Christine Allen, Ryan M. Barber, Zulfiqar A. Bhutta, Austin Carter, Daniel C. Casey, et al. 2016. "Global, regional, and national life expectancy, all-cause mortality, and cause-specific mortality for 249 causes of death, 1980–2015: A systematic analysis for the Global Burden of Disease Study 2015." *The Lancet* 388 (10053): 1459–1544. https://doi.org/10.1016/S0140-6736(16)31012-1.

Weaver, Lesley Jo, and K. M. Narayan. 2008. "Reconsidering the history of type 2 diabetes in India: emerging or re-emerging disease?" *Natl Med J India* 21 (6): 288–91.

West, Christina E, Harald Renz, Maria C Jenmalm, Anita L Kozyrskyj, Katrina J Allen, Peter Vuillermin, Susan L Prescott, Charles MacKay, Seppo Salminen, and Gary Wong. 2015. "The gut microbiota and inflammatory noncommunicable diseases: associations and potentials for gut microbiota therapies." *Journal of Allergy and Clinical Immunology* 135 (1): 3–13.

Winskill, Peter, Alexandra B Hogan, Julie Thwing, Lazaro Mwandigha, Patrick GT Walker, and Ben Lambert. 2021.

"Health inequities and clustering of fever, acute respiratory infection, diarrhoea and wasting in children under five in low-and middle-income countries: a Demographic and Health Surveys analysis." *BMC medicine* 19 (1): 1–11.

World Bank. 2022. "Life Expectancy at Birth, total (years) - Low income." World Bank. Accessed 01/01/2023. https://data.worldbank.org/indicator/SP.DYN.LE00.IN?locations=XM.

Yasunaga, Jun-Ichirou, and Masao Matsuoka. 2018. "Oncogenic spiral by infectious pathogens: Cooperation of multiple factors in cancer development." *Cancer Science* 109 (1): 24–32. https://doi.org/https://doi.org/10.1111/cas.13443. https://onlinelibrary.wiley.com/doi/abs/10.1111/cas.13443

Zijdeman, Richard, and Filipa Ribeira da Silva. 2015. Life Expectancy at Birth (Total). IISH Data Collection.

PART 3

The Third Epidemiological Transition

CHAPTER 5

New and Converging Infections

"... the role of the infinitely small appeared to me to be infinitely great"

Louis Pasteur (1882)[1]

In the early months of the COVID-19 pandemic, the term "unprecedented" was often used to describe the outbreak in popular and political discourse.[2] Yet despite its apparent novelty, the disease is a classic example of many novel infections that have emerged over the past several decades. Like most novel pathogens, the associated virus, SARS-CoV-2, had already been circulating in the host population for some time before it was first detected. In early December 2019, the first patients were admitted to hospitals in the Chinese city of Wuhan with respiratory distress due to a severe pneumonia of unknown cause (Wong et al. 2020). The Chinese government reported a cluster of infections from a novel coronavirus to the World Health organization on December 31st (World Health Organization 2020). Even then, retrospective testing would later find cases from mid-November of that year, and epidemiological models estimate the first undetected infections occurred as early as September 2019 (Bryner 2020; Wong et al. 2021a). There may have been several thousand cases by the time the world became aware of this deadly new pathogen.

Some reports suggest that the Chinese government may have delayed the reporting of COVID-19, much like what happened during the severe acute respiratory syndrome (SARS) outbreak in 2002–2004 (McMullen 2021). Regardless of whether this is correct or not, it is likely that an even larger delay was caused by a shortcoming that China commonly shares with most other nations: the insufficient provision of health resources to their most vulnerable and isolated communities. Infectious diseases are especially prevalent among the

poor, and new pathogens are easily camouflaged in the mix. When these same communities lack access to medical resources, it can be months or even years before the pathogen is detected. HIV-1 is a prime example; the virus had been circulating for over 20 years in Sub-Saharan Africa before the biomedical establishment became aware of its existence, and only then after it appeared in a cluster of urban American patients (CDC 1981; Zhu et al. 1998). Even when a new pathogen is detected, it can take years before significant resources are brought to bear on the problem. World leaders paid little attention to the Ebola virus for nearly two decades, despite nine major outbreaks, until related viruses were found in US and European primate research facilities (Barrett 2015; Garrett 1994). For COVID-19, the delay amounted to months rather than years. But even a few weeks would have been crucial for containing the spread of a deadly infection before it became a global pandemic.

With early detection in mind, the SARS and Middle East respiratory syndrome (MERS) outbreaks should have been sufficient warning that conditions were ripe for the appearance of another pathogenic coronavirus. All three pathogens—SARS-CoV, MERS-CoV, and SARS-CoV-2—evolved from zoonotic viruses from which bats are the most likely reservoir (Kesheh et al. 2021). Bats are also the most likely reservoir for three other coronaviruses associated with up to 30 percent of milder upper respiratory infections (cf. the common cold) in humans. This is troubling, given the size, diversity, and mobility of bat species. As the second largest mammalian order, *Chiroptera*, includes over 1,400 bat

Emerging Infections. Second Edition. Ron Barrett, Molly K. Zuckerman, Matthew R. Dudgeon, with George J. Armelagos, Oxford University Press.
© Ron Barrett, Molly K. Zuckerman, Matthew R. Dudgeon (2024). DOI: 10.1093/oso/9780192843135.003.0006

species, many of whom frequently move back and forth between wild and domesticated environments (Jones et al. 2009). In the course of these movements, bat species probably transmitted the SARS viruses to peri-domestic food animals, such as civets and pangolins, and the MERS virus to fully domesticated dromedary camels (Paules et al. 2020). In all three outbreaks, human subsistence practices linked to global trade networks helped to bring deadly new pathogens to our doorstep.

Ten weeks after the initial public report, the World Health Organization determined that the COVID-19 outbreak had become a global pandemic (Wong et al. 2021b). The velocity and reach of the virus also seemed unprecedented, but many other infectious diseases have had similar trajectories (Markel 2004). We need only look at all the human influenza epidemics, seasonal as well as pathogenic, that have occurred since the nineteenth century (Wille and Holmes 2021). Yet now that the majority of the world population lives in dense urban centers, all of them linked to complex networks of migration, travel, and trade, the wave velocities of infectious disease epidemics have increased substantially in recent decades (Hazarie et al. 2021). With these dynamics in mind, it is worth noting that the first reported cases of COVID-19 were located in a city of 12 million people that serves as a major hub for international trade. Wuhan is but one example of many twenty-first century "settlements" that have become giant incubators situated at the intersections of microbial superhighways.

These global networks are permeated with vulnerable populations. As such, the vulnerable are hardly "marginalized" in the geographic sense of the term. The same can be said for their heightened burdens of infection, which in a pandemic become everyone else's problems as well. COVID-19 revealed these problems with significantly higher rates of infectivity and mortality among the poor, elderly, ethnic, and racial minorities, and people with non-communicable diseases (Kompaniyets et al. 2021; Mude et al. 2021; Pijls et al. 2021; Rossen et al. 2021). Thus, the pandemic can be more accurately described as a global syndemic. Tragically, the international response to COVID did not account for its syndemic nature, and societies that were at the highest risk for infection were the lowest

priority for vaccination. This proved advantageous for the virus, which has evolved new variants in vulnerable populations at a faster rate than its human hosts can develop new medicines.

With COVID-19 and the other pathogenic coronaviruses, we see how human modes of subsistence, settlement, and social organization have played major roles in our exposure to infectious diseases. These same themes apply to over 335 species of viruses, bacteria, and parasites that were newly discovered between 1940 and 2004 (Jones et al. 2008). Of course, we must also factor in variable periods between first infections and first discoveries, and we must also consider detection bias when discoveries increase with improved surveillance, especially in nations with better developed public health systems. Yet regardless of delays and biases, phylogenetic comparisons of newly identified strains indicate that most of these pathogens are indeed newcomers to human populations (Scarpino 2016).

When we include new variants to this growing list of novel pathogens, the numbers grow into the thousands (Allen et al. 2017). New strains of existing infections are especially challenging because they have had time to evolve traits that increase their prevalence in human hosts. These traits include, but are not limited to, drug resistance and evasion from innate, acquired, and vaccine-triggered immune defenses. We will address issues of antimicrobial resistance in Chapter 6 but for now it should be noted that the rates at which these novel infections are appearing has increased in the last few decades. Diagnostic of this is a significant increase in the uniqueness, diversity, and total number of infectious disease outbreaks from 1980 to 2013 (Smith et al. 2014).[3] Since then, we have seen seven Ebola outbreaks, the arrival of MERS, and, of course, the COVID-19 pandemic.

These growing threats of new, recurring, and drug-resistant infections constitute the US Institute of Medicine's definition of emerging infectious diseases, a problem that has continued well into the twenty-first century (Lederburg et al. 1992; Morens and Fauci 2013). When viewed from an even broader anthropological time frame, we recognize a significant deviation from the declining infections of the Second Epidemiological Transition and its associated patterns. This deviation also presents features that distinguish it from the previous two transitions: a greater number of synergistic interactions between acute infections and chronic non-communicable diseases, a demographic shift to increasingly older host populations, and the globalization of our interconnections into a single human disease ecology. These major changes constitute the Third Epidemiological Transition that we are experiencing today.

In this chapter, we examine how these factors contribute to the emergence of novel human infections as well as newer variants of our longstanding diseases. Because most of these diseases originate in non-human animal species, we begin by unpacking the biosocial forces that drive the entry and evolution of zoonotic pathogens in human host populations. We then turn to familiar themes of subsistence with respect to hunting and agriculture but in the modern context of global supply chains, habitat displacements, and industrial methods of food production. We consider how the world's disease ecologies have converged, not only through our extensive networks of transport and trade but also through the synergies between infectious and non-infectious diseases, especially among poor, elderly, and socially marginalized populations. In the last section, we will examine how these human vulnerabilities create opportunities, not only for spillover and spread but also for the evolution of traits that determine their levels of morbidity and mortality once they have infected us.

5.1 Zoonotic spillover

Among the 335 novel infections described above, more than 60 percent originated in non-human animal species (Jones et al. 2008). This has brought increasing attention to the process known as spillover. There is some variation in the ways that disease biologists have operationalized this term, but in its general sense spillover describes an adaptive process by which a pathogen that is found in one or more reservoir host species acquires the ability to sustain infection in a new host species (Becker et al. 2019; Sokolow et al. 2019). The new species can be any manner of organism: an animal, plant, or even a bacterium. From our anthropocentric perspective, we are selfishly interested in the

ways that zoonotic infections become human infections. Accordingly, we will operationally define our selfish topic of interest as *zoonotic spillover*, and use it interchangeably with the term *spillover* for the sake of convenience.

Spillover is a process, not a singular event. A zoonotic pathogen must somehow overcome a series of potential barriers to successfully invade and gain permanent entry into a human host population. There are different models to describe these barriers, each having its own series of stages or steps (Anderson and May 1986; Wolfe 2011). Yet at the most basic level, all of these barriers fall into three broad categories: between humans and animals (interspecies), within humans (intra-human), and between humans (inter-human) (Gortazar et al. 2014). The first are interspecies barriers between infected animals or vectors and potential human hosts. To overcome these barriers, humans and animals must somehow be brought close enough together, often enough, and for long enough to allow for the physical possibility of cross-species transmission.

At the macro level, the particular circumstances of human–animal interactions shape the proximity, duration, and frequency of their exposure to one another (Plowright et al. 2017). These circumstances can include human subsistence practices such as hunting, herding, and farming. They can also include animal subsistence behaviors, including the opportunistic consumption of livestock, crops, and, in the particular case of microbial subsistence, our own body tissues. Along with subsistence, humans and animals can be brought together by cohabitation, territorial competition, or simply intersecting paths within locally shared environments. All these circumstances can lead to more proximate transmission events, such as a cow shedding intestinal bacteria in an upstream defecation, a mosquito sharing parasites during a blood meal, or a butcher transferring viruses with the slip of a knife.

At the micro level, it is common to think of transmission solely as a characteristic of the agent or the disease itself: HIV/AIDS is a blood-borne disease, Zika is a vector-borne disease, and so forth. Pathogen characteristics, such as the environmental resilience of a protein capsid or a lipid membrane, can profoundly influence transmission modes. For instance, the Ebola virus quickly degrades outside particular physiological environments, which restricts its transmission within the medium of mammalian body fluids, whereas most influenza viruses are environmentally much hardier, allowing them to survive on fomite surfaces for extended periods of time (Vetter et al. 2016; Wille and Holmes 2021). But the physiological responses of animals and vectors also play important roles. These include common physical symptoms, such as diarrhea and coughing, that can expel significant quantities of infected material into local environments. They also include biobehavioral responses, such as the neuropathies of rabid mammals and the alimentary obstructions of plague-infected insects, both of which can increase the frequency and intensity of biting activity (Barrett 2008; Wolfe 2011).

Even when accounting for these macro- and micro-level issues, we must recognize that transmission merely allows for human exposure to the pathogen. It does not guarantee the invasion, colonization, and proliferation of the pathogen in the fertile territories of particular human tissues and cells. Here the pathogen must overcome significant intra-human barriers. Skin, epithelial tissues, and cellular membranes present physical barriers to entry. Tears, oils, and digestive fluids present chemical barriers. Immune cells and proteins threaten survival, and other microbial species compete for limited resources.

Pathogens must overcome or avoid these intra-human barriers using specific molecular processes. They breach boundaries through the interaction of surface proteins coming together like keys into locks, and they form defenses by the assembly of specific protein-mediated structures. Bacteria suppress competitors through natural antibiosis, and viruses exploit the replication mechanisms of host cells. All these processes are ultimately determined by genetic coding, and while the genome of a zoonotic pathogen may be adapted to the infection of one or more animal host species, it may not be adapted as well, or at all, to the barriers particular to human hosts. If the pathogen species is not already adapted to a given barrier, then it must undergo some degree of evolutionary change. This entails a series of mutations leading to an accumulation of genetically coded traits that confer reproductive benefits in the new environment of the human host.

Some pathogens have intrinsic characteristics that allow them to evolve more quickly than others. Viruses, for example, tend to have simpler and cruder replication mechanisms than those of bacteria or parasites, making more errors when copying their genomes for the next generation. The genomes of some viruses are comprised of RNA instead of DNA, a much more reactive molecule that is itself prone to higher mutation rates. And viruses with more than one genetic segment, such as influenza, can reshuffle these segments into new combinations when more than one variety infects the same cell (Wille and Holmes 2020).

Although not as dynamic as viruses, bacteria can also evolve more quickly through mechanisms of horizontal gene transfer (HGT), incorporating small DNA segments from other bacteria of the same or different species, or from bacteria-infecting (bacteriophage) viruses. Many of these segments contain genes that confer virulence traits or antibiotic resistance, issues that we will address later in this chapter and the next. HGT also occurs in some protozoan parasites (Sibbald et al. 2020).

Recalling the metaphor of soil and seed in Chapter 3, it is important to note that spillover is not determined by pathogen characteristics alone. Exposure events and the health of the potential human host often play essential roles in this process. Regarding exposure, the rate at which a pathogen species evolves spillover traits increases with exposure to the human host environment. This is sometimes referred to as *pathogen pressure*, which is determined by the number of zoonotic pathogens available to a potential human host at a given moment in time and space. Pathogen pressure is a particular form of selection pressure that increases opportunities for random mutations and gene transfers that may lead to beneficial molecular traits (Plowright et al. 2017). And as we have seen in previous chapters, under-nutrition and comorbid medical conditions suppress the immune system, reducing intra-human barriers to spillover and allowing pathogens to gain an initial foothold in vulnerable reservoir populations where it can further evolve more efficient adaptations for colonizing healthier human hosts.

Inter-human barriers can present major challenges to zoonotic spillover. Simply put, they entail navigating through an additional gauntlet of intra-human barriers, any of which can pose different challenges for exit than for entry. If the person who is initially infected has diminished host barriers, as previously described, then the threshold will be higher for onward transmission to a healthier population. Once again, physiological responses to the infection can enable or inhibit transmission, but these responses may be very different in human hosts than in other species. And finally, another series of circumstances must somehow enable the kinds of social interactions that allow infected people to transmit the pathogen to one another. Because of these and other inter-human barriers, any single instance of human infection can nevertheless prove to be a dead end for a zoonotic pathogen. Successful spillover requires sustained human-to-human transmission.

Epidemiologically, we can observe these dead ends in a phenomenon known as "viral chatter." This term is adopted from signals intelligence agencies that monitor radio chatter for characteristic patterns that might reveal useful information (Wolfe 2011). In the case of viral chatter, the patterns take the form of limited and sporadic human outbreaks of an otherwise zoonotic infectious disease. These often occur when a zoonotic pathogen is initially capable of animal-to-human infection but is not yet capable, or not fully capable, of onward transmission from human to human.

We have seen viral chatter in the transmission of simian retroviruses to primate hunters in West and Central Africa, which may explain the phylogenetic evidence that HIV-1 and HIV-2 made at least 10 incursions into the human population for a century prior to the arrival of the AIDS pandemic (Wolfe et al. 2004; Wolfe 2011). We have also seen chatter in some highly pathogenic avian influenza strains that infected human individuals without onward transmission (Wang et al. 2021). Early outbreaks of Nipah virus were solely caused by animal–human transmission and only later found to have limited transmission between humans (Singh et al. 2019). In the year leading up to the MERS epidemics, the virus was primarily attributed to camel-to-human infections and a few limited hospital clusters, though interview data for initial cases were limited (Gossner et al. 2014). These examples reveal transitional moments in the coevolution of pathogens and their future human hosts.

Spillover processes are well illustrated by a human cholera infection. The bacterial pathogen, *Vibrio cholerae*, has remarkable swimming abilities, and it can survive in a variety of aquatic environments, ranging from open seas to open sewers, nearly any pool of water with sufficient salinity, warmth, and nutrients (Faruque et al. 2003). There are many serotypes and strains of *V. cholerae*, and while their ingestion may cause varying degrees of human illness, only a few varieties cause the cholera disease itself. It appears that most of these bacteria make their livings on the exoskeletons of marine crustaceans, zooplankton especially. In these primary host environments, *V. cholerae* break down chitin, a principal component of the exoskeletons that is indigestible to most other animals. By digesting chitin, *V. cholerae* increase the bioavailability of a major global carbon source (Pruzzo et al. 2008). It is likely that one or more of these zoonotic strains were the evolutionary ancestors of those associated with human cholera.

As it turns out, aquatic *V. cholerae* are somewhat pre-adapted to the lower guts of land animals. The same protein structure that allows the bacteria to latch onto crustaceans also allows them to latch onto the epithelial lining of human intestines, making it very difficult for the host to expel them. But for the bacteria to reach this environment, they must first overcome a number of interspecies and intra-human barriers. The journey from mouth to intestine is perilous, and only a very small percentage survive. The stomach is especially good at destroying microorganisms with a highly acidic gastric fluid that activates enzymes for breaking down the proteins and lipids of cellular membranes. Even then, the few bacteria that survive this onslaught must be undamaged enough to swim against convective currents of food and water and resist the propulsive motility of the gut, until an even smaller number eventually find purchase on the appropriate tissue attachment point (Muanprasat and Chatsudthipong 2013).

To breach these barriers, *V. cholerae* must enter the human mouth in large numbers: for disease-producing strains, the minimum infective dose is around 400–600 million bacteria, though this can vary by strain and host vulnerability (Cash et al. 1974a, 1974b). This is not a large number in microbial terms, but it can be particularly difficult for *V. cholerae* to achieve because although they are good swimmers, these bacteria live and reproduce as films on host and particle surfaces. The water has to be lively, or dirty, or both. Climate change has helped produce these numbers by raising average sea surface temperatures. This has resulted in massive coastal algae blooms, the scales of which can only be appreciated with satellite imagery (see Figure 5.1). The zooplankton thrive on the algae and *V. cholerae* thrive on the zooplankton. From the coasts, the bacteria migrate into brackish estuaries, and from there, abject poverty and poor infrastructure help to bring *V. cholerae* to human drinking water (Balasubramanian et al. 2021).

With sufficient starting numbers, *V. cholerae* can find its way to the human intestine. And when the numbers are even higher, the bacteria can apply pathogen pressure to further the evolution of spillover traits. This best explains two major events in the evolution of *V. cholerae*, both of which resulted from the horizontal transfer of genetic segments from viral infections acquired by the bacteria themselves (Das et al. 2016). One segment enhances the latching ability of *V. cholerae* to a specific binding site in the small intestine, an area of the lower gut with far fewer numbers of competing bacteria. The other segment produces a combination of toxins that result in a massive efflux of water and electrolytes from the inner body to the inner lumen of the intestine. Awash with its preferred environment of salty fluids, this toxigenic *V. cholerae* latches tightly onto the intestinal wall while its microbial competitors are flushed away. Meanwhile, the human host dehydrates at rates of up to one liter an hour, often dying within a day of initial infection (Muanprasat and Chatsudthipong 2013).

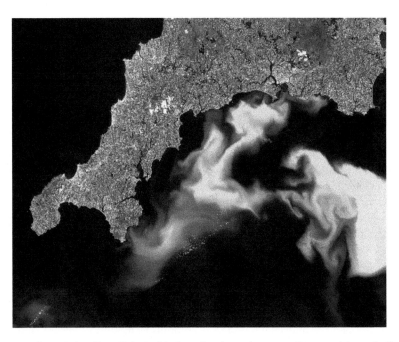

Figure 5.1 Landsat image of a 1999 algae bloom in the English Channel on the southern coast of Devon and Cornwall. Often triggered by rising sea surface temperatures, these massive blooms typically accompanied by increased populations of V. cholera bacteria, though only a few serotypes are known to cause disease in humans.

Source: USGS courtesy of Steve Groom.

Rapid dehydration is the primary hazard and chief hallmark of cholera disease.

In many instances, it is not in the interest of the pathogen to kill off its host so quickly. But like their marine ancestors, toxigenic *V. cholerae* are quite capable of surviving on their own, especially in the sewage and other contaminated water sources that are often found in impoverished human communities. Under these conditions, the rapid shedding of pathogens by dying patients increases their concentration in surrounding environments, thus greatly assisting *V. cholerae* in overcoming significant inter-human barriers to onward transmission. These conditions can also increase pathogen pressure toward the evolution of even more virulent strains; we saw this with the emergence of a virulent new serotype, O139 Bengal, in the early 1990s, which may have evolved as a result of recombination with non-toxic strains (Faruque et al. 2003). If so, then we should be watching for the chatter of other *V. cholerae* species that are currently producing only sporadic and attenuated infections in humans (Vezzulli et al. 2020). The same advice holds for the global surveillance of other zoonotic infections when they make early appearances in human populations (CDC 2021).

5.2 Subsistence and stereotypes

More than 70 percent of novel spillover infections originate from wild animal populations (Jones et al. 2008). Given the thousands of years that humans have been living with domesticated animals and acquiring their diseases, it makes sense that most novel infections of zoonotic origin would arise from wild animals with which we previously had less contact. It is also understandable that this would bring international attention to atypical human subsistence practices, such as the so-called bushmeat hunting that occurs in West and Central Africa and the sale of unusual meat products in East and Southeast Asian "wet markets." Yet although there are good reasons for examining these practices to determine whether or how they may increase human exposure to new pathogens, it is nevertheless important that we take a systematic approach to these issues, undistorted by popular myths, exotic stereotypes, xenophobia, and blame. These

distortions are not only damaging to subject communities and their cultural traditions, they also cloud our ability to fully understand the complex biocultural factors surrounding the origins of new and recurring epidemics.

In the early years of the AIDS pandemic, distorted views were often more contagious than the virus. One example of this concerned the putative origins of the disease. In the United States, early data found an unusually high prevalence among Haitian immigrants (Farmer 1992). This led epidemiologists to consider whether the virus originated in Haiti. In the absence of better data, it was reasonable to test this hypothesis. Unfortunately, however, some irresponsible professionals embellished this hypothesis with speculations that Voodoun religious rituals were responsible for the initial human exposure. There was no evidence for this, but Voodoun played into racist stereotypes of Haiti as a dark country where a new and exotic disease arose from exotic cultural practices. Adding further insult to injury, the popular press got hold of this stereotype and ran with it. One report stated that AIDS among Haitians

"was a clue from the grave, as though a zombie, leaving a trail of unwinding bandages and rotting flesh, had come to the hospital's Grand Rounds to pronounce a curse."
(Abbott 1988, cited in Farmer 1992).

Today, there is overwhelming evidence that AIDS originated on the African continent. Furthermore, its later appearance in Haiti was initially among young adult males engaged in low-income labor in the capital city of Port-au-Prince (Farmer 1992; Pape et al. 2008). Combined with ethnographic accounts of these men having to engage in commercial sex exchange out of economic desperation, the evidence suggests that HIV was bought to Haiti by international sex tourism and soon transmitted throughout the country, though labor migration between Haiti and West Africa may have also played a role. Before the world was aware of the virus, its transmission was amplified and accelerated under conditions of severe poverty. By the time the virus was detected, the prevalence was significantly higher among Haitians than North Americans and Europeans. Ironically, the societies that incorrectly pointed to Haiti as the original source of HIV/AIDS were probably the same ones who brought the virus there in the first place.

Closer to issues of food and cultural differences, ceviche was blamed for the inland spread of cholera during a 1991 epidemic in Peru. The marinated shellfish in Peruvian ceviche was thought by many health officials to harbor the *Vibro* bacilli that had entered the capital city of Lima from its coastal estuaries, and attempts were made to ban local sales (Lynn 1991). Yet later testing found that the low pH of the lime marinade in ceviche samples destroyed more than 99.5 percent of the pathogen within a few minutes (Mata et al. 1994). Far from being an exotic vector of cholera transmission, Peruvian ceviche actually played a protective role against the disease. As with London in the mid-nineteenth century, Lima's inadequate plumbing and drainage turned out to be the primary conduits for the inland spread of cholera, yet in the case of Peru, the distractors were those of stigma rather than miasma.

In 2009, another food source was mistakenly blamed during the H1N1 influenza pandemic. Initial forecasts predicted that this particular strain would be significantly more virulent than those of typical seasonal influenzas, and many governments around the world were bracing for a pandemic similar to the one we are currently experiencing. Unfortunately, this strain was also known as a "swine flu" because some of its genetic sequences originated in viruses that were found in pigs at some earlier point their evolution (Mena et al. 2016). Yet this strain was a mix of different sequences that had originated from other viruses, and although there were some instances of human-to-pig transmission, none were detected in the other direction. Nevertheless, many governments banned the import, export, and sale of pork products, and Egypt culled nearly all its pig population (Leach and Tadros 2014). The mistake proved costly to ethnic minority communities that relied on pork for their sustenance and income, and it disrupted urban systems for the management of organic waste.

Keeping these examples in mind, we should endeavor to avoid any short-sighted stereotypes when considering the culinary origins of novel infections. A case in point: "bushmeat" simply refers to the meat of terrestrial wild animals, though historically the term was used by British colonists to describe animals consumed by their African subjects which they did not consider as proper "game" (Allen 1843). Recently, Nigerian novelist Chika Unigwe characterized the cultural distinction between bushmeat and game:

Years ago, I was enjoying my bushmeat in an Australian restaurant in Belgium and said as much when my dinner companion gently reminded me that what I was eating was "game" and not bushmeat, and I had been invited out to "enjoy game." Apparently, bushmeat is what you get in a small, ramshackle affair by the roadside in Nsukka, paired with palm wine and most often eaten by hand, not meat carefully paired with a Pinot Noir or a Shiraz in a restaurant where the silverware is so shiny and so smudge free you can use it to fix your makeup
(Unigwe, cited in Edoro 2017).

In addition to its colonial and class distortions, "bushmeat" is rendered meaningless when paired with the term *hunting*. With the exception of poaching, a practice with a word of its own, it is difficult to imagine why anyone would hunt a domesticated animal. So it would be redundant to call the practice "wild animal hunting" just as it would to call it "bushmeat hunting," except that the latter makes this common activity sound more exotic and primitive.

Likewise, a "wet market" simply refers to a place where vendors sell fresh fruit, vegetables, and meat along with other dry goods. In this respect, wet markets are no different than farmer's markets (see Figure 5.2). In some societies, live animals are slaughtered at these markets. Yet this practice in itself does not bring new pathogens into human populations, and in communities that cannot afford refrigerated transport, the best way to avoid decay and contamination is to keep the animals alive as long as possible before sale.

Many societies rely on the hunting and trade of meat for food security and economic survival (Nasi et al. 2011). And while it is still important to examine how some of these practices may be linked to epidemiological outcomes, the task is more effective when we focus more precisely on the factors that increase risk of disease exposure. Here, we can take a lesson from another AIDS risk factor: sex between cis-gendered males. Epidemiological risk factors are nothing more than statistical associations, and any causal inferences must be tested

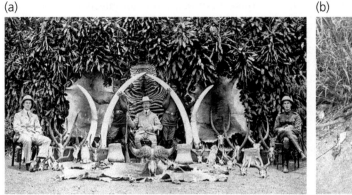
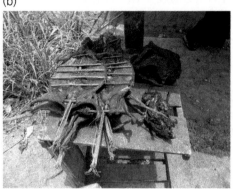

Figure 5.2 Two very different images of wild game displays that could both be attributed to "bushmeat hunting." a. Hunting trophies displayed by British Governor Sir Henry Hesketh Bell in Uganda, 1908. b. Wild animal meat sold for food at a roadside stand in Ghana, 2013.
Source: Wikiseal. CCA-SA 3.0 unported.

before considering their validity. It would be easy to infer that male homosexuality is itself a cause of AIDS, but further studies find that unprotected anal sex presents minimal barriers to blood-borne transmission of the virus, thus explaining the statistical association. Maintaining that homosexuality itself causes AIDS, as many people still do, is not only harmful to gay and bisexual communities but it impedes our scientific understanding of a deadly infectious disease.

When examining unfamiliar subsistence practices, it is important that we first define our terms in a manner best suited to our research aims rather than our potential biases. Throughout this book, we have seen how human subsistence entails complex arrays of cultural beliefs, behaviors, materials, and relationships both social and environmental. From these arrays, we must sort out potential disease determinants, locate these determinants within larger chains of causality, and then try to understand the broader ecological and political-economic contexts in which they occur. Accomplishing these scientific aims requires careful framing of research questions and hypotheses, which are in turn, shaped by the way the problems are defined.

5.3 New pathogens and hunting

The most promising starting points for examining the potential links between human subsistence and zoonotic spillover are those practices that expose people to wild animal reservoirs. Hunting increases opportunities for direct exposure between people and potential host species. So does territorial expansion into new wilderness areas, but with the added risk of indirect exposure via domesticated and peri-domesticated species. These expansions often occur in the context of commercial agriculture, large-scale resource extraction, and the building of associated roads and settlements. Quite often, all these practices are interconnected.

Hunting is a broad category of methods for the deliberate exploitation of wild animal resources. These methods typically include some form of stalking, which entails tracking the animals over the course of hours or days, and often involves moving through wilderness areas where the hunter is exposed to multiple species in addition to the intended prey. If the hunt entails live capture or trapping then there is the additional risk of biting and clawing. If, however, the animal is to be killed then this part of the activity can present different exposure risks, depending on factors such as the hunter's skill and technique, the nature of the prey, and the presence of competing predators.

In most cases, the greatest risk for pathogen exposure occurs after the animal is killed. The butchering process entails hard labor and the use of sharp implements that are soon covered in blood and body fluids, tools that can cut into the human body at least as easily as they cut into an animal body.

This experience is well-described by a poet whose father taught her how to process a freshly killed elk:

This labor will make you sweat. Your knife will do the cutting, but your arms will do the work. The skin is taut, connected by strong, white sinew. It will resist you. It was designed to resist you, to cling to the bones and muscle, to be the boundary. Dig your fingers into the cut your knife made, nails sinking into fatty mats of heat and fur. Rip.

(Coleman 2020).

One need not have first-hand experience to know that self-lacerations are common and easy when working with sharp objects and food; time in the kitchen will inevitably provide these experiences, even for the staunchest vegetarian. Yet, in the particular case of meat, even the smallest laceration by a contaminated blade can present a river of opportunity for a blood-borne pathogen to flow from the interior of an infected animal to the interior of a human body. Moreover, the risk of self-injury increases with the resistance of the tissue; for instance, the disarticulation of joints is especially risky, as is the skinning process. For a hunter, this risk may be increased if at least some of the butchering occurs at the site of the kill, as often happens for the sake of easy and/or concealed transport. Under these conditions, the hunter may have to sacrifice safety for speed, knowing that authorities may be alerted to the sound of a firearm, or predators to the scent of a freshly opened carcass. Butchering, of course, can also occur in multiple stages at different locations. Even then, safety may also give way to speed if the secondary locations include a fast-moving marketplace, a busy restaurant, or a family home with a heavy burden of care.

Having dissected the activity itself, we turn to the nature of the prey. As we discussed earlier, "bushmeat" simply refers to the meat that people derive from terrestrial wild animals, a very broad category that includes up to 500 species in Sub-Saharan Africa, 400 species in South and Southeast Asia, and 200 species in South America (Cawthorn and Hoffman 2015. Among these many different animals, non-human primates pose some of the greatest risks for zoonotic spillover. Comprising about 0.5 percent of all vertebrate species, non-human primates have been the earlier hosts and ongoing reservoirs of 20 percent of major human infections (Wolfe et al. 2007). These include new infections such as HIV, Ebola, and Hepatitis B, as well as older vector-borne infections such as malaria, dengue, and yellow fever. Furthermore, these spillover infections can happen in both directions; humans have also transmitted diseases to non-human primates, often with devastating consequences for already endangered animal populations (Wolfe 2011).

With respect to hunting as a risk factor for spillover, the key issue is not the activity in general but rather the processing and consumption of those species with whom we are most closely related. Humans are members of the primate order, bipedal apes with similar immune systems and physiological vulnerabilities to those of our evolutionary cousins. Because of this, a potential pathogen that has successfully negotiated the infective barriers of a host monkey or ape, is more likely to successfully negotiate the barriers of a human being. And seeing as how our simian cousins live in local environments that are different than our own, wilderness areas we abandoned millions of years ago that have since continued their own evolutionary trajectories, the microbiomes of non-human primates are more likely to include potential pathogens to whom we have not been previously exposed. Through the butchering and consumption of non-human primates, we are exposing ourselves to familiar bodies with unfamiliar microbes, an ideal situation for the emergence of novel human infections.

Humans have probably been consuming other primates since the time before our hominoid ancestors diverged from the most recent common ancestor of chimpanzees and bonobos (Wolfe 2011). Today, however, primate hunting has risen far above sustainable levels due to increased human populations, expansion into wilderness areas, food and economic insecurity, and market demand for specialty meats as well as animal products for traditional medicines (Cawthorn and Hoffman 2020; Nasi et al. 2011). Although primate carcasses comprise a minority of the wild animal meat sold in markets, their value has made them a prime target for opportunistic as well as professional hunting. Along with other anthropogenic threats such as habitat destruction, climate change, and pollution, the hunting of non-human primates has contributed to substantial declines of many endangered primate species around the world (Estrada et al. 2017).

Wild species are a primary source of animal protein for many poor and rural-based communities, and non-human primates can meet this need when alternatives are neither available nor affordable (Nasi et al. 2011). Under these conditions, food insecurity is the major driver for hunting. In places like the Congo Basin, home to the greatest diversity of non-human primates, food insecurity is increased by the frequency and severity of droughts, disruptions of food transport networks by political conflicts, and the diversion of smaller-scale subsistence-based agriculture to larger-scale commercial crops (Wallace 2016). In coastal West Africa, large-scale commercial fishing depletes local fish, resulting in increased consumption of wild terrestrial meat (Brashares et al. 2004). Reminiscent of the conditions during the First Epidemiological Transition, these communities may have adequate overall caloric intake, but they are often undernourished with respect to essential amino acids and trace elements (Cawthorn and Hoffman 2020). The consumption of primates and other wild animals can fill this critical nutritional gap. Somewhat paradoxically, these practices contribute to overall host immunity against infectious diseases, even as they increase the risk of exposure to new and deadly pathogens.

Economic insecurity is the other major driver, and wild meat presents lucrative opportunities for impoverished rural communities. A survey of 2,000 households in Ghana, Cameroon, Tanzania, and Madagascar finds that although wild meat consumption is inversely proportional to income in rural populations, it actually increases with the wealth of urban populations (Brashares et al. 2011). Wild meat is a necessity in the first instance, a luxury item in the second. Yet if the urban and international demand is high enough, then the potential income returns can exceed the nutritional value of the catch; it can also provide for other important family needs, such as school fees and major ceremonial expenses such as funerals and marriages (Cawthorn and Hoffman 2015; Grande Vega et al. 2013).

As mentioned earlier, primates typically comprise less than 20 percent of the wild meat sold in markets worldwide, but their monetary value is often much higher than that of other species (Estrada et al. 2017). This is due in large part to their demand as specialty foods, but body parts are also sold for medicinal purposes in many parts of Asia, and to a lesser extent for ritual purposes and trophies. Although the commodity chains can be complex, in many instances hunters can obtain a significant percentage of the final market price (Cowlishaw et al. 2005; Tagg et al. 2018). Along these chains, hunters can also incur the highest risk for disease transmission as the carcasses are often butchered on site for ease of transport and to reduce detection by authorities.

Regardless of whether it is for protein or profit, the hunting and butchering of non-human primates presents a major pathway for the entry of new pathogens into the human population. This has been the case for several retroviruses, such as Simian Foamy Virus and several T-lymphotrophic viruses, primate pathogens that have displayed chatter in rural West African communities who regularly engage in these practices (Wolfe 2011). These same communities are found to have a large number of previously undetected varieties of HIV, a finding that indicates what these viruses may have looked like in an initial human host population before their descendants spread to the rest of the world (Carr et al. 2010).

Returning to the issue of drivers, it is important to note that the increased hunting of primates and other high risk wild animals correlates geographically and temporally with large-scale resource extraction by multinational companies (Cawthorn and Hoffman 2015; Estrada et al. 2017). For instance, industrial logging of tropical timber has created roads deep into animal habitats and populated their shrinking peripheries with migrant workers and support communities that often engage in supplemental hunting (Wolfe et al. 2011). The same dynamics can be seen with the expansion of commercial agriculture in neotropical areas (Estrada et al. 2017). In addition to furthering the human encroachment of primate habitats, agriculture on the edges of new wilderness areas increases human–animal conflicts related to crop raiding, and non-human primates are no less opportunistic than their human cousins. Opportunistic subsistence occurs in both directions when human and non-human primates are brought together.

5.4 New pathogens and large-scale agriculture

Notwithstanding the interactions between human and non-human primates, the large-scale production of domesticated meat, dairy, and eggs may be an even larger conduit for zoonotic spillover. Being part of the greater enterprise of industrial agriculture, these industries do not have the same exotic ring as neotropical hunting. Yet for all their technologies and neat packaging, these industries are the world's primary source for meat and animal products. Global terrestrial meat production has tripled in the last 50 years to more than 330 million tonnes per year (Food and Agriculture Organization of the United Nations, 2020; see Figure 5.3). During the same period, global egg and milk production have doubled to more than 90 and 800 million tonnes per year, respectively. Recall from

Chapter 2 that today's agriculture (industrial and otherwise) accounts for approximately 38 percent of the world's habitable land mass; more than three-quarters of this land is used for livestock and feed production (Ritchie and Roser 2019). Given the lessons of the First Epidemiological Transition, we should not be surprised that this massive scale of agricultural activity would be a primary contributor to newly emerging infections, and as we will see in Chapter 6, to the accelerated evolution of antimicrobial resistance.

During the Neolithic, the domestication of animals brought new pathogens into contact with ancient human populations. After thousands of years, these same pathogens have become familiar figures of our ecological history. Although or adaptations to these diseases have not always been effective, nor have they been socially well distributed, human populations have had time to develop some degree of host immunity, protective behaviors, and medicinal responses. During this same period, our domesticated plants and animals have also adapted

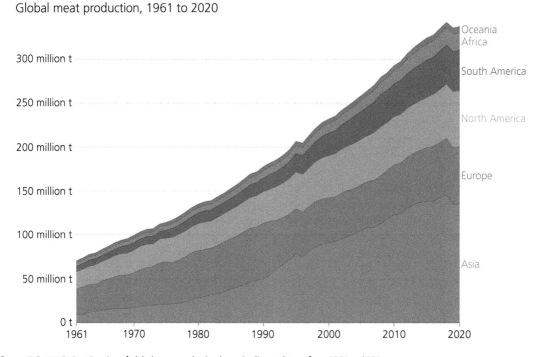

Global meat production, 1961 to 2020

Figure 5.3 UN FAO estimation of global meat production by major livestock type from 1961 to 2020.

Source: U.N. Food and Agriculture Organization via Our World in Data. CCA-BY.

to one another as well as to their respective microbiomes. This includes cross-species adaptations in the transitional areas (a.k.a. edges) between domestic and wild environments.

These adaptations are less frequent when domestication expands into new and previously uninhabited environments or when new subsistence practices change longstanding ecological relationships within and between existing environments. Such expansions and changes were implicated in the multiple, chatter-like introductions of Nipah Virus (NiV) into human populations (Singh et al. 2019). NiV infection in humans typically leads to encephalitis and cerebral atrophy with severe neurological symptoms and a case fatality ranging from a very high 32 percent to an exceptionally high 92 percent. The best-known wild animal reservoirs of NiV are four species of large fruit bats belonging to the *Pteropus* genus. Many of these bats in outbreak regions have tested positive for the virus and, quite worryingly for onward transmission, the infection does not appear to cause them any symptoms.

This was the case for fruit bats that were captured from the areas surrounding the first human outbreaks in rural Malaysia, where the majority of 283 patients had been working in large-scale pig farms. According to a detailed study by an interdisciplinary team that included the Henipavirus Ecology Research Group, the anthropogenic culprit was the intensification of dual-use pig and mango farming (Pulliam et al. 2012). The index farm included 30,000 pigs and 400 mango trees in close proximity to each other. Fruit bats ate the fruit and littered the grounds with leftovers, urine, and guano, which were probably consumed by the pigs. NiV produces severe respiratory symptoms in pigs, so transmission to humans could have happened via droplets or aerosol, but it may also have happened from handling and slaughtering, much like with hunting.[4] In these outbreaks, domesticated mangos and pigs were key intermediaries in the transmission of a previously unknown and very deadly virus from wild bats to humans.

From 2001 to 2004, Bangladesh experienced 33 Nipah outbreaks for a total of 157 patients, and while these may seem like relatively small numbers, it is of particular concern that 22 percent of these

cases were the result of human-to-human transmission (Islam et al. 2016). Also worrying is that the zoonotic transmission to humans did not involve any intermediate animals but only the sap of the date palm tree. While the virus can remain viable in fruit and juice for three days, its viability extends to seven days in date palm sap (Singh et al. 2019). Another team of interdisciplinary researchers found that infected patients had consumed the sap as a traditional drink, which had been contaminated by the secretions and excretions of infected *Peteropus* fruit bats while consuming the sap-laden bark shavings from the trees (Islam et al. 2016).

In addition to their sap, date palms provide an excellent roosting habitat for fruit bats who, in turn, make excellent reservoirs for the Ebola virus (EBV). Returning to the West African Ebola outbreak of 2014, it is notable that this region has seen a major expansion of internationally financed commercial palm oil production, placing increasing numbers of bats in proximity to a rapidly increasing human population (Wallace 2016). Other bat genera are also reservoirs of the EBV, including the insectivorous species that transmitted the virus to humans, leading to the first known human Ebola epidemic in 1976 (WHO 1978). As it turned out, the index cases were workers in a factory that produces cloth from raw cotton grown in the area; here, the bats were roosting on the ceiling, but they were also feasting on the cotton-associated insects (Williams et al. 2021).

Returning to domestic meat production, it is worth examining the role of the poultry and pork industries in the evolution and transmission of highly pathogenic influenza viruses from wild birds to humans. Most of these viruses belong to the A serotype, which is subtyped according to two surface proteins, hemagglutinin (H) and neuraminidase (N), that respectively allow the pathogen to enter and exit host cells. These same proteins function as antigens detected by host immune systems, so they are of particularly relevance for vaccine development. Within these H and N subtypes, particular influenza lineages (sub-taxa) are classified according to a set of genetic, epidemiological, and/or disease characteristics chosen by an international committee.[5] Less formally, these types and subtypes may also be grouped according to animal host categories (non-Linnean) in which they are commonly associated, or from which they are thought to have originated: avian, swine, horse, human, and so forth. Yet although different varieties will infect different species, including humans, all influenza A viruses can be found in birds. As such, they are all essentially "avian influenzas," even if they bear a different animal label.

Wild aquatic birds are the primary animal reservoirs for influenza A. These include migratory birds such as ducks, geese, and swans, and shorebirds such as gulls and terns. The prevalence of influenza among these animals can exceed 20 percent during the spring and autumn migration seasons, though most common influenza varieties produce little, if any, clinical signs of sickness (Wille and Holmes 2020). As disease carriers with global mobility, avian waterfowl are the ideal vectors for the spread of the influenza virus, infecting other wild bird species, domesticated animals, and human populations.

Furthermore, by carrying the greatest variety of influenza viruses, avian waterfowl also provide ideal opportunities for pathogen evolution. Most of the transmission between birds occurs via the fecal-oral route, usually in shared waters around nesting and breeding areas as well as migration stopover points (Blagodatski et al. 2021). These intra- and interspecies transmissions are aided by several pathogen characteristics. The first of these is the resilience of the influenza virus, which can remain viable for a week in freshwater and feces at room temperature (20° C) and more than a month at near freezing temperatures (Joseph et al. 2016). The second is the high mutability of its RNA genome, and the inability of its replication enzymes to detect and eliminate (i.e., proofread) these mutations when they occur. These mutations can express themselves as changes in the H and N surface proteins detected by immune systems, a process known as antigenic drift. And finally, the influenza A genome is composed of multiple segments, and when two or more varieties infect the same host, these segments can reassort to produce new combinations of H and N surface proteins, a process known as antigenic shift. These drifts and shifts make influenza a rapidly moving target, evolving quickly into new varieties which, in addition to the recirculation of previous varieties, requires that we develop new vaccines every year.

The H1N1 virus responsible for the pandemic of 1918 (a.k.a. the "1918 flu" or "Spanish flu") is the archetypical example of a highly pathogenic influenza. It is conservatively estimated to have killed 50 million people in three waves occurring between the spring seasons of 1918 and 1919 (Johnson and Mueller 2002). Within this 16-month time frame, the 1918 flu was the largest known infectious disease pandemic in human history. It also resulted in unusually high mortality among otherwise ablebodied young adults; in contrast, most seasonal influenza deaths occur among very young and older populations and people with comorbid medical conditions. Given that a new variety may someday have the same devastating effects, researchers are watching the evolution of likely candidates. Reconstruction of the 1918 H1N1 virus revealed that it was closely related to a classic swine variety, though it also contained an important avian (poultry) gene (Xu et al. 2010). With this precedent in mind, new and recurring swine influenza A viruses (swIAVs) are a priority for global surveillance.

Ninety years later, the "Swine flu" pandemic of 2009 reminds us of an swIAV's pathogenic potential. Its estimated mortality was less than two interim pandemics, the so-called "Hong Kong flu" of 1957–1958 (H2N2), and "Asian Flu" of 1968 (H3N2).[6] Each of these outbreaks resulted in approximately 1 million deaths (CDC 2019a; 2019b). Nevertheless, the global health impact of the 2009 pandemic was substantial; the US Centers for Disease Control and Prevention estimates that it was responsible for the deaths of up to 575,000 people, more than 80 percent of whom were under 65 years of age (CDC 2019c). The virus, H1N1pdm, appears to have emerged from the reassortment of at least three other influenza lineages, and of particular concern, two of these were swIAVs (Christman et al. 2011; Gibbs et al. 2009).

Pigs are considered to be ideal mixing vessels for influenza because their tissue receptors are susceptible to infection by avian, human, or swine lineages (Chauhan and Gordon 2020). This constitutes a large variety of influenza viruses that can potentially coinfect the same pig and reassort into an exponentially larger variety of new pathogens with the potential to infect human populations. With this risk in mind, national health authorities often recommend or require a variety of biosafety[7] measures for the raising and slaughter of pigs, such as covered pens with bird nets, air circulated through high-efficiency, particulate-absorbing (HEPA) filters, and widely spaced and segregated facilities[8] (Alarcon et al. 2021). Small-scale and family-based producers, so-called backyard farms, typically cannot afford these kinds of measures. Because of this, policy-makers often focus their attention on the biosecurity shortcomings of small-scale producers whenever there is a new outbreak (Wallace 2014).

There is evidence, however, that the international trade of live pigs by large-scale producers may play a greater role than small-scale producers in the global introduction of new influenza variants. With respect to H1N1pdm, retrospective serological studies suggest the virus originated in Mexican pig farms (Chauhan and Gordon 2020; Gibbs et al. 2009). Yet even if this is correct, the geographic origin of a virus with multiple recent ancestors does not tell us enough about the preceding chain of events. The two swIAVs thought to be ancestral to H1N1pdm, a European lineage and a North American lineage, were predominantly segregated within their respective continental pig populations in the years before 2009 (Christman et al. 2011). Something must have united these viruses across nations and continents. Although it is possible that the viruses migrated via the travel of infected human hosts, the transport of live pigs across nations and continents is the more likely determinant.

In the 1980s and 1990s, several influenza variants were introduced into Mexico through the importation of live pigs from Europe and the United States (Mena 2016). This is consistent with a larger global trend that was found in a spatial analysis of 18 swIAV lineages between 1970 and 2014 (Nelson et al. 2015). Among these 18 lineages, 11 migrated to the Asian continent from Europe and North America while only two migrated in the other direction. This trend may seem surprising given that the large majority of domestic swine reside in Asian countries. China alone has over 450 million pigs, more than all other major countries combined, but the same analysis finds only one swIAV migration

from China and only two migrations between Asian countries. These findings are consistent with the fact that although Asian countries produce the majority of the world's pork, they do not export as many live pigs as do European and North American countries (Nelson et al. 2015).

In addition to swine influenza viruses, several subtypes of avian influenza viruses (AIAVs) have received considerable global attention. Thus far, AIAVs have only sporadically infected people without any sustained human-to-human transmission. As such, these outbreaks can be considered the viral chatter of zoonotic pathogens in the early stages of potential spillover. However, among the 22 recorded outbreaks of avian influenza among humans between 1959 and 2019, 10 were highly pathogenic. These were H5 and H7 lineages that infected a total of approximately 2,500 people in 17 countries with case fatality rates between 40 and 60 percent (Wang et al. 2021). Although these outbreaks were sporadic and limited, their mortality rates were far greater than those caused by any other influenza virus, including that of the 1918 pandemic.

With mortality in mind, the chief concern is that a highly pathogenic avian influenza virus will eventually complete the spillover process and produce a catastrophic human pandemic. The most likely routes for this to occur is through the interfaces between wild birds and domesticated poultry. Migratory waterfowl are the ultimate reservoirs of these viruses, but recent evidence suggests that infection with highly pathogenic strains may impede wild bird migrations, and hence, the range at which they can spread disease (Blagodatski et al. 2021). A study of highly pathogenic H5N1 outbreaks between 1996 and 2006 finds that they are more closely correlated with transport routes for poultry and related products than with the migration routes of wild birds (Gauthier-Clerc et al. 2007). Supporting this evidence, most human outbreaks have occurred in the context of much larger poultry outbreaks, and most cases have occurred among commercial poultry workers (Dinh et al. 2006; Wang et al. 2021). Finally, it has been observed that influenza viruses evolve more rapidly in domesticated poultry than in wild birds due to greater frequencies of reassortment events (Wille and Holmes

2020). Although these viruses originate in wild birds, domesticated poultry appear to be the main mixing vessels and primary conduits to human infection.

As with the swine influenzas, avian influenza outbreaks often bring disproportionate attention to small-scale farmers as well as rural families with "backyard" animals. The majority of these outbreaks have been confined to poultry, and when they have occurred in large-scale facilities, small-scale producers are still often blamed based on the premise that they lack sufficient biosecurity measures regarding ventilation, water, and feed (Wallace 2014). However, a 2014–2015 outbreak of H5N2 among 50 million poultry in 15 US states brings this premise into question. The outbreak occurred in 211 commercial flocks but it only occurred in 21 backyard flocks, the inverse of what would be expected if the latter flocks were more vulnerable (USDA 2016). There are unconfirmed accounts that the initial infections occurred among birds in close vicinity to air inlets, animal studies have demonstrated airborne transmission of H5N2, and an analysis of airflow for large poultry houses in one state demonstrated how commercial flocks could be infected by sustained exposure to air-borne particulate matter from their outside environments (Zhao et al. 2019). This air-borne exposure not only explains the transmission of influenza between poultry houses but it also allows for viral transmission from wild birds to large-scale commercial poultry flocks.

The increased scale and intensity of commercial animal husbandry may also play a role in in the spillover of pathogenic coronaviruses into the human population. Several insectivorous bat species are known to carry coronaviruses similar to SARS-CoV and MERS-CoV, suggesting that these mammals may be the original reservoirs for the human disease-causing pathogens (Wong et al. 2019). However, during the 2003 SARS epidemic, field investigations focused more on potential intermediate hosts with greater interface between wild and human environments, especially in the live animal markets of southern China, where handlers were found to have unusually high frequencies of antibodies to the virus relative to the general population (Shi and Hu 2008). Subsequently, public health authorities gave particular attention

to wildlife markets, game farms, and restaurants that served specialty meats (Bell et al. 2004). Several mammalian species tested positive to a very similar virus, and in particular, the masked palm civet (*Paguma larvata*) was found to have antibodies indicative of SARS-CoV exposure. The discoveries led to a series of animal bans and quarantines, as well as the culling of many civet populations (Shi and Hu 2007).

These events received a great deal of attention by the international media, which generated many stories of wild civets sold in "wet markets" (Person et al. 2004). Yet later investigations indicate that civets had only recently been infected by SARS-CoV, and vaccine studies have found a much wider range of wild and domestic species that could serve as zoonotic reservoirs (Shi and Hu 2007). Even among the civets, tests of farm-raised animals showed more indications of viral exposure than those captured in the wild. It should also be noted that the civet trade is not restricted to China; there are a growing number of civet farms in Southeast Asia where the animals continue to be raised for meat production, and for processing a highly expensive specialty coffee known as *kopi luwak* (a.k.a. "civet coffee"), the beans of which are modified in the digestive tracts of the animals, often under inhumane conditions when produced commercially (D'Cruze et al. 2014).

Since MERS was first identified in 2012, over 2,500 cases have been detected in 27 countries, including larger outbreaks in South Korea and along the Arabian peninsula (Rabaan et al. 2021). Dromedary camels (*Camelus dromedarius*) have been identified as a major intermediate host, with serological evidence of viral exposure among animals in North and East Africa as well as the Middle East (Gossner et al. 2014). Retrospective testing of archived serum has revealed camel exposure in Egypt, Sudan, and Somalia as early as 1983; the gap between exposure and discovery is explained by the fact that the virus produces only mild symptoms in the animals (Müller et al. 2014). Not surprisingly, camel workers are at higher risk for infection, but the majority of cases have been attributed to human-to-human transmission in hospital settings, and many camel herders show signs of previous exposure without recalling any major illnesses (Alshukairi et al. 2018; Rabaan et al. 2021). These findings indicate that at least some of these communities were previously infected with either an attenuated form of MERS-CoV, or a related (and perhaps ancestral) virus that provided some level of cross-immunity.

As in the case of civets, it may be difficult to associate camels with the recurring themes of large-scale domestic animal production. Yet many of these themes emerge in the work of Bernard Faye, a veterinarian from the United Nations Food and Agriculture Organization who has consulted on camel production issues in 45 countries. Faye has calculated that the world camel population has more than doubled since 1961 to about 40 million animals (2016; 2020). As in past millennia, camels are utilized for a variety of services, including transport, draught labor, sport, and leisure. Additionally, camels are a source of hide, wool, dung, urine, and meat. But of all camel products, their milk has become an increasingly valuable commodity in international markets, and camelids are able to produce more milk than cattle when feed quality is low. Because of this, camels have been increasingly used for intensive dairy production in arid environments, which has increased the concentration of camel populations in production facilities near urban areas. The last 50 years has also seen a major increase in in the international trade in live camels; as a prime example, breeders in North and East Africa are the main suppliers of new camels to the Middle East. Faye also suggests that climate change may further expand intensive camel farming with the desertification of many regions in the world. Given these trends, we may see additional MERS outbreaks in future years.

The same themes of domestic animal production guide much of the current research into the origins of SARS-CoV-2 and its introduction into the human population, though it should also be mentioned that the possibility of a laboratory accident has not been definitively ruled out. Spillover continues to be the predominant and most parsimonious hypothesis, and once again, bats are considered a likely wild animal reservoir for the virus. Closely related coronaviruses have been detected in several species of horseshoe bats (genus *Rhinophilus*) located in the region where the first human cases of COVID-19 were detected, though support for this particular origin requires further sampling of other species and regions (Zhou et al. 2021).

While bat-to-human transmission is always a possibility, bats were not sold at the animal markets in the vicinity of the first detected human outbreak. As with the SARS virus, it is more likely that the COVID virus was transmitted from bats to humans via one or more intermediate host species whose products were sold in the markets. With this hypothesis in mind, much of the initial research focused on pangolin anteaters (*Manis javanica*) which carry a few of the same COVID-like viruses as do the horseshoe bats; these animals were sold at the markets for meat and medicinal purposes (Liu et al. 2020). However, later studies have raised questions about the specific evolutionary relationships between these viruses, and other candidate host species are being examined, including civet cats, foxes, minks, and racoon dogs, all of which were also sold at the markets (Holmes et al. 2021).

It took more than 10 years to identify the likely animal reservoir and intermediate host species for the SARS virus, and without adequate environmental sampling, it is possible that we may never ascertain (or rule out) the particular zoonotic origins of SARS-CoV-2 with the same level of probability. Yet even if this information was available tomorrow, it would only reveal the proximate players of interspecies transmission. Larger contextual questions would still remain. Why, for instance, have there been only two East Asian coronavirus spillover events over the course of 20 years, despite the continued activity of animal markets during the interim period?

In an attempt to address this larger question, a joint team of virologists from the United Kingdom and China have looked to major ecological events preceding and surrounding the initial COVID-19 outbreak in Wuhan City (Lytras et al. 2021). One notable event was a 2019 outbreak of African swine fever virus (ASFV) in China that led to the culling of around 150 million pigs. This, in turn, reduced pork supplies by 11.5 million tonnes and raised meat prices substantially. Given heavy consumer demand for pork in China, these investigators hypothesize that consumption shifted to alternative meat sources, thus increasing the trade in animal products with a higher risk for coronavirus transmission. Alternatively, a substantial increase in cold-chain transport of frozen meat from other regions, partly in response to the ASFV outbreak, may have brought infected carcasses into the Wuhan markets. These hypotheses bear further investigation, but in the interim, they prompt us to consider the potential roles of large-scale food production in the spillover of novel pathogens from animal to human populations.

5.5 Connectivity and converging infections

Examining the role of food production in the emergence of highly pathogenic avian influenzas, Mike Davis, an urban theorist and historian, states that "the superurbanization of the human population . . . has been paralleled by an equally dense urbanization of its meat supply." He then asks: "Could production density become a synonym of viral density?" (Davis 2006: 84).

The answer is yes, if the previous case studies are representative, and it can also be a synonym of bacterial density amid the rising tide of new pathogens entering the human population. At the time that Davis was studying the commercial poultry industry, there were about 12 billion chickens in East Asia alone, 70 percent of which lived in high-density commercial poultry cages that provided an average of only 300 square centimeters per bird. These practices continue today and they are by no means limited to East Asia, nor are they limited to poultry. High livestock densities are a common feature throughout the world's large-scale meat producers, and when domestic food animals are associated major disease outbreaks, many governments respond with regulations that favor this kind of large-scale production (Wallace 2016).

As for the humans, the majority of the world's 7 billion plus people live in urban centers with population densities greater than 1500 per square kilometer (Pesaresi et al. 2016) (see Figure 5.4). Both humans and their domesticated food animals have been increasingly squeezed into crowded

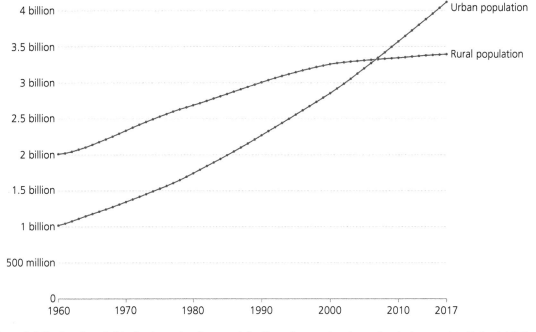

Figure 5.4 Number of people living in urban and rural areas as defined by each country based on each nation's census data. National definitions of urban centers vary, and this method of estimation used by the United Nations, is believed by some to undercount actual urban populations.

Source: U.N. Population Division via Our World in Data. CCA-BY.

settlements, subjected to physical and psychological stressors, and dosed with an abundance of antimicrobial drugs. With the exception of the drugs, which will be addressed in Chapter 6, our current situation is reminiscent of the First Epidemiological Transition. The scales of these settlement trends are far greater, however, and both human and animal populations are far more connected, both to ourselves and to each other, than at any other time in the past.

This connectivity has profound epidemiological implications as the world's health problems converge into a single disease ecology. In the year prior to the COVID-19 pandemic, the commercial airline industry flew an average 100,000 routes a day, carrying upwards of 4.4 billion people a year to destinations around the world (Mazareanu 2021).[9] These numbers give weight to the oft-cited dictum that even the most distant outbreaks are only a plane flight away (see Figure 5.5). Outbreaks can also spread via 103 million kilometers of paved roads, 1.3 million kilometers of rail, and the sea routes of 50,000 merchant ships bearing the flags of 150 countries (de Loisy 2021). With these extensive networks, there is little wonder that a pathogenic virus could spread throughout the world in only a few months.

As we saw in the previous section, many animal species and their products move along these networks, as do their pathogen stowaways. This includes wild as well as domesticated animals, which explains why some hunting practices currently pose a global health threat, despite the fact that people have continuously engaged in these subsistence activities for hundreds of millennia. There is little doubt that Paleolithic foragers faced many of the same risks for novel infections as the so-called bushmeat hunters of today, but now the hunters and their game are connected to major population centers via far-reaching supply chains and transport corridors. Adding to the problem, shrinking habitats are increasing the density of wild animal populations, even as their total numbers are declining. As with any potential host species, higher population densities in wild animals increases transmission opportunities for more acute and virulent pathogens. Furthermore, since shrinking habitats also bring different wild species

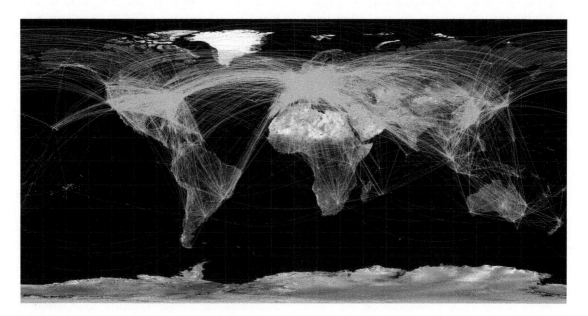

Figure 5.5 Global commercial air routes in 2013. This map does not depict the actual number of flights, which average about 50 thousand at any given moment.

Source: Josulivan59. Wikimedia commons. CCA 3.0 unported.

closer together, the opportunities for transmission between them is higher (Maria Gomez et al. 2013; Wolfe 2011). For these reasons, hunting has never been riskier for pathogen spillover. The same risks apply to the expansion of farms, resource extraction enterprises, and human settlements into new wilderness areas.

The nature of human host populations has also changed. Following the Second Epidemiological Transition, chronic non-communicative diseases (NCDs) have become the leading cause of death throughout most of the world. Low-income societies experienced this transition differently than high-income societies—with weaker declines in infectious diseases despite strong increases in non-communicable diseases. Low-income societies have also become aging societies as part of the global demographic shift toward increasing percentages of elderly people. As we learned in the previous chapter, this aging trend has more to do with earlier fertility declines in urban environments than greater numbers of people living to older ages. Growing percentages of older people present a major challenge for all societies as they try to address the rising vulnerability of frail elderly in their populations. They are especially challenging in poor societies that lack sufficient resources for prevention, treatment, and care (United Nations 2019).

In the previous chapter, we referred to this dilemma as the worst-of-all-worlds syndrome. We also examined synergistic relationships between infectious diseases (IDs) and NCDs in the context of poverty and structural violence. Once considered a temporary delay in the Second Transition of underdeveloped societies, these syndemics have nevertheless persisted, despite the industrial development of low- and middle-income countries (LMICs). Today, these persistent syndemics have affected societies both rich and poor through the global spread of new and recurring infections. The global impact of these syndemic diseases are a characteristic feature of the Third Epidemiological Transition.

These characteristics are tragically illustrated by the major coronavirus outbreaks of the early twenty-first century. In the regions most affected by the SARS epidemic, the highest case fatality rates, excluding health workers, were among patients over 60 years of age with at least one pre-existing diagnosis of heart disease, chronic obstructive pulmonary disease (COPD), chronic kidney disease (CKD), or diabetes (Booth et al. 2003; Chen et al. 2005; Leung et al. 2004). During the initial MERS outbreak, 95 percent of the first detected cases were comorbid with most of the same chronic conditions[10] (Assiri et al. 2013). Within this vulnerable cohort, the highest mortality was once again among patients over 60 years of age, though it should be noted that, in later months, the distributions of MERS-related morbidity and mortality shifted to younger ages (Lim et al. 2013). Perhaps even more troubling, this demographic shift may have been the result of MERS-CoV becoming better adapted to its new human host populations.

As with SARS and MERS, the COVID-19 pandemic has underscored the synergies between infectious and noncommunicable diseases, though it has done so at a very large scale. Numbers vary by country and population sample, but most studies find that patients hospitalized for COVID-19 have a significantly higher risk for progression to severe disease and death if they are elderly, obese, or have a pre-existing diagnosis of heart disease, COPD, active cancer, or diabetes with complications (Bae et al. 2021; Booth et al. 2021). A study of more than 500,000 hospitalized COVID-19 patients in the United States finds that 89 percent were comorbid with at least one of nine medical conditions that are strongly associated with disease progression and death, the most common being heart disease, diabetes, obesity, and lipid metabolic disorders (Kompaniyets et al. 2021). The same study reveals a dose-response effect such that the risk of COVID-related death increases substantially with the total number of these non-communicable diseases. Unfortunately, chronic non-communicable diseases tend to cluster together, so we can expect the dose-response to be high among these vulnerable patients.

As we learned in Chapter 4, non-communicable diseases have become increasingly prevalent in low and middle-income countries, and it is here where we often see syndemic clusters of poverty, depression, and diabetes (Mendenhall et al. 2017; Weaver and Mendenhall 2014). Likewise, food insecurity clusters with chronic conditions such as diabetes, heart disease, dyslipidemia, and kidney disease, sometimes in the absence of obesity (Weaver and

Fasel 2018). Similarly, these syndemics are also found among racial and ethnic minority communities in high-income countries such as the United States and the United Kingdom where they combine with discrimination and distrust to produce disproportionately high rates of COVID infection, hospitalization, and death (Mude et al. 2021; Pijls et al. 2021; Rossen et al. 2021). These represent major vulnerabilities for the entry and spread of new pathogens into a globally connected human host population.

5.6 Virulence and vulnerability

We live in a sea of microbes, but we are only threatened by those that are able to cause disease. This disease-causing ability is usually described as the *pathogenicity* or *virulence* of a microorganism. Although pathogenicity and virulence are sometimes used interchangeably, there are also disciplinary and individual differences in the ways that these terms are defined, so it important to note these definitions when examining source literature on the topic. Based on recent common usage, pathogenicity often describes a few discrete categories of disease-causing ability. For instance, one could say that a bacterial strain is either pathogenic, highly pathogenic, or non-pathogenic to human hosts. Yet if the strain is indeed pathogenic (hence a pathogen) then it is likely to evolve variations in its disease-causing traits that can result in a continuum of greater or lesser harm. To address these variations, and their evolution, in a better way the term "virulence" is more often used to describe the *degree* to which a pathogen causes harm, as measured by the associated morbidity and mortality in an infected host species or population.

We will use this latter definition as we examine the evolution of virulence, yet as with other disease characteristics, virulence is not simply a set of genetic traits that lie solely within a pathogen. It is closely intertwined with other variables such as transmission, competition, coinfection, and of course, reproduction. And as with the other disease phenomena we have studied, these variables entail a broader set of coevolutionary relationships between pathogen species, animal and human host species, and their surrounding environments.

Lastly, it should be clear by now that whenever human hosts are involved, the environments are social as well as biological.

Building on the earlier work of other microbiologists, Louis Pasteur and colleagues published a classic study demonstrating that the virulence of a single microbial species could increase or decrease (attenuate) in subsequent generations, based on changing environmental conditions (Mendelsohn 2002). The intended aim of the study was to develop new and better vaccines, but the findings raised a broader question: what are the conditions in which we can predict the changing virulence of an evolving pathogen in a given host population?

This question is especially relevant for novel infectious diseases such as COVID-19. In less than two years following the first appearance of SARS-CoV-2, the World Health Organization identified five additional variants of concern (WHO 2022). Among these, the Omicron variant has turned out to be significantly attenuated (i.e., less virulent) in comparison to the earlier Delta variant, even when accounting for age, comorbidity, and vaccination status (Fernandes et al. 2022). We could reasonably ask whether Omicron is indicative of an evolutionary trend toward the further attenuation of future variants. Yet at the same time, we could also ask whether this is a one-off event, and that a more virulent form of SARS-CoV-2 will emerge at some future date.

For much of the twentieth century, the Attenuation Hypothesis predicted that newly emerging pathogens tend to be virulent when they first appear in a species, but they eventually become attenuated as they co-adapt with their hosts (Alizon et al. 2009). The underlying reason for this prediction was that, assuming no other changes in transmissibility or dormancy, it is not in the evolutionary interest of the pathogen to kill its host and thus destroy its source of sustenance before infecting another host (Smith 1904). To turn an old phrase: one should not bite too hard on the hand that feeds you, especially if you are a pathogen and your meal is the hand itself.

Attenuation increases opportunities for further transmission because the host is more likely to remain mobile and remain contagious for a longer period of time. Recalling the lessons of Chapter 1, this explains the selection for chronic, less virulent infections in Paleolithic foraging populations. In these small and geographically scattered groups, it took more time for people to come into contact with one another compared to the larger and denser populations of the Neolithic. A highly virulent pathogen could become extinct if it killed off one group before it had a chance to infect another, so it was in the evolutionary interest of these pathogens to keep their Paleolithic hosts healthy enough, and for long enough, to walk long distances and interact with other susceptible hosts.

By this same logic, attenuation may have been a successful strategy for migrating populations after the First Epidemiological Transition. The smallpox virus may have been a good candidate for this— *Variola* having major and minor varieties. During the European invasions of Americas in the fifteenth and sixteenth centuries, the minor variety would have been the more likely stowaway on the long journeys to the New World, especially if it could hide undetected in an asymptomatic carrier (Watts 1997). Yet even if we could confirm that this occurred, it would be belied by the increased virulence of the treponemal bacteria that caused syphilis after it spread in Europe (Arora et al. 2016; Harper et al. 2011). Unfortunately, we do not see a consistent trend toward attenuation in our long-standing infectious diseases, and there are multiple instances of increasing virulence among newer infections (Geoghagen and Holmes 2018). Even Pasteur's early experiments did not support this simple claim (Mendelsohn 2002).

In the 1980s, evolutionary biologists focused in earnest on the fitness trade-offs between the virulence and transmissibility of pathogens (Anderson and May 1986; Ewald 1983; Ewald 1994). These studies built on a basic Trade-off Hypothesis that is best explained at the extremes of virulence and attenuation. Highly virulent pathogens are those that replicate faster, with the benefit that they generate larger population sizes that can improve transmission at a given moment. However, larger pathogen populations also produce greater harm to the host, which shortens the time to immobility or death, thereby reducing the overall time window for transmission. In contrast, highly attenuated pathogens reproduce more slowly, with the benefit of increasing the transmission window by

extending the mobility and viability of the host. However, this also comes at the cost of smaller population sizes for further transmission. These scenarios sound much like the Classical Greek myth of Icarus, in which his father warns him not to fly too high or too low with his newly fashioned wings because disaster awaits at both extremes.

Somewhere between the extremes, the basic Trade-off Hypothesis predicts that new pathogens will evolve to balance their competing fitness costs and benefits, eventually arriving at intermediate levels of virulence and transmissibility. For several decades, the coevolution of the myxoma virus (MYXV) and European rabbits was thought to be the best studied example of the trade-off model. Relatively benign in American rabbit species, MYXV causes lethal systemic response in the European species. In the nineteenth century, European rabbits were introduced to Australia, where they quickly overpopulated many rural areas. In an effort to control the population, the Australian government deliberately introduced a single MYXV variety to the rabbits in the 1950s; this gave researchers a rare opportunity to monitor the evolutionary trajectory of a somewhat controlled outbreak. Initially, the virus was highly virulent with a nearly 100 percent case fatality ratio. A few years later, however the ratio declined to between 50 and 75 percent (Fenner 1983). This appeared to support the case for intermediate virulence as predicted by the trade-off model.

For a while, this was thought to be the end of the myxoma-rabbit "experiment," and there was little follow-up data to update the story. Meanwhile, the Trade-off Hypothesis did not account for host evolution, and by the 1990s the rabbits had become increasingly resistant to the virus. In the context of this selective pressure, later varieties of MYXV had evolved a novel trait that shuts down the rabbit immune system entirely (Kerr et al. 2017). Once again, these infections have become highly lethal to the rabbits, but rather than dying from the old symptoms of myxomatosis they die instead of septic shock as their bodies are overrun with unchecked viral particles. They also die of secondary opportunistic infections, much like with AIDS in humans. Moreover, these highly virulent strains are overrunning those with intermediate virulence because the immunosuppression extends the period of infectivity in rabbits. More rabbits die, but the dying process is slow enough for them to infect other rabbits with larger quantities of the virus. In this scenario, virulence and transmissibility work hand-in-hand ... thus far.

Whatever the future may hold for Australia's rabbits, the scenario is nevertheless an artificial (albeit poorly controlled) experiment involving an invasive virus within an invasive host population. Finding the evidence for changing virulence in a natural outbreak is far more difficult, and the data obtained for novel human infections are not sufficient to account for the many selection variables (Geoghegan and Holmes 2018; Lipsitch and Moxon 1997). The Trade-off Hypothesis is no longer applied in its basic form. However, it is often a launching point for the development of more complex models that incorporate variables such as coinfection, host resistance and recovery times, horizontal gene transfer, and changing conditions at different stages of an epidemic (Alizon et al. 2009; Visher et al. 2021). Rather than predicting a generalized outcome, these models consider how multiple variables can shift or remove selection pressures to maintain, attenuate, or even increase the virulence of evolving pathogens.

Increasing virulence is especially troubling so it is worth examining some of the instances in which this has occurred. Beginning with a longstanding disease, bubonic plague demonstrates how virulence can further interhost transmission between different host species. The disease is caused by the bacterium *Yersinia pestis*, a mostly zoonotic (*enzootic*) pathogen that typically circulates between biting insects and rodents in many parts of the world. The bacterium occasionally becomes "epizootic," infecting a small number of human individuals each year. In rare instances, it can cause larger outbreaks, which are usually self-limiting and usually associated with acute environmental disruptions (Barrett 2006). Either way, the human hosts can usually be cured of the infection with a course of commonly available antibiotics.

The insect hosts are not so lucky, especially the rat flea (*Xenopsylla cheopis*), which typically contracts the disease by dining on the blood of its infected namesake. Once inside the flea, *Y. pestis* multiplies rapidly in the gut until forms a large bolus that completely prevents the entry of any more food. Starving and ravenous, the flea bites even more animals whilst regurgitating bacteria, thereby rapidly transmitting large quantities of the pathogen. As in the case of the recent MYXV variants in rabbits, increased virulence *Y. pestis* in biting insects is linked with increased transmissibility, except that in the latter case the transmission is between animal host species.

We are not likely to shed tears over the deaths of fleas and rats, but the same virulence strategy can also apply to human hosts. Paul Ewald, an evolutionary biologist, compared the mortality rates for human infections that were transmitted between humans via insect vectors with those that were transmitted directly from human to human (Ewald 1983). He found a higher proportion of diseases with greater than 1 percent mortality rates among the vector-borne infections than among directly transmitted infections. Based on these data, Ewald hypothesized that evolution favors increasing virulence for pathogens that can survive in multiple species and are therefore less constrained by the death of a single type of host.

As with the previous hypotheses, it is important that we do not overgeneralize Ewald's Virulence Hypothesis. Its predictions are contradicted in some cases. For example, *Y. pestis* is far more virulent in its pneumonic form, which is directly transmitted via respiratory droplets, than in its bubonic form as a vector-borne pathogen. And we must still recognize that there are many, largely unmeasured factors that can impact virulence levels. Like the basic forms of the other hypotheses, the Virulence Hypothesis is perhaps best approached as a heuristic model toward the development of a more complex theory.

Mindful of these disclaimers, there is a further extension of the Virulence Hypothesis that bears further consideration for the purposes of this book. The hypothesis also extends to pathogens that can live outside the human host. As a prime example, *V. cholerae* can take advantage of its ability to survive independently in nutrient rich waters by causing its human host to expel large quantities of progeny into the surrounding environment. This is especially the case if that environment is a sewage-contaminated slum or refugee camp. Based on this reasoning, different levels of environmental contamination—as mediated by factors such as poverty, conflict, or displacement—can select for varieties of *V. cholerae* with greater or lesser virulence.

Essentially, the contaminated water, food, or fomites act much like insect vectors, serving as avenues of escape and vehicles for the further transmission of the pathogen from a debilitated or dying host. Ewald refers to these contaminated media as "cultural vectors," insofar as the contamination itself is the product of human activity. Applying this Cultural Vectors Hypothesis, he further argues that in the 1960s, the less virulent (*el tor*) variety of cholera overtook the more virulent (classic) variety in many low-income countries because their water quality had been improved, whereas the classic variety persisted where this intervention had not occurred, although the supporting evidence for this argument is too crude to establish a causal relationship. Yet if one could be established, then the Cultural Vectors Hypothesis would be a substantial update to John Snow's work on the topic. Improving water and other living conditions would not only reduce infectious diseases but it would also attenuate their pathogens along the way.

Earlier in this chapter we discussed some of the factors that can influence whether exposure to a pathogen leads to host infection. The same factors can apply to virulence insofar as they influence different stages in the transmission process, such as dispersion from the initial host, translocation to another susceptible host, and colonization within that host. Likewise, the state of human hosts and their surrounding environments are bound to place selection pressure on the evolution of pathogen traits that affect their virulence. We may lack some of the details and diagnostics but it is unlikely to be a coincidence that H1N1, the most virulent form of human influenza, emerged on the heels of the First World War (Crosby 2003). Nor is it a likely coincidence that O139, the most virulent form of cholera, emerged in one of the world's poorest societies (Faruque et al. 2003). And after first detecting all five SARS-CoV-2 variants of concern in the least vaccinated parts of the world, we should not be surprised if something more virulent emerges under similar conditions at a later date. Whatever the future

holds for evolutionary forecasting, the models will have to address the relationships between pathogen virulence and human vulnerability.

Notes

1. Pasteur originally wrote a similar phrase in the preface of his book on silkworm disease. This quotation was a restatement of that phrase during an 1882 interview about rabies that was translated to English by John Illo (1996).

2. As an indication of this, there was a greater than 75 percent increase in the use of the term "unprecedented" in worldwide Google searches conducted during the week of March 8–14, 2020, compared with the same searches over a five-year period (2017–2021). This is the same week that the World Health Organization officially declared COVID-19 a global pandemic. https://trends.google.com/trends/explore?date=today%205-y&=unprecedented.

3. The same study finds an overall decrease in per capita cases, but undetected cases are common in epidemics and more so in underserved populations. This could be accounted for with broader measures of excess mortality in those societies and years in which the epidemics had substantial demographic impact and then compared to determine the secular trend.

4. Interestingly, the first outbreak may have primed the pig population for a longer, second outbreak that could cycle among pigs for up to two years by carrier animals with partial or temporary immunity (Pulliam et al. 2021).

5. The International Committee on the Taxonomy of Viruses (ICTV) determines the official nomenclature. As with other taxonomic categories, the official name of a viral lineage does not encompass all its characteristics, and a viral lineage can be named for a characteristic shared by other lineages bearing a different name. For the purposes of this book, it is best to simply regard these viral names as unique identifiers.

6. The problematic terms "Asian Flu" and "Hong Kong Flu" arose in the popular media. We

include them only for the purpose of historical reference. Even with respect to formal terminology, it should be noted that, beginning with the identification of COVID-19, the ICTV no longer includes putative geographic origins as part of viral nomenclature.

7. We use the term "biosafety" instead of "biosecurity" to minimize ambiguity. Biosecurity is a general term that refers to any measure taken to prevent the spread of pathogens to human, animal, or plant life. Although it is more commonly used in the context of agricultural and laboratory safety measures, its military associations can be distracting.

8. It should be noted that recommendations for the spacing of facilities may not include those for the further spacing of animals within those facilities.

9. Commercial passenger air traffic declined about 50 percent during the first year of the COVID-19 pandemic and has since been slowly recovering.

10. COPD was not listed among the comorbid conditions in this initial patient cohort, however it did appear in later case groups (Alraddadi et al. 2016).

References

Alarcon, Laura Valeria, Alberto Allepuz Alberto, and Enric Mateu. 2021. "Biosecurity in pig farms: A review." *Porcine Health Management* 7 (1). https://doi.org/10.1186/s40813-020-00181-z

Alizon, Samuel, Amy Hurford, Nicole Mideo, and Minus Van Baalen. 2009. "Virulence evolution and the trade-off hypothesis: history, current state of affairs and the future." *Journal of Evolutionary Biology* 22 (2): 245–259. https://doi.org/10.1111/j.1420-9101.2008.01658.x

Allen, Toph, Kris A. Murray, Carlos Zambrana-Torrelio, Stephen S. Morse, Carlo Rondinini, Moreno Di Marco, Nathan Breit, Kevin J. Olival, and Peter Daszak. 2017. "Global hotspots and correlates of emerging zoonotic diseases." *Nature Communications* 8. https://doi.org/10.1038/s41467-017-00923-8

Allen, William. 1843. "Excursion up the River of Cameroons and to the Bay of Amboises." *The Journal of the Royal Geographical Society of London* 13: 1–17.

Alraddadi, Basem M., John T. Watson, Abdulatif Almarashi, Glen R. Abedi, Amal Turkistani, Musallam Sadran, Abeer Housa et al. 2016. "Risk factors for primary Middle East respiratory syndrome coronavirus illness in humans, Saudi Arabia, 2014." *Emerging infectious diseases* 22 (1): 49.

Alshukairi, Abeer N., Jian Zheng, Jingxian Zhao, Atef Nehdi, Salim A. Baharoon, Laila Layqah, Ahmad Bokhari et al. 2018. "High prevalence of MERS-CoV infection in camel workers in Saudi Arabia." *Mbio* 9 (5). https://doi.org/10.1128/mBio.01985-18

Anderson, R.M., and R.M. May. 1986. "The invasion, persistence and spread of infectious diseases within animal and plant communities." *Philosophical Transactions of the Royal Society of London Series B-Biological Sciences* 314 (1167): 533–570. https://doi.org/10.1098/rstb.1986.0072

Arora, Natasha, Verena J. Schuenemann, Guenter Jaeger, Alexander Peltzer, Alexander Seitz, Alexander Herbig, Michal Strouhal et al. 2016. "Origin of modern syphilis and emergence of a pandemic Treponema pallidum cluster." *Nature Microbiology* 2 (1). https://doi.org/10.1038/nmicrobiol.2016.245

Assiri, Abdullah, Jaffar A. Al-Tawfiq, Abdullah A. Al-Rabeeah, Fahad A. Al-Rabiah, Sami Al-Hajjar, Ali Al-Barrak, Hesham Flemban et al. 2013. "Epidemiological, demographic, and clinical characteristics of 47 cases of Middle East respiratory syndrome coronavirus disease from Saudi Arabia: a descriptive study." *Lancet Infectious Diseases* 13 (9): 752–761. https://doi.org/10.1016/S1473-3099

Bae, Sung A., So Ree Kim, Mi-Na Kim, Wan Joo Shim, and Seong-Mi Park. 2021. "Impact of cardiovascular disease and risk factors on fatal outcomes in patients with COVID-19 according to age: A systematic review and meta-analysis." *Heart* 107 (5): 373. https://doi.org/10.1136/heartjnl-2020-317901

Balasubramanian, Deepak, Sebastian Murcia, C. Brandon Ogbunugafor, Ronnie Gavilan, and Salvador Almagro-Moreno. 2021. "Cholera dynamics: Lessons from an epidemic." *Journal of Medical Microbiology* 70 (2). https://doi.org/10.1099/jmm.0.001298

Barrett, Ron. 2008. "The 1994 Plague in Western India: Human Ecology and the Risks of Misattribution." In *Terrorism, War, or Disease? Unraveling the Use of Biological Weapons*, edited by A. Clunan and P. Lavoy, 49–71. Stanford: Stanford University Press.

Barrett, R. 2015. "The Specter of Ebola: Epidemiological Transitions vs. the Zombie Apocalypse." In *New Directions in Biocultural Anthropology*, edited by M.K. Zuckerman and D. Martin, 277–293. New York: Wiley-Blackwell.

Becker, Daniel J., Alex D. Washburne, Christina L. Faust, Erin A. Mordecai, and Raina K. Plowright. 2019. "The problem of scale in the prediction and management of pathogen spillover." *Philosophical Transactions of the Royal Society B: Biological Sciences* 374 (1782). https://doi.org/10.1098/rstb.2019.0224

Bell, Diana, Scott Roberton, and Paul R. Hunter. 2004. "Animal origins of SARS coronavirus: Possible links with the international trade in small carnivores." *Philosophical Transactions of the Royal Society B: Biological Sciences* 359 (1447): 1107–1114. https://doi.org/10.1098/rstb.2004.1492

Blagodatski, Artem, Kseniya Trutneva, Olga Glazova, Olga Mityaeva, Liudmila Shevkova, Evgenii Kegeles, Nikita Onyanov et al. 2021. "Avian influenza in wild birds and poultry: Dissemination pathways, monitoring methods, and virus ecology." *Pathogens* 10 (5): 630. https://doi.org/10.3390/pathogens10050630

Booth, Adam, Angus Bruno Reed, Sonia Ponzo, Arrash Yassaee, Mert Aral, David Plans, Alain Labrique et al. 2021. "Population risk factors for severe disease and mortality in COVID-19: A global systematic review and meta-analysis." *PloS One* 16 (3). https://doi.org/10.1371/journal.pone.0247461

Booth, Christopher M., Larissa M. Matukas, George A. Tomlinson, Anita R. Rachlis, David B. Rose, Hy A. Dwosh, Sharon L. Walmsley et al. 2003. "Clinical features and short-term outcomes of 144 patients with SARS in the greater Toronto area." *Journal of the American Medical Association* 289 (21): 2801–2809. https://doi.org/10.1001/jama.289.21.JOC30885

Brashares, Justin S., Peter Arcese, Moses K. Sam, Peter B. Coppolillo, Anthony RE Sinclair, and Andrew Balmford. 2004. "Bushmeat hunting, wildlife declines, and fish supply in West Africa." *Science* 306 (5699): 1180–1183. https://doi.org/10.1126/science.1102425

Brashares, Justin S., Christopher D. Golden, Karen Z. Weinbaum, Christopher B. Barrett, and Grace V. Okello. 2011. "Economic and geographic drivers of wildlife consumption in rural Africa." *Proceedings of the National Academy of Sciences* 108 (34): 13931–13936.

Bryner, Jeanna. 2020. "1st known case of coronavirus traced back to November in China." *Live Science* (March 14, 2020).

Carr, Jean K., Nathan D. Wolfe, Judith N. Torimiro, Ubald Tamoufe, E. Mpoudi-Ngole, Lindsay Eyzaguirre, Deborah L. Birx et al. 2010. "HIV-1 recombinants with multiple parental strains in low-prevalence, remote regions of Cameroon: Evolutionary relics?" *Retrovirology* 7. https://doi.org/10.1186/1742-4690-7-39

Cash, R.A., S.I. Music, J.P. Libonati, J.P. Craig, N.F. Pierce, and R.B. Hornick. 1974a. "Response of man to infection with Vibrio-cholerae. 2. Protection from illness afforded by previous disease and vaccine." *Journal of Infectious Diseases* 130 (4): 325–333. https://doi.org/10.1093/infdis/130.4.325

Cash, R.A., S.I. Music, J.P. Libonati, M.J. Snyder, R.P. Wenzel, and R.B. Hornick. 1974b. "Response of man to infection with Vibrio-cholerae. 1. Clinical, serologic, and bacteriologic responses to a known inoculum." *Journal of Infectious Diseases* 129 (1): 45–52. https://doi.org/10.1093/infdis/129.1.45

Cawthorn, Donna-Maree, and Louwrens C. Hoffman. 2015. "The bushmeat and food security nexus: A global account of the contributions, conundrums and ethical collisions." *Food Research International* 76: 906–925. https://doi.org/10.1016/j.foodres.2015.03.025

CDC. 1981. "Kaposi's sarcoma and pneumocystis pneumonia among homosexual men—New York City and California." *Morbidity and Mortality Weekly Report* 30: 305–308.

CDC. 2019a. "1957–1958 Pandemic (H2N2 virus)." Centers for Disease Control and Prevention. https://www.cdc.gov/flu/pandemic-resources/1957-1958-pandemic.html

CDC. 2019b. "1968 Pandemic (H3N2 virus)." Centers for Disease Control and Prevention. https://www.cdc.gov/flu/pandemic-resources/1968-pandemic.html

CDC. 2019c. "2009 H1N1 Pandemic (H1N1pdm09 virus)." Centers for Disease Control and Prevention. https://www.cdc.gov/flu/pandemic-resources/2009-h1n1-pandemic.html

CDC. 2021, "CDC stands up new disease forecasting center." https://www.cdc.gov/media/releases/2021/p0818-disease-forecasting-center.html

Chauhan, Ravendra P., and Michelle L. Gordon. 2020. "A systematic review analyzing the prevalence and circulation of influenza viruses in swine population worldwide." *Pathogens* 9 (5): 355. https://doi.org/10.3390/pathogens9050355

Chen, Kow-Tong, Shiing-Jer Twu, Hsiao-Ling Chang, Yi-Chun Wu, Chu-Tzu Chen, Ting-Hsiang Lin, Sonja J. Olsen et al. 2005. "SARS in Taiwan: An overview and lessons learned." *International Journal of Infectious Diseases* 9 (2): 77–85. https://doi.org/10.1016/j.ijid.2004.04.015

Christman, Mary C., Ambreen Kedwaii, Jianpeng Xu, Ruben O. Donis, and Guoqing Lu. 2011. "Pandemic (H1N1) 2009 virus revisited: An evolutionary retrospective." *Infection Genetics and Evolution* 11 (5): 803–811. https://doi.org/10.1016/j.meegid.2011.02.021

Coleman, Janna. 2020. "My Father's Guide To Field Dressing An Elk." *The Rumpus*. https://therumpus.net/2020/07/my-fathers-guide-to-field-dressing-an-elk/

Cowlishaw, G., S. Mendelson, and J.M. Rowcliffe. 2005. "Structure and operation of a bushmeat commodity chain in southwestern Ghana." *Conservation Biology* 19 (1): 139–149.

Crosby, Alfred W. 2003. *America's Forgotten Pandemic: The Influenza of 1918*. 2nd ed. Cambridge: Cambridge University Press.

D'Cruze, N., J. Toole, K. Mansell, and J. Schmidt-Burbach. 2014. "What is the true cost of the world's most expensive coffee?" *Oryx* 48 (2): 170–171.

Das, Bhabatosh, Gururaja P. Pazhani, Anirban Sarkar, Asish K. Mukhopadhyay, G. Balakrish Nair, and Thandavarayan Ramamurthy. 2016. "Molecular evolution and functional divergence of Vibrio cholerae." *Current Opinion in Infectious Diseases* 29 (5): 520–527. https://doi.org/10.1097/qco.0000000000000306

Davis, Mike. 2006. *The Monster at our Door: The Global Threat of Avian Flu*. New York: Owl Books.

de Loisy, Nicholas. 2021. *Transportation and the Belt and Road Initiative*. Hong Kong: Supply Chain Management Outsource Ltd.

Dinh, Pham Ngoc, Hoang Thuy Long, Nguyen Thi Kim Tien, Nguyen Tran Hien, Hoang Van Tan, Nguyen Binh Nguyen, Phan Van Tu et al. 2006. "Risk factors for human infection with avian influenza A H5N1, Vietnam, 2004." *Emerging Infectious Diseases* 12 (12): 1841–1847.

Edoro, Ainehi. 2017. Why I no longer use the term "game" for bushmeat—Chika Unigwe. *Brittle Paper*. https://brittlepaper.com/2017/08/longer-term-game-bushmeat-chika-unigwe/. Accessed 09/18/2023.

Estrada, Alejandro, Paul A. Garber, Anthony B. Rylands, Christian Roos, Eduardo Fernandez-Duque, Anthony Di Fiore, K. Anne-Isola Nekaris et al. 2017. "Impending extinction crisis of the world's primates: Why primates matter." *Science Advances* 3 (1). https://doi.org/10.1126/sciadv.1600946

Ewald, Paul W., 1983. Host-parasite relations, vectors, and the evolution of disease severity. *Annual Review of Ecology and Systematics*, 14 (1): 465–485.

Ewald, Paul W. 1994. *Evolution of Infectious Disease*. New York: Oxford University Press.

Farmer, P. 1992. *AIDS and Accusation: Haiti and the Geography of Blame*. Berkeley: University of California Press.

Faruque, Shah M., David A. Sack, R. Bradley Sack, Rita R. Colwell, Yoshifumi Takeda, and G. Balakrish Nair. 2003. "Emergence and evolution of Vibrio cholerae O139." *Proceedings of the National Academy of Sciences of the United States of America* 100 (3): 1304–1309. https://doi.org/10.1073/pnas.0337468100

Faye, B. 2016. "The camel, new challenges for a sustainable development." *Tropical Animal Health and Production* 48 (4): 689–692. https://doi.org/10.1007/s11250-016-0995-8.

Faye, B. 2020. "How many large camelids in the world? A synthetic analysis of the world camel demographic changes." *Pastoralism-Research Policy and Practice* 10 (1). https://doi.org/10.1186/s13570-020-00176-z

Fenner, Frank. 1983. "Biological control as exemplified by smallpox eradication and myxomatosis." *Proceedings of the Royal Society B: Biological Sciences* 218: 259–285.

Fernandes, Queenie, Varghese Philipose Inchakalody, Maysaloun Merhi, Sarra Mestiri, Nassiba Taib, Dina Moustafa Abo El-Ella, Takwa Bedhiafi et al. 2022. "Emerging COVID-19 variants and their impact on SARS-CoV-2 diagnosis, therapeutics and vaccines." *Annals of medicine* 54 (1): 524–540.

Food and Agriculture Organization of the United Nations. 2020. "FAOSTAT—Crops and livestock products." UN FAO. https://www.fao.org/faostat/en/#data/QCL

Garrett, L., 1994. *The coming plague: newly emerging diseases in a world out of balance*. Farrar, Straus and Giroux.

Gauthier-Clerc, M., C. Lebarbenchon, and F. Thomas. 2007. "Recent expansion of highly pathogenic avian influenza H5N1: A critical review." *Ibis* 149 (2): 202–214. https://doi.org/10.1111/j.1474-919X.2007.00699.x

Geoghegan, Jemma L., and Edward C. Holmes. 2018. "The phylogenomics of evolving virus virulence." *Nature Reviews Genetics* 19 (12): 756–769. https://doi.org/10.1038/s41576-018-0055-5

Gibbs, Adrian J., John S. Armstrong, and Jean C. Downie. 2009. "From where did the 2009 'swine-origin' influenza A virus (H1N1) emerge?" *Virology Journal* 6. https://doi.org/10.1186/1743-422x-6-207

Gortazar, Christian, Leslie A. Reperant, Thijs Kuiken, Jose de la Fuente, Mariana Boadella, Beatriz Martinez-Lopez, Francisco Ruiz-Fons et al. 2014. "Crossing the interspecies barrier: opening the door to zoonotic pathogens." *PloS Pathogens* 10 (6). https://doi.org/10.1371/journal.ppat.1004129

Gossner, C., N. Danielson, A. Gervelmeyer, F. Berthe, B. Faye, K. Kaasik Aaslav, C. Adlhoch et al. 2014. "Human–dromedary camel interactions and the risk of acquiring zoonotic Middle East Respiratory Syndrome coronavirus infection." *Zoonoses and Public Health* 63 (1): 1–9. https://doi.org/10.1111/zph.12171

Grande Vega, Maria, Bruno Carpinetti, Jesus Duarte, and John E. Fa. 2013. "Contrasts in livelihoods and protein intake between commercial and subsistence bushmeat hunters in two villages on Bioko Island, Equatorial Guinea." *Conservation Biology* 27 (3): 576–587. https://doi.org/10.1111/cobi.12067

Harper, Kristin N., Molly K. Zuckerman, Megan L. Harper, John Kingston, and George J. Armelagos. 2011. "The origin and antiquity of syphilis revisited: An appraisal of Old World Pre-Columbian evidence for treponemal infection." *Yearbook of Physical Anthropology* 54: 99–133.

Hazarie, Surendra, David Soriano-Panos, Alex Arenas, Jesus Gomez-Gardenes, and Gourab Ghoshal. 2021.

"Interplay between population density and mobility in determining the spread of epidemics in cities." *Communications Physics* 4 (1). https://doi.org/10.1038/s42005-021-00679-0

Holmes, Edward C., Stephen A. Goldstein, Angela L. Rasmussen, David L. Robertson, Alexander Crits-Christoph, Joel O. Wertheim, Simon J. Anthony et al. 2021. "The origins of SARS-CoV-2: A critical review." *Cell* 184 (19): 4848–4856. https://doi.org/10.1016/j.cell.2021.08.017

Illo, J., 1996. "Pasteur and rabies: an interview of 1882." *Medical history*, 40 (3): 373–377.

Islam, M. Saiful, Hossain M.S. Sazzad, Syed Moinuddin Satter, Sharmin Sultana, M. Jahangir Hossain, Murshid Hasan, Mahmudur Rahman et al. 2016. "Nipah Virus transmission from bats to humans associated with drinking traditional liquor made from date palm sap, Bangladesh, 2011–2014." *Emerging Infectious Diseases* 22 (4): 664–670. https://doi.org/10.3201/eid2204.151747

Johnson, Npas, and J. Mueller. 2002. "Updating the accounts: global mortality of the 1918–1920 'Spanish' influenza pandemic." *Bulletin of the History of Medicine* 76 (1): 105–115. https://doi.org/10.1353/bhm.2002.0022

Jones, G., D.S. Jacobs, T.H. Kunz, M.R. Willig, and P.A. Racey. 2009. "Carpe noctem: The importance of bats as bioindicators." *Inter-Research* 8: 93–115.

Jones, K.E., N.G. Patel, M.A. Levy, A. Storeygard, D. Balk, J.L. Gittleman, and P. Daszak. 2008. "Global trends in emerging infectious diseases." *Nature* 451 (7181): 990–993.

Joseph, Udayan, Yvonne C.F. Su, Dhanasekaran Vijaykrishna, and Gavin J.D. Smith. 2017. "The ecology and adaptive evolution of influenza A interspecies transmission." *Influenza and Other Respiratory Viruses* 11 (1): 74–84. https://doi.org/10.1111/irv.12412

Kerr, Peter J., Isabella M. Cattadori, June Liu, Derek G. Sim, Jeff W. Dodds, Jason W. Brooks, Mary J. Kennett et al. 2017. "Next step in the ongoing arms race between myxoma virus and wild rabbits in Australia is a novel disease phenotype." *Proceedings of the National Academy of Sciences of the United States of America* 114 (35): 9397–9402. https://doi.org/10.1073/pnas.1710336114

Kesheh, Mina Mobini, Parastoo Hosseini, Saber Soltani, and Milad Zandi. 2021. "An overview on the seven pathogenic human coronaviruses." *Reviews in Medical Virology*. https://doi.org/10.1002/rmv.2282

Kompaniyets, Lyudmyla, Audrey F. Pennington, Alyson B. Goodman, Hannah G. Rosenblum, Brook Belay, Jean Y. Ko, Jennifer R. Chevinsky et al. 2021. "Original research underlying medical conditions and severe illness among 540,667 adults hospitalized with COVID-19, March 2020–March 2021." *Preventing Chronic Disease* 18. https://doi.org/10.5888/pcd18.210123

Leach, Melissa, and Mariz Tadros. 2014. "Epidemics and the politics of knowledge: Contested narratives in Egypt's H1N1 response." *Medical Anthropology* 33 (3): 240–254. https://doi.org/10.1080/01459740.2013.842565

Lederburg, Joshua, Robert E. Shope, and Stanley. C. Oaks. 1992. *Emerging Infections: Microbial Threats to Health in the United States*. Washington, DC: Institute of Medicine, National Academy Press.

Leung, Gabriel M., Anthony J. Hedley, Lai-Ming Ho, Patsy Chau, Irene OL Wong, Thuan Q. Thach, Azra C. Ghani et al. 2004. "The epidemiology of severe acute respiratory syndrome in the 2003 Hong Kong epidemic: An analysis of all 1755 patients." *Annals of Internal Medicine* 141 (9): 662–673.

Lim, Poh Lian, Tau Hong Lee, and Emily K. Rowe. 2013. "Middle East Respiratory Syndrome coronavirus (MERS CoV): Update 2013." *Current Infectious Disease Reports* 15 (4): 295–298. https://doi.org/10.1007/s11908-013-0344-2

Lipsitch, Marc., and E. Richard. Moxon. 1997. "Virulence and transmissibility of pathogens: What is the relationship?" *Trends in Microbiology* 5 (1): 31–37. https://doi.org/10.1016/s0966-842x

Liu, Ping, Jing-Zhe Jiang, Xiu-Feng Wan, Yan Hua, Linmiao Li, Jiabin Zhou, Xiaohu Wang et al. 2020. "Are pangolins the intermediate host of the 2019 novel coronavirus (SARS-CoV-2)?." *PloS Pathogens* 17 (6). https://doi.org/10.1371/journal.ppat.1009664

Lynn, B. 1991. "Cholera epidemic worsens in Peru and doctors criticize president." *Associated Press News*, February 28.

Lytras, Spyros, Wei Xia, Joseph Hughes, Xiaowei Jiang, and David L. Robertson. 2021. "The animal origin of SARS-CoV-2." *Science* 373 (6558): 968. https://doi.org/10.1126/science.abh0117

Maria Gomez, Jose, Charles L. Nunn, and Miguel Verdu. 2013. "Centrality in primate-parasite networks reveals the potential for the transmission of emerging infectious diseases to humans." *Proceedings of the National Academy of Sciences of the United States of America* 110 (19): 7738–7741. https://doi.org/10.1073/pnas.1220716110

Mata, L., M. Vives, and G. Vicente. 1994. "Extinction of Vibrio-cholerae in acidic substrata—Contaminated fish marinated with lime juice (ceviche)." *Revista De Biologia Tropical* 42 (3): 479–485.

Markel, Howard 2004. *When Germs Travel: Six Epidemics That Invaded America Since 1900 and the Fears They Unleashed*. New York: Pantheon.

Mazareanu, E. 2021. "Global air traffic—Scheduled passengers 2004–2021." *Statistica*. https://www.statista.

com/statistics/564717/airline-industry-passenger-traffic-globally/

McMullen, Jane. 2021. "Covid-19: Five days that shaped the outbreak." *BBC News*.

Mena, Ignacio, Martha I. Nelson, Francisco Quezada-Monroy, Jayeeta Dutta, Refugio Cortes-Fernandez, J. Horacio Lara-Puente, Felipa Castro-Peralta et al. 2016. "Origins of the 2009 H1N1 influenza pandemic in swine in Mexico." *Elife* 5. https://doi.org/10.7554/eLife.16777

Mendelsohn, J. Andrew. 2002. "'Like all that lives': Biology, medicine and bacteria in the age of Pasteur and Koch." *History and Philosophy of the Life Sciences* 24 (1): 3–36. https://doi.org/10.1080/03919710210001714293

Mendenhall, Emily, Brandon A. Kohrt, Shane A. Norris, David Ndetei, and Dorairaj Prabhakaran. 2017. "Non-communicable disease syndemics: poverty, depression, and diabetes among low-income populations." *Lancet* 389 (10072): 951–963.

Morens, David M., and Anthony S. Fauci. 2013. "Emerging infectious diseases: Threats to human health and global stability." *PloS Pathogens* 9 (7). https://doi.org/10.1371/journal.ppat.1003467

Muanprasat, Chatchai, and Varanuj Chatsudthipong. 2013. "Cholera: Pathophysiology and emerging therapeutic targets." *Future Medicinal Chemistry* 5 (7): 781–798. https://doi.org/10.4155/fmc.13.42

Mude, William, Victor M. Oguoma, Tafadzwa Nyanhanda, Lillian Mwanri, and Carolyne Njue. 2021. "Racial disparities in COVID-19 pandemic cases, hospitalisations, and deaths: A systematic review and meta-analysis." *Journal of Global Health* 11. https://doi.org/10.7189/jogh.11.05015

Müller, Marcel A., Victor Max Corman, Joerg Jores, Benjamin Meyer, Mario Younan, Anne Liljander, Berend-Jan Bosch et al. 2014. "MERS coronavirus neutralizing antibodies in camels, Eastern Africa, 1983–1997." *Emerging infectious diseases* 20 (12): 2093.

Nasi, Robert, A. Taber, and Nathalie Van Vliet. 2011. "Empty forests, empty stomachs? Bushmeat and livelihoods in the Congo and Amazon Basins." *International Forestry Review* 13 (3): 355–368. https://doi.org/10.1505/146554811798293872

Nelson, Martha I., Cecile Viboud, Amy L. Vincent, Marie R. Culhane, Susan E. Detmer, David E. Wentworth, Andrew Rambaut et al. 2015. "Global migration of influenza A viruses in swine." *Nature Communications* 6. https://doi.org/10.1038/ncomms7696

Organization, World Health. 2022. "Tracking SARS-CoV-2 variants." World Health Organization. https://www.who.int/en/activities/tracking-SARS-CoV-2-variants/

Pape, Jean William, Paul Farmer, Serena Koenig, Daniel Fitzgerald, Peter Wright, and Warren Johnson. 2008. "The epidemiology of AIDS in Haiti refutes the claims of Gilbert et al." *Proceedings of the National Academy of Sciences of the United States of America* 105 (10): E13–E13. https://doi.org/10.1073/pnas.0711141105

Paules, Catharine I., Hilary D. Marston, and Anthony S. Fauci. 2020. "Coronavirus infections—more than just the common cold." *Journal of the American Medical Association* 323 (8): 707–708. https://doi.org/10.1001/jama.2020.0757

Person, Bobbie, Francisco Sy, Kelly Holton, Barbara Govert, Arthur Liang, SARS Community Outreach Team, Brenda Garza et al. 2004. "Fear and stigma: The epidemic within the SARS outbreak." *Emerging Infectious Diseases* 10 (2): 358–363. https://doi.org/10.3201/eid1002.030750

Pesaresi, Martino, Michele Melchiorri, Alice Siragusa, and Thomas Kemper. 2016. *Atlas of the Human Planet 2016: Mapping Human Presence on Earth with the Global Human Settlement Layer. European Commission—DG Joint Research Centre* (Luxemburg: Publications Office of the European Union).

Pijls, Bart G., Shahab Jolani, Anique Atherley, Raissa T. Derckx, Janna I.R. Dijkstra, Gregor H.L. Franssen, Stevie Hendriks et al. 2021. "Demographic risk factors for COVID-19 infection, severity, ICU admission and death: A meta-analysis of 59 studies." *BMJ Open* 11 (1). https://doi.org/10.1136/bmjopen-2020-044640

Plowright, Raina K., Colin R. Parrish, Hamish McCallum, Peter J. Hudson, Albert I. Ko, Andrea L. Graham, and James O. Lloyd-Smith. 2017. "Pathways to zoonotic spillover." *Nature Reviews Microbiology* 15 (8): 502–510. https://doi.org/10.1038/nrmicro.2017.45

Pruzzo, Carla, Luigi Vezzulli, and Rita R. Colwell. 2008. "Global impact of Vibrio cholerae interactions with chitin." *Environmental Microbiology* 10 (6): 1400–1410. https://doi.org/10.1111/j.1462-2920.2007.01559.x

Pulliam, Juliet R.C., Jonathan H. Epstein, Jonathan Dushoff, Sohayati A. Rahman, Michel Bunning, Aziz A. Jamaluddin, Alex D. Hyatt et al. 2012. "Agricultural intensification, priming for persistence and the emergence of Nipah virus: A lethal bat-borne zoonosis." *Journal of the Royal Society Interface* 9 (66): 89–101. https://doi.org/10.1098/rsif.2011.0223

Rabaan, Ali A., Shamsah H. Al-Ahmed, Ranjit Sah, Mohammed A. Alqumber, Shafiul Haque, Shailesh Kumar Patel, Mamta Pathak et al. 2021. "MERS-CoV: Epidemiology, molecular dynamics, therapeutics, and future challenges." *Annals of Clinical Microbiology and Antimicrobials* 20 (1). https://doi.org/10.1186/s12941-020-00414-7

Ritchie, Hannah, and Max Roser. 2019. "Urbanization." Our World in Data. https://ourworldindata.org/urbanization

Rossen, Lauren M., Farida B. Ahmad, Robert N. Anderson, Amy M. Branum, Chengan Du, Harlan M. Krumholz, Shu-Xia Li et al. 2021. "Disparities in excess mortality associated with COVID-19-United States, 2020." *Morbidity and Mortality Weekly Report* 70 (33): 1114–1119.

Scarpino, S.V. 2016. "Evolution and Emergence of Novel Pathogens." In *Encyclopedia of Evolutionary Biology*, edited by R.M. Kliman, 77–82. Cambridge MA: Academic Press.

Shi, Zhengli, and Zhihong Hu. 2008. "A review of studies on animal reservoirs of the SARS coronavirus." *Virus Research* 133 (1): 74–87. https://doi.org/10.1016/j.virusres.2007.03.012

Sibbald, Shannon J., Laura Eme, John M. Archibald, and Andrew J. Roger. 2020. "Lateral gene transfer mechanisms and pan-genomes in eukaryotes." *Trends in Parasitology* 36 (11): 927–941. https://doi.org/10.1016/j.pt.2020.07.014

Singh, Raj Kumar, Kuldeep Dhama, Sandip Chakraborty, Ruchi Tiwari, Senthilkumar Natesan, Rekha Khandia, Ashok Munjal et al. 2019. "Nipah virus: Epidemiology, pathology, immunobiology and advances in diagnosis, vaccine designing and control strategies—A comprehensive review." *Veterinary Quarterly* 39 (1): 26–55. https://doi.org/10.1080/01652176.2019.1580827

Smith, Katherine F., Michael Goldberg, Samantha Rosenthal, Lynn Carlson, Jane Chen, Cici Chen, and Sohini Ramachandran. 2014. "Global rise in human infectious disease outbreaks." *Journal of the Royal Society Interface* 11 (101). https://doi.org/10.1098/rsif.2014.0950

Smith, Theobald. 1904. "Some problems in the life history of pathogenic microorganisms." *Science* 20: 817–832. https://doi.org/10.1126/science.20.520.817

Sokolow, Susanne H., Nicole Nova, Kim M. Pepin, Alison J. Peel, Juliet R.C. Pulliam, Kezia Manlove, Paul C. Cross et al. 2019. "Ecological interventions to prevent and manage zoonotic pathogen spillover." *Philosophical Transactions of the Royal Society B-Biological Sciences* 374 (1782). https://doi.org/10.1098/rstb.2018.0342

Tagg, N., N.J. Maddison, J. Dupain, L. Mcgilchrist, M. Mouamfon, G. Mccabe, M.M. Ngo Badjeck et al. 2018. "A zoo-led study of the great ape bushmeat commodity chain in Cameroon." *International Zoo Yearbook* 52 (1): 182–193.

United Nations. 2019. *Patterns and Trends in Household Composition and Size: Evidence from a United Nations Dataset*. New York: United Nations, Department of Economic and Social Affairs, Population Division.

USDA. 2016. *Final Report for the 2014–2015 Outbreak of Highly Pathogenic Avian Influenza (HPAI) in the United States*. Washington, DC: United States Department of Agriculture, Veterinary Services, Surveillance, Preparedness, and Response Services, Animal and Plant Health Inspection Service.

Vezzulli, Luigi, Craig Baker-Austin, Alexander Kirschner, Carla Pruzzo, and Jaime Martinez-Urtaza. 2020. "Global emergence of environmental non-O1/O139 Vibrio cholerae infections linked with climate change: A neglected research field?" *Environmental Microbiology* 22 (10): 4342–4355. https://doi.org/10.1111/1462-2920.15040

Visher, Elisa, Claire Evensen, Sarah Guth, Edith Lai, Marina Norfolk, Carly Rozins, Nina A. Sokolov et al. 2021. "The three Ts of virulence evolution during zoonotic emergence." *Proceedings of the Royal Society B: Biological Sciences* 288 (1956). https://doi.org/10.1098/rspb.2021.0900

Vetter, Pauline, William A. Fischer II, Manuel Schibler, Michael Jacobs, Daniel G. Bausch, and Laurent Kaiser. 2016. "Ebola virus shedding and transmission: Review of current evidence." *Journal of Infectious Diseases* 214: S177–S184. https://doi.org/10.1093/infdis/jiw254

Wallace, Robert G. 2016. *Big Farms Make Big Flu: Dispatches on Infectious Disease, Agribusiness, and the Nature of Science*. New York: Monthly Review Press.

Wang, Dayan, Wenfei Zhu, Lei Yang, and Yuelong Shu. 2021. "The epidemiology, virology, and pathogenicity of human infections with avian influenza viruses." *Cold Spring Harbor Perspectives in Medicine* 11 (4). https://doi.org/10.1101/cshperspect.a038620

Watts, S. 1997. *Epidemics and History: Disease, Power, and Imperialism*. New Haven: Yale University Press.

Weaver, Lesley Jo, and Emily Mendenhall. 2014. "Applying syndemics and chronicity: Interpretations from studies of poverty, depression, and diabetes." *Medical Anthropology* 33 (2): 92–108. https://doi.org/10.1080/01459740.2013.808637

Weaver, Lesley Jo, and Connor B. Fasel. 2018. "A systematic review of the literature on the relationships between chronic diseases and food insecurity." *Food and Nutrition Sciences* 9: 519–541.

Wille, M., and E.C. Holmes. 2021. "The Ecology and Evolution of Influenza Viruses." In *Influenza: The Cutting Edge*, edited by G. Neumann and Y. Kawaoka, 201–219. Cold Spring Harbor: The Cold Spring Harbor Press.

Williams, Evan P., Briana M. Spruill-Harrell, Mariah K. Taylor, Jasper Lee, Ashley V. Nywening, Zemin Yang, Jacob H. Nichols et al. 2021. "Common themes in zoonotic spillover and disease emergence: lessons learned from bat- and rodent-borne RNA viruses." *Viruses-Basel* 13 (8): 1509.

Wolfe, Nathan D. 2011. *The Viral Storm: The Dawn of a New Pandemic Age*. New York: Henry Holt and Company.

Wolfe, Nathan. D., Claire P. Dunavan, and Jared Diamond. 2007. "Origins of major infectious diseases." *Nature Reviews* 447: 279–283.

Wolfe, Nathan D., A. Tassy Prosser, Jean K. Carr, Ubald Tamoufe, Eitel Mpoudi-Ngole, J. Ndongo Torimiro, Matthew LeBreton, et al. 2004. "Exposure to nonhuman primates in rural Cameroon." *Emerging infectious diseases* 10 (12): 2094.

Wong, Antonio C.P., Xin Li, Susanna K.P. Lau, and Patrick C.Y. Woo. 2019. "Global epidemiology of bat coronaviruses." *Viruses-Basel* 11 (2): 174.

Wong, Antonio C.P., Xin Li, Susanna K.P. Lau, and Patrick C.Y. Woo. 2020. *Novel Coronavirus (2019-nCoV) Situation Report 1.* Geneva: World Health Organization.

Wong, Antonio C.P., Xin Li, Susanna K.P. Lau, and Patrick C.Y. Woo. 2021a. *WHO-convened Global Study of Origins of SARS-CoV-2: China Part.* Joint WHO-China Study Geneva: World Health Organization.

Wong, Antonio C.P., Xin Li, Susanna K.P. Lau, and Patrick C.Y. Woo. 2021b. "Listings of WHO's response to COVID-19." Geneva: World Health Organization. https://www.who.int/news/item/29-06-2020-covidtimeline

World Health Organization. 1978. "Ebola haemorrhagic fever in Sudan, 1976." *Bulletin of the World Health Organization* 56 (2): 247–270.

Xu, Rui, Damian C. Ekiert, Jens C. Krause, Rong Hai, James E. Crowe, Jr., and Ian A. Wilson. 2010. "Structural basis of preexisting immunity to the 2009 H1N1 pandemic influenza virus." *Science* 328 (5976): 357–360. https://doi.org/10.1126/science.1186430

Zhao, Yang, Brad Richardson, Eugene Takle, Lilong Chai, David Schmitt, and Hongwei Xin. 2019. "Airborne transmission may have played a role in the spread of 2015 highly pathogenic avian influenza outbreaks in the United States." *Scientific Reports* 9. https://doi.org/10.1038/s41598-019-47788-z

Zhou, Hong, Jingkai Ji, Xing Chen, Yuhai Bi, Juan Li, Qihui Wang, Tao Hu et al. 2021. "Identification of novel bat coronaviruses sheds light on the evolutionary origins of SARS-CoV-2 and related viruses." *Cell* 184 (17): 4380-+. https://doi.org/10.1016/j.cell.2021.06.008

Zhu, T, B.T. Korber, A.J. Nahmias, E. Hooper, P.M. Sharp, and D.D. Ho. 1998. "An African HIV-1 sequence from 1959 and implications for the origin of the epidemic." *Nature* 391 (6667): 594–597.

CHAPTER 6

Inevitable Resistance

It is not difficult to make microbes resistant to penicillin in the laboratory...and the same thing has occasionally happened in the body.

Sir Alexander Fleming (1945). Nobel lecture.

It is hard to imagine what the world would be like without antimicrobial medicines, the drugs that directly kill or inhibit the growth of most bacteria, many parasites, and fungi, and in recent years, some viruses as well. Eighty-five years ago, a single scratch could result in a "staph" or "strep" infection for which there was no cure, and doctors could do little more than prescribe nutrition, fluids, and rest for major diseases such as tuberculosis (TB), typhoid, and plague. Today, we routinely treat and cure these and many other infections with antimicrobial medicines. Global consumption of antibiotics is more than 35 billion doses a year (Klein et al. 2018). Once hailed as miracle drugs, antimicrobials are now key components of the WHO Essential Medicine List and Model Formulary (World Health Organization 2020). They are routine aspects of clinical treatment in wealthier societies and a primary means of survival in poorer societies bereft of healthy living conditions and access to professional medical services.

Despite advancements in drug development, there are worrisome signs that this antimicrobial era may soon be drawing to a close. Many pathogens are evolving drug resistance faster than we can find new drugs that work against them. While the development of antimicrobial resistance comes as recent news in the popular media, biologists and physicians have been aware of the threat for many decades. Depending on whether one takes an evolutionary or clinical viewpoint, it could be argued that the history of antimicrobial resistance is as

long, or as short, as the history of the antimicrobials themselves.

From an evolutionary perspective, microbes have been competing with each other for more than a billion years. Under a million millennia of selective pressure, microbial species have evolved the ability to produce chemical toxins and protein armaments that inhibit, destroy, and even re-program their competitors. These chemical compounds have served as the molecular starting points for the development of our antimicrobial drugs. With the exception of some dye-based synthetic compounds (the "sulfa drugs"), most first-generation antibiotics, such as penicillin, are derived directly from the natural substances themselves.

It should also be noted that, given a billion years of microbial competition, we should also expect many species have evolved ways to defend themselves by resisting or evading these chemical assaults. We have been identifying antibiotic resistant bacteria in natural settings for some time, but these discoveries have been complicated by questions about how much of the resistance was the result of human contact. Such controversies have largely been laid to rest in recent years with the discoveries of at least 24 resistant organisms in very remote environments such as those found deep within unexplored caves and under the receding ice sheets of Antarctica (Scott et al. 2020). Given these natural, and most likely ancient precedents, it is no surprise that pathogens in environments well-trodden by humans have evolved defenses against our pharmacological efforts to combat them.

Emerging Infections. Second Edition. Ron Barrett, Molly K. Zuckerman, Matthew R. Dudgeon, with George J. Armelagos, Oxford University Press.
© Ron Barrett, Molly K. Zuckerman, Matthew R. Dudgeon (2024). DOI: 10.1093/oso/9780192843135.003.0007

Yet from a clinical viewpoint, we are nevertheless taken aback by the pace of the resistance. Three years after penicillin was first introduced as the "Magic Bullet" and "Wonder Drug" against major bacterial infections, resistant strains of *Staphylococcus aureus* appeared in British and North American hospitals (Zaman 2020). In the next decade, resistance in *Streptococcus pneumoniae* was detected and the first strains of methicillin-resistant *Staphylococcus aureus* (MRSA) appeared among hospitalized patients. Similarly, the first drug-resistant strains of *Mycobacterium tuberculosis*, and its cousin, *M. leprae*, were detected within a decade after antibiotics were introduced for TB and leprosy control.

Today, many pathogen species are resistant to multiple antimicrobial drugs and some are extensively drug resistant. Once confined to clinical settings, an increasing number of infections caused by these pathogens are now endemic to communities around the world. Unless they are soon brought under control, infections caused by vancomycin-resistant *Enterococci* (VRE), drug-resistant *N. gonorrhoeae*, and multidrug- and extensively drug-resistant *M. tuberculosis* (MDR-TB and XDR-TB, respectively) could become major pandemics (CDC 2019; WHO 2020).

The problem has been popularly framed as an interspecies arms race between humans and microbes in which the odds favor the smaller and more numerous combatants. In biosocial terms, it is a problem of host–pathogen evolution in which the rate of genetic adaptation among pathogens exceeds the rate of cultural adaptation among their human hosts. Yet however the problem is framed, it appears that resistance is inevitable as the human world moves toward a post-antimicrobial era in which our best defenses against infectious diseases in the twenty-first century will be little different than those of the nineteenth century.

6.1 Ancient and traditional antimicrobials

Long before modern vaccines and antibiotics, societies around the world used a variety of traditional medicines for the treatment and prevention of infectious diseases (Plotkin 2005). Many of these medicines did have some efficacy, and some have since been adopted into the pharmacopeia of Western biomedicine. More than a thousand years before Edward Jenner gave his first vaccination, Indian Ayurvedic physicians, and priests of the smallpox goddess, Shitala Ma, inoculated people by scratching their skin with scab preparations obtained from those infected with a milder strain of the virus, *Variola minor*. A similar practice was described in traditional Chinese medical texts. This method, known as variolation, conferred partial immunity to the deadlier strain of the virus, *Variola major* (Boylston 2012).

The British royal family began variolating its members in the early eighteenth century, after which the practice was quickly adopted in Europe and North America. One well-publicized study at the time showed that people who had been variolated were 10 times more likely to survive a *V. major* infection than those who were not (Klebs 1913). As a child, Jenner himself was inoculated using this ancient technique, which he later improved by substituting *V. minor* for a cowpox preparation (Hopkins 2002). Jenner received worldwide recognition for this improved method, which became known as vaccination.

Yet even then, Jenner's "discovery" was based on earlier ethnomedical knowledge. English dairy farmers had long known about the protective effects of cowpox (Jenner 2020 [1798]). One of these farmers, Benjamin Jesty, vaccinated his family and two of his children twenty five years before Jenner's experiments. The Jennerian Society would later recognize Jesty was the first person to "personally institute . . . the vaccine pock inoculation, . . . (and) provide decisive proofs of the permanent anti-variolous effects of the Cow Pock" (Gross and Sepkowitz 1998: 58). The Jennerian Society invited Jesty to London, commissioned a portrait of him, and gave him a small monetary award. Having thus been recognized, Jesty returned to his farm.

Variolation was also practiced throughout China for at least a dozen centuries as one of many traditional Chinese medicines for boosting immunity and fighting fever-related diseases (Plotkin 2005). These traditional medicines included *Qinghao*, a tea prescribed for intermittent fevers. *Qinghao* was rediscovered in the 1960s by a joint team of Chinese pharmacologists and textual scholars who were seeking to develop new biomedicines from ancient remedies (Hsu and Barrett 2009). One of *Qinghao*'s major ingredients was an extract of *Artemisia annua*—also known as "sweet worm-wood" or "Sweet Annie"—a turquoise, fern-like herb with a camphor scent that is commonly found in temperate regions around the world.

Further testing of the wormwood extract allowed for the isolation of a particular compound that is highly effective for treating malaria, schistosomi-asis, and other parasitic infections. The discovery of this substance, known as artemisinin, led to a Nobel Prize for Tu Youyou of China (Fu 2015). Presently, the World Health Organization (WHO) recommends artemisinin as a first-line therapy for *Plasmodium falciparum* malaria, one of the deadliest and most prevalent forms of the disease. It should be noted, however, that because of the recent emer-gence of partially resistant *Plasmodium* parasites, artemisinin is currently being used in combination with other antimicrobial medications (World Health Organization 2015).

In addition to the use of antimicrobial herbs, some ancient societies ingested what we would con-sider to be a proper antibiotic today. In the late 1970s, Deborah Martin was conducting her doc-toral research in biological anthropology, examin-ing bone remodeling in order to improve her under-standing of the health of Sudanese Nubians who lived along the Nile River between 350 and 550 CE. At one point, she needed a standard light micro-scope to check her measurements on some very thin sections of bone. None was available at that moment so she resorted to an ultraviolet microscope and was surprised to see an unusual yellow-green glow. With further chemical analysis, the source of that glow would prove to be tetracycline molecules bound to the calcium within the tissue (Bassett et al. 1980). The discovery was like unwrapping a mummy, only to find the corpse wearing earphones and a pair of sunglasses.

There is, however, a reasonable explanation for this discovery. Tetracycline is a naturally occur-ring substance excreted by soil microbes, proba-bly as an adaptive mechanism for gaining advan-tage over competing species through a mechanism called antibiosis, the namesake of modern antibi-otics. Even so, Martin's discovery was met with some disbelief. Because of its natural origins, the tetracycline in the Nubian skeletons could have resulted from process known as taphonomic infil-tration: post-mortem contamination by invading microorganisms that occurred as the body decom-posed, or during the centuries of burial in the ground (Piepenbrink et al. 1983).

It turned out that taphonomic contamination was not the probable cause of tetracycline in these ancient Nubians. The analysis of collagen and osteons indicated excellent preservation of these remains, with natural mummification that resisted invading organisms. Furthermore, closer examina-tion revealed patterns of deposition that are consis-tent with long-term tetracycline ingestion by living people (Nelson et al. 2010). Moreover, these patterns clearly indicate long-term tetracycline consumption during the formative stages of bone development in the early years of life. Similar evidence has been found in neighboring societies: a 2,000-year-old Jor-danian population, and a group of Egyptians that lived during the Roman occupation between 400 and 500 CE (Armelagos et al. 2001).

Although we know these societies consumed tetracycline, we can only hypothesize their means or motives for doing so. Bread and beer are plausi-ble vehicles. Both were staple foods, the beer having been brewed for nutrition rather than intoxication. Some ancient Egyptian and Nubian recipes include steps that could easily lead to the molding of grains similar to the blue, penicillin-like streaks found on certain cheeses. Two undergraduates at Emory Uni-versity demonstrated how these recipes could pro-duce tetracyclines by experimentally adding *Strep-tomyces* organisms at various stages of the cooking process (Armelagos et al. 2001). As to motives, some Egyptian texts prescribe beer as a treatment for a variety of ills to include gum disease, vaginitis, and wound infections. However, they do not describe a specific kind of yeast, one that would have been bacterially contaminated and traceable to the tetra-cycline found in those skeletons.

We should not be surprised by these discover-ies of ancient treatments. Throughout the world's diverse ecosystems, biologists have identified hun-dreds of plant and animal substances with antimi-crobial activities (Górniak et al. 2019; Rios and Recio 2005). It is reasonable to expect that people who lived in and near these environments would have made similar discoveries through trial and error over many generations, even if they did not have accurate explanations for how they worked.

Indeed, pharmaceutical companies often bank on this expectation. Rather than conduct exhaustive, "brute-force" searches of all the world's flora and fauna, which would be very impractical and expensive, these companies send field researchers to far corners of the globe to gather ingredients used in traditional medicines. The ingredients are then brought back to the laboratory, where their constituent compounds are extracted, isolated, and tested for biomedical efficacy. These activities are collectively known as pharmacognosy, or by the more popular terms, "bioprospecting" and "medicine hunting" (cf. Reid 1993). Over the years, the hunting has proven to be quite successful. Of the 210 small molecule drugs in the WHO's List of Essential Medicines, 139 of these substances have been derived or modified from natural sources (Jones et al. 2006). Many of these substances have been used as ingredients for traditional medicines.

That said, pharmacognosy has significant shortcomings. There are a problems with attribution and intellectual property rights. All too often, traditional healers and their communities do not receive sufficient credit or economic benefit from these discoveries, if any recognition at all (Wilcox et al. 2015). Additionally, because of its focus on finding individual (patentable) molecules, pharmacognosy rarely considers the broader contexts in which traditional medicines are used (Etkin and Elisabetsky 2005). The contexts include the interactions of therapeutic substances with other elements of the healing process, not just the pharmacological ones, and the role of these therapies in particular belief systems and social relationships. Such investigations are usually made by ethnopharmacologists, specially trained ethnographers who attempt to bridge our cultural and biological understandings of traditional healing. It should also be noted that unlike the pharmacognocist, the ethnopharmacologist typically operates outside the financial interests of the pharmaceutical industry.

It is difficult to summarize the findings of ethnopharmacology without running the risk of overgeneralization. That said, we can identify a few common themes in these studies of traditional healing systems, even if the themes are by no means universal. Some follow the predictions above: that societies who develop biologically effective medicines have typically done so after observing the effects of different substances on the human body over the course of many generations. Another is that the accumulated wisdom of these observations need not rely on biomedical beliefs about why these medicines work.

Indeed, the same can be said for biomedicine itself. In most industrialized countries, years of research and bureaucratic hurdles are required to approve a biomedicine for official use. But these efforts are focused on demonstrating the efficacy, safety, and relative risks of a candidate drug compared with other treatments. They are not as focused on the reasons why that drug works the way it does. Browse any biomedical drug reference, and you will find approved medications for which the mechanisms of action are not yet known. In these cases, biomedicine relies on empirical observations independent of its own causal theories. The empiricism may be more systematic, but the overall approach is similar to the trial and error of many non-biomedical healing traditions.

Lastly, an important theme of this chapter is that traditional medicines are frequently based on extensive ecological knowledge. In Chapter 1, we saw how the subsistence practices of foraging societies require detailed knowledge of flora and fauna in order to meet people's nutritional needs in diverse and changing environments. The same could be said for the environmental knowledge required to meet people's therapeutic needs. Brent Berlin's comprehensive study of traditional taxonomies reflects this kind of ecological knowledge, with foraging societies describing a greater number and variety of taxa than agricultural societies in the same local environments (Berlin 1992). Many of these taxa are, in turn, associated with health and disease categories within belief systems that emphasize people's relationships to one another and the species around them—Indigenous theories of human ecology.

Human ecology is also a frequently occurring theme among major textual healing traditions

(Hsu and Barrett 2009). Indian Ayurvedic medicine considers human health characteristics based on factors such as seasonal climates, personal habits, and interpersonal relationships, as well as the different balances of humor-like *doshas* that govern all living creatures in the middle world. Traditional Chinese medicine accounts for similar health factors in the context of five winds, dynamic balances of *yin* and *yang*, and flows of *qi* energy that permeate the natural and supernatural alike. Tracing its origins to Classical Greece, the Islamic healers of *Unaani Tib* maintain their emphasis on human physical constitutions based on the particular social and physical environments in which people were raised, principles reflected in the writings of Galen and Hippocrates.

Hippocrates is often attributed to the aphorism: "It is more important to know what sort of person has a disease than what disease has a person." Although apocryphal, this exemplifies the Hippocratic approach to healing by which the physician must examine more than just the patient's body but also his or her personal relationships with surrounding physical, biological, and social environments (Lawrence et al. 2017). Because of this, Hippocrates and his co-authors are often considered to be founding philosophers of a human ecology of health, not just of Western biomedicine per se. Unfortunately, however, biomedicine has since narrowed much of its attention to pathogens and bodies while searching for singular causes of individual diseases, often at the expense of understanding broader environmental relationships.

6.2 From soil and seed to magic bullets

Writing in the last years of the nineteenth century, Timothy McGillicuddy, a New York obstetrician, employed an agricultural metaphor to describe the ecology of a TB infection. In deference to Germ Theory, he acknowledged the recently discovered mycobacteria to be the "seed" of the disease, stating that *M. tuberculosis* had been "defined and described until there is no more doubt as to its nature and characteristics than there is about a grain of wheat." But as with the wheat grain, this microorganism "does not always sprout where it falls; if the tubercle bacillus attacked everyone exposed to its influence, the

[human] race would have been exterminated ere this. Not only seed but soil is essential to the crop" (McGillicuddy 1898: 1396).

By the time of McGillicuddy's writing, seed and soil were popular metaphors among an increasing number of European and North American physicians who had recently converted from Miasma Theory to Germ Theory but who also continued to recognize the importance of pre-existing health conditions and surrounding environments for the development of infectious diseases (Barnes 1995). As we saw in Chapter 3, contagionists and anticontagionists had been waging a hard-fought battle since the mid-nineteenth century—a conflict fueled by social and economic considerations as much as the ambiguity of scientific evidence (Ackerknecht [1948] 2009). By the 1880s, Germ Theory was prevailing within the Western biomedical community, but despite the growing academic emphasis on the microscopic seeds of infection, the clinical practice of biomedicine was still firmly rooted in the soil of sanitary reform.

We now know that Germ Theory is not exclusive of sanitary practice. Indeed, the discovery of pathogens further supported the virtues of clean environments for preventing disease transmission. As such, the recognition of both seed and soil could have informed a new holistic approach to infection, one that considered the interactions between microscopic and macroscopic worlds. But these metaphors did not signal a holistic perspective so much as a disjuncture between theory and practice. Seed and soil informed different kinds of medical activities. One was more academic and better geared to further research. The other was more applied and better geared to clinical practice.

On the academic side, microbiologists were discovering new pathogens at every turn. But on the clinical side, Germ Theory offered little new for the practice of medicine until well into the twentieth century. Robert Koch discovered *M. tuberculosis* 16 years before Dr. McGillicuddy wrote about the soil and seed of consumption, but it would be another 40 years before the development of effective biomedicines for this disease. In the absence of such developments, McGillicuddy believed that the best therapy was to cleanse the body of contaminants and provide exercise, rest, and good nutrition. He felt the latter was especially important, stating an old maxim: "If you take care of the stomach, the lungs will take care of themselves" (1898: 1397). Recalling the lessons of Chapter 3, McKeown would have approved of these measures, as they were largely responsible for the decline of infectious diseases from the beginning of the Second Epidemiological Transition to the end of the Second World War (1988).

In the early twentieth century, biomedical attention began shifting from the interactions of seed and soil to the characteristics of the seeds alone. This arose with the discoveries of new medicines that were selectively toxic to microbial pathogens but did little or no harm to human tissue cells. The clues to these discoveries appeared as soon as the first microbiologists began identifying bacterial species and associating them with specific diseases. In 1887, a year after Robert Koch first demonstrated Germ Theory with his early anthrax experiments, Louis Pasteur observed that the causative bacteria, *Bacillus anthracis*, could be inhibited in the presence of unspecified bacteria found in soil and putrefied animal blood (Sams et al. 2014). Ten years later, Rudolph Emmerrich and Oscar Löw discovered that a bluish substance produced by *Pseudomonas aeruginosa* could inhibit the growth of several disease-causing bacteria. Emmerich later found that animals infected with streptococci bacteria did not develop cholera (Aminov 2017).

Paul Ehrlich was an early leader in these discoveries. Guided by Koch's success in identifying *M. tuberculosis*, Ehrlich focused on selective staining techniques for visualizing particular microorganisms. From this, he hypothesized that the unique characteristics of bacterial walls allowed them to absorb, or adhere to, certain stains and dyes while the cells of surrounding human tissues could not. Ehrlich reasoned that some of these stains and dyes might also be selectively toxic to bacteria, thereby killing pathogens while leaving the host unharmed. Inspired by the self-guided projectiles of Norse mythology, Ehrlich dubbed these selective toxins *Magic Bullets* (Winau et al. 2004).

The Magic Bullet approach became famous with the early successes of Ehrlich and his colleagues, many of whom were working for the pharmaceutical divisions of German dye companies (Amyes 2001). Ehrlich developed an arsenic-based compound known as Salvarsan (a.k.a. Arsphenamine or Compound 606) which had more success against syphilis and African trypanosomiasis than any previous treatment (Williams 2009). Ehrlich's former assistant, Julius Morgenroth, discovered a quinine-derived dye, known as Optochin, that not only stained *Streptococcus pneumoniae* but also inhibited the growth of this and other bacterial pathogens. Yet although these and other early synthetic drugs appeared promising, they also carried significant side effects. Salvarsan injections were intensely painful, and the drug often led to skin reactions and sometimes, kidney damage (Guy 1919). Optochin carried a high risk for blindness (von Hippel 1916).[1] For many patients, there was little 'magic' in these 'bullets'.

The first major success came with a synthetic red dye derivative with the trade name Prontonsil, a sulfonamide that proved even more effective against *S. pneumonia* than Optochin, but without the same degree of side effects. Following on the heels of Erlich and Morgenrath, Gerard Domagk discovered its antimicrobial properties in the mid-1930s while working as a managing chemist for Bayer (Lesch 2006). After a long series of methodical trials, Prontosil became a widely used antimicrobial medication, made famous for saving the life of Franklin Roosevelt's son. Perhaps more importantly, it became the prototype for an entire class of medications known as "sulfa drugs" that we continue to use today.

Prontosil was biomedicine's first effective antimicrobial drug, but penicillin proved an even greater success by curing more gram-positive bacterial infections with even fewer side effects, except for the allergic reactions that occurred in 8 to 12 percent of patients. The story of penicillin has been well documented, and important elements of the story are widely known: Alexander Fleming's "accidental" discovery, the initial resistance to his finding within the scientific community, the subsequent decade in which it was ignored, its reinvestigation by Edward Florey and Ernst Chain, the search and selection for a more productive strain, a moldy cantaloupe, early treatments for victims of the Coconut Grove Fire, and of course, the Nobel Prize (Goldsworthy and McFarlane 2002; Lax 2004).

Heroic narratives notwithstanding, penicillin represented an entirely different approach to antimicrobial discovery. Instead of searching for drug compounds among synthetic dyes and stains, the discovery of penicillin proved that humans could harness the naturally occurring weapons that microorganisms deploy against each another. These natural weapons were often secreted by fungi against bacteria in a process that microbiologists refer to as antibiosis. As such, penicillin became the first true "antibiotic" in the strictest sense of the word. It also became the poster drug for Magic Bullet medicine.

Following the Second World War, penicillin became widely distributed among the public, to whom it was touted as a "Wonder Drug" that could cure all manner of human diseases, including the scourges of baldness and bad breath. There was even a penicillin lipstick for those concerned about "hygienic kissing" (Brown 2004). But aside from the surrounding hype and quackery, penicillin proved effective against many staphylococcal and streptococcal infections. Even today, it is the preferred treatment for primary syphilis. All told, penicillin is thus far responsible for saving more than a 100 million lives (Amyes 2001).

No drug is free from the risk of side effects. In the case of penicillin, the risk has been epistemological as well as physiological—the history of penicillin has fundamentally affected biomedical approaches to illness and healing. The success of penicillin enshrined the Magic Bullet concept in the teaching and practice of biomedicine, displacing other more holistic approaches that address the soil as well as the seeds of human infectious diseases. Since then, the majority of medical research funding (public and private) has been devoted to the molecular characteristics of pathogens over the state of human hosts and their surrounding environments. Moreover, the language used to think about these problems has become increasingly militaristic, such that medicines are seen as weapons for destroying enemy diseases. As a result, biomedical approaches to disease have often reduced complex relationships of humans with each other and their socio-economic environments to biological problems with single causes and convenient solutions. At the same time, most biomedical research has focused attention and resources on laboratory investigation at the molecular level of pathogens, pharmaceuticals, and their interactions with human cells and signaling pathways, at the expense of investigating the social and ecological determinants of human health and disease.

The eminent microbiologist, Rene Dubos, referred to this reductive approach as the "Doctrine of Singular Etiology." He believed this doctrine was largely responsible for the naïve optimism that biomedical science would eventually cure all human ills, infectious diseases among them (Dubos 1987). As an alternative to this approach, Dubos promoted an ecological view of humans and microbes as participants in a complex web of interactions. Some of these interactions are commensal, insofar as the microorganism derives benefit without affecting its human host; this is the case for many species of microbes that live in our digestive tracts or on the surface of our skin and mucous membranes. Under healthy conditions, these microflorae coexist, cooperate, and compete with one another to maintain a certain balance of their respective populations. They can also aid the host in digestion or act as immune defenses by keeping pathogenic organisms in check.

Disease occurs when these ecological balances are disrupted, either by an external change in the host's surrounding environment or an internal change within the host that may involve diet, stress, the presence of non-infectious diseases, or the presence of other pathogens. Under these conditions, protective microbial populations may decline, or their relationship to the host shifts from commensalism or mutualism, to parasitism and potential disease.

Infectious diseases are not a simple matter of a single species of pathogen invading a generic human host in an environmental vacuum. Like McGillicuddy, many nineteenth-century physicians understood this, evoking the concept of soil and seed to wed the new Germ Theory to sanitary medicine. In defense of present-day biomedicine, at least some twenty-first-century clinicians understand this as well, but many others are either distracted by the latest Magic Bullets, or perhaps more often, their practices are constrained by the structural barriers of health and insurance systems that were built on the Doctrine of Singular Etiology.

The ecological approach has also proven effective in medical research. Dubos applied it in his laboratory experiments, which led to his developing a methodology for isolating and identifying antibiotic-producing organisms amid the many microbial species living in soil and other natural sources. Most notably, Dubos' method was applied or adapted to the discovery of nearly every core antibiotic molecule since erythromycin (Amyes 2001). The approach was also a forerunner to the many recent microbiome studies aimed at understanding interactions among myriad populations of different bacteria, fungi, protozoa, and viruses that live in and on the bodies of humans and other animals—microscopic ecosystems that are more diverse and complicated than any major rainforest in the macro world (Gilbert et al. 2018).

Lastly, Rene Dubos' ecological consideration of pathogen–pathogen interactions, as well as those of pathogen pathology, laid much of the groundwork for our thinking about syndemics today. It is ironic that for the breadth of his thinking, Rene Dubos would be best known for his contributions to antibiotic discovery, focusing attention on the medicinal products of his ecological ideas while ignoring the ideas themselves.

6.3 The human use of antibiotics today

The evolution of antimicrobial resistance is as old as life itself, but humanity is currently accelerating the process. The speed of this evolution can be observed with a simple laboratory experiment by covering an agar plate (a.k.a. Petri dish) with a thin layer of antibiotic. We then use a sterilized wire loop to inoculate the plate with a small spot of pure bacterial culture and streak it across the surface in a series of squiggly lines to spread them out. Depending on the drug and the bacterial species, we might expect the antibiotic to kill all the bacteria on the plate, or at least inhibit them from growing any further. But after incubating the plate overnight, we often discover colonies of the same bacteria growing on the plate. These new colonies are resistant to that antibiotic.

That initial "spot" typically contains about a billion bacterial cells. So even if there is only a one-in-a-100-million chance that any single bacterium would win the lottery by possessing a rare advantageous trait, or new mutation, that would allow it to survive the antibiotic, we could reasonably predict about 10 lottery winners among a billion bacteria. Those 10 lucky bacteria would then multiply exponentially, producing trillions of bacteria in less than a day

This one-day experiment is a quick way to demonstrate the rapid evolution of antimicrobial resistance under the selective pressure of an antibiotic. It is important to note, however, that the antibiotic did not *cause* the mutations that led to the resistance trait. That trait arose through random mutation. Rather, the antibiotic *selected* for the resistance trait by allowing those particular varieties of bacteria to reproduce while other varieties could not, thus increasing the frequency of resistance in the population. When this happens in nature, the process is known as natural selection. When it happens in a laboratory, a hospital, or at home, then the process is known as artificial selection.

We perform an artificial selection experiment every time we use an antibiotic, and we accelerate the experiment even further when we misuse an antibiotic. Here, the misuse usually falls into one of two categories: ineffective use and overuse. (Ventola 2015). Ineffective use occurs when the type or dose of an antibiotic does not completely kill or inhibit the particular species or strain associated with the infection, or when the course of an antibiotic is sporadic, too short, or prematurely terminated.

Yet unlike the bacteria we described in the previous laboratory experiment, pathogenic bacteria do not usually become resistant with a single mutation. If that were the case, our antibiotics would not have been effective in the first place. Instead, most pathogens acquire resistance in a series of mutations that confer partial resistance with each stage. The under-use of antibiotics increases the odds of these stepwise mutations by allowing some partially resistant (a.k.a. incompletely sensitive) organisms to survive that might otherwise be killed with a sufficient dose of medication over a subscribed period of time. The surviving generation might then require a larger or stronger dose of the antibiotic, or else it will have the opportunity to play the lottery once again; some of those survivors may acquire even further resistance, and so the cycle continues.

Microbiologists can measure degrees of resistance according to the amount of antibiotic it takes to prevent visible growth in *in vitro* culture, using a measure known as the minimum inhibitory concentration (MIC) (see Figure 6.1). Under the selective pressure of an antibiotic, the MIC increases to a breakpoint beyond which the dose is toxic to the human host. When that happens, the pathogen is considered fully resistant to the antibiotic.

Solving the problems of ineffective use is often more challenging than may first appear. Underuse may be a matter of educating health providers and their patients, but education is not a simple matter of pouring knowledge into an empty vessel (Rodriguez 2012). For education to be effective, it must be meaningful and relevant to people's beliefs and practices, which may sometimes be more accurate or more effective than those of biomedicine (Kleinman 1989). All too often, patients

have histories of distrust or miscommunication with their providers, requiring a slow rebuilding of these relationships over time.

Even when these factors are addressed, poor access to medical resources often results in self-medication when antibiotics can be readily obtained without a prescription in local community pharmacies along with free advice from whomever is working behind the counter (Kamat and Nichter 1998; Sakeena et al. 2018). This pattern is commonly seen in low- and middle-income countries throughout the world, where infections of the gut, bladder, and upper respiratory tract are a regular part of daily life. In these instances, self-medication most often involves the use of broad-spectrum antibiotics (Auta et al. 2019).

Similar factors apply to the over-use of antibiotics, but this problem is often harder to identify and define due to incomplete reporting, undocumented

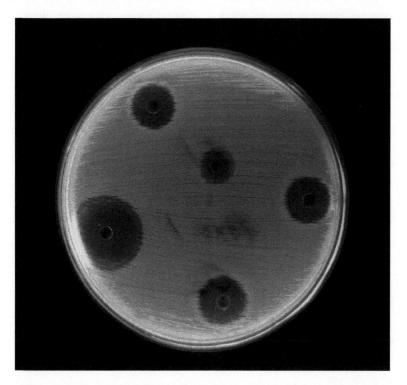

Figure 6.1 A drug sensitivity test, with five antibiotic substances placed on an agar plate that has been covered with *Staphylococcus aureus* bacteria. The clear circles around the drugs indicate areas of inhibition against the bacteria. The concentration of the drug diminishes as it diffuses from the center, until reaches the minimum inhibitory concentration (MIC) where it can no longer prevent bacterial growth. More sensitive bacteria leave wider rings, while more resistant bacteria would leave no clear rings at all.

Source: Don Stalons. CDC Public Health Image Library #2641.

use without a prescription, and the inability to determine, at a population level, which instances of prescribed use were appropriate. Yet even with these challenges, we could still argue that the massive scale of their adoption by human societies constitutes over-use on a global scale. From 2000 to 2015, global antibiotic consumption increased 65 percent, from 21.1 to 34.8 billion defined daily doses (DDDs) (Klein et al. 2018). The increases occurred throughout the 65 participating countries, but once again, the highest increases occurred in low- to middle-income countries.

Responding to these trends, the WHO launched the Global Antimicrobial Surveillance System (GLASS) to monitor resistant infections and antimicrobial consumption; they also launched an AWaRe database to classify antibiotics based on priority of use and potential for resistance (WHO 2018).

Unfortunately, these monitoring efforts reveal that more than 40 percent of countries are consuming an increasing percentage of broader spectrum antibiotics with higher potentials for resistance (Klein et al. 2020). This trend is especially troubling when we consider that many of these medicines are intended as second- and third-line treatments for infections that are already resistant to the older drugs.

Considering the short history of antimicrobial medicines, these trends are especially alarming. Figure 6.2 shows the emergence of resistant strains only a few years after the discovery and adoption of major antibiotics. It is also alarming to note that many of these earlier resistant strains emerged at a time when antibiotics were not as accessible as they are today, but even the lesser use of these medications brought resistance anyway.

This situation would not be so bad if the rate of our technical achievements outpaced the evolution of our pathogens. Unfortunately, this has not been the case. At present, there are microbes with one or more resistance mechanisms to every major class of antibiotics. Even more troubling, it has been more than thirty years since a truly new antibiotic class was discovered (WHO 2017). Among the existing drug classes, there are several dozen potential medications in the research pipeline, but science moves slowly, and even these medicines will not fully address the growing threat

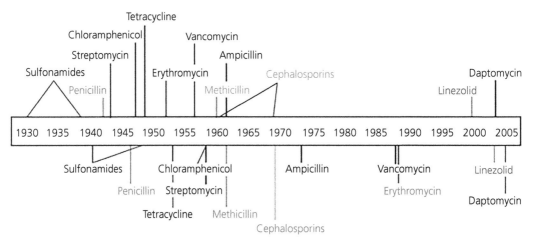

Figure 6.2 Timeline illustrating the rate of antibiotic development from 1940 to 2000. The rate of antibiotic development has tapered in recent decades while that of antibiotic resistance has increased.

Source: Clatworthy, Ann, Emily Pierson & Deborah T Hung (2007) Nature Chemical Biology 3, 541 - 548 Published online: 20 August 2007 doi:10.1038/nchembio.2007.24.

of antimicrobial resistance. Thus far, pathogens are adapting at a much faster rate than their human hosts.

In an effort to decrease global antibiotic consumption, the WHO recommends curtailing use for prophylaxis and for typically self-resolving infections such as non-febrile diarrhea or pediatric ear infections (World Health Organization 2015). Prophylactic use may be the easiest to forego, as patients are not yet faced with difficult symptoms. But it may be more difficult to avoid antibiotics for minor infections, especially for the impoverished majority of the world that lacks either the time or the money to give up days of productive work when quick relief, or in some cases, the perception of relief, can be found with a few generic pills costing less than half the daily wage of an unskilled laborer.

Another major form of over-use is the consumption of antibiotics that have no efficacy against the infection, such as when an antibiotic for one class of bacteria is used for another, or quite commonly, when it is used against viruses for which it has no effect whatsoever. These behaviors are certainly wasteful and possibly detrimental to a patient who might otherwise find a better treatment. Yet in terms of resistance, they might seem relatively harmless insofar as they could do no worse for an already resistant pathogen. Not so, especially when we recall the phenomenon of horizontal gene transfer from the previous chapter.

In the same ways that many bacteria can transfer genes for virulence, they can also transfer genes for antibiotic resistance between one another. As with virulence genes, resistance genes can be encoded into plasmids, transposable sequences, and even viruses that infect bacteria. Now consider that antibiotics not only create a selective environment for pathogens but also for many species of commensal bacteria in our bodies. Some of these commensal species evolve antibiotic resistant genes which they can then transfer to potential pathogens. Others pass these genes on, having acquired them from previous infections, or from other resistant microflora that had been growing in antibiotic laden foods—a topic which we will turn to shortly. In the interim, it is important to note that the genes for pathogen resistance can often be passed horizontally between strains and species of bacteria, and the spread of these genes is strongly mediated by the ways we use and misuse these medications.

6.4 Antibiotics in commercial agriculture

Stuart Levy taught antibiotic resistance with a tomato. A physician and leading researcher on the topic, Levy had his medical students conduct an experiment in which they sliced a tomato with a sterile knife, briefly touched the knife to an agar plate covered with nutrients, and then incubated the plate overnight at body temperature. By the next morning, the plate was speckled with colonies of bacteria from the tomato, 10 percent of which were resistant to one or more antibiotics without the selective presence of any additional drugs in the first place (Levy 2002).

In a field study of Boston food markets, Levy and his colleagues found 10,000 to 100,000 antibiotic-resistant bacteria for each gram of vegetable they sampled. While none of these bacteria were harmful, 10 to 20 percent were capable of colonizing human intestines, where they could transfer these resistance genes to other potentially pathogenic species (Levy 2002). In a larger study, the introduction of three common antibiotics induced resistance among bacteria found in lettuce plant roots and their surrounding soil, from which 56 antibiotic resistance genes were identified with activity against 14 antimicrobial drug families (Cerqueira et al. 2020). In both studies, resistance levels were far greater than those found in wild plant environments.

How did this resistance arise? It might have been because of the antibiotics used in commercial crop production. Human antibiotics are routinely combined with insecticides and herbicides, and then sprayed on commercial fruit trees and vegetables in the United States. Recently, the US Environmental Protection Agency recently approved the use of over a million pounds a year of human antibiotics for citrus trees alone, the equivalent of 450 million daily human doses (US EPA 2018a; 2018b). These antibiotics include tetracycline and streptomycin compounds that are commonly used to treat human infections

Even larger quantities are used on livestock for commercial meat production. In the United States, about nine times more antibiotics are administered to domesticated animals than humans, mostly in the form of sub-therapeutic doses that are 1 to 10 percent of the amount needed to cure most infections (Rohr et al. 2019). The United States is not alone in these practices; most of the world's large-scale animal growers treat their livestock with low-dose antibiotics (see Figure 6.3).

For more than half a century, the primary aim of antibiotic use in livestock has not been to prevent or treat infections but to accelerate animal growth. The use of antibiotics as growth promoters was discovered by accident in the 1950s. Chickens that had been fed a vitamin B12 supplement put on more weight at faster rates than those that were not. However, it turned out that the supplement was contaminated with tetracycline and the latter was responsible for the accelerated growth. The most accepted explanation for this phenomenon is that the antibiotic suppresses large quantities of commensal bacteria that help digest plant cellulose in exchange for their share of the meal. But commercial feed does not require such digestion, so the bacteria become a liability. Suppress these bacteria and the animals obtain more energy per meal, thereby resulting in faster growth (Amyes 2001).

The commercial agriculture industry is highly competitive and farmers operate on narrow profit margins. A few days difference in growth rates can spell success or ruin for a farmer or commodities trader. Consequently, antibiotic growth factors have become essential ingredients of food production. Beginning with the Swann Report, written by Stuart Levy's research team in 1969, major studies about the impact of these practices on the emergence of drug-resistant bacteria eventually led many countries, including the United Kingdom and the European Union, to pass regulations against using antibiotics as growth factors if they are commonly prescribed for human patients (Zaman 2020).

The United States, however, was much slower to pass these regulations, so it is not surprising that by the late 1980s, the rate of tetracycline resistance in the *E. coli* of food producing animals in the United States was 96 percent, and the rate for ampicillin resistance was 77 percent (Amyes 2001). These antibiotics, and their sister compounds, are among the most commonly prescribed medications for human patients around the world. Their use as animal growth factors could render them ineffective at a much faster rates than if they were solely used for human infections.

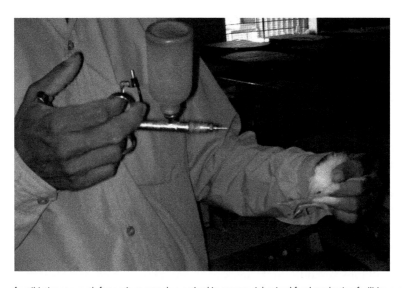

Figure 6.3 The use of antibiotics as growth factors is commonly practiced in commercial animal food production facilities around the world. Here we see the administration of antibiotics to a baby chick in a commercial poultry facility in India.
Source: Photograph by Ron Barrett

More recently, the US Food and Drug Administration (US FDA), in consultation with the Center for Veterinary Medicine, has issued agriculture industry guidelines for phasing out the use of human antibiotics for "production purposes" (US FDA 2013). And although these guidelines are non-binding recommendations, the industries have been largely responsive. However, the guidelines still allow for the prophylactic use of these drugs when there is a risk of specific infections, and given the living conditions of most commercial livestock, these risks are very high. European Union regulations have a similar loophole, and in many low- and middle-income countries, the guidelines and regulations are absent altogether.

The health implications of these practices are starkly apparent. About 15 percent of all poultry, turkey, ground beef, and large-scale commercial poultry are infected with salmonella (NACMCF 2019). Most of these strains have little or no effect on the animals. Nevertheless, some of these strains are resistant to as many as five different antibiotics. These strains can be passed to humans through the consumption of meat and eggs, causing severe and sometimes life-threatening infections. *Campylobacter* species, which are a leading cause of human food-borne infections, are also commonly found in poultry with resistance rates up to 18 percent (Economou and Gousia 2015). MRSA is also commonly found in nasal swabs of cattle, and resistant gram-negative bacteria are increasingly prevalent among cattle, chicken, and pigs. The latter are especially troubling, given their propensity for the horizontal transfer of resistance genes to other bacterial species, including commensal flora in the human gut.

Even the agricultural use of non-human antibiotics can pose significant risks. Many of these molecules resemble their human counterparts, and many resistance mechanisms apply to similar molecules. Case in point: strains of vancomycin-resistant *Enteroccocus faecium* were found in Danish farm animals that had been taking avoparcin (Bager et al. 2000). Although avoparcin is a non-human antibiotic growth factor, the molecule is very similar to that of vancomycin. This finding is particularly troubling because vancomycin is often reserved as an antibiotic of last resort for infections that might otherwise be incurable, such as MRSA. Similarly, the use of ciprofloxin-like growth factors has resulted in cipro-resistant *Camphylobacter* strains in commercial poultry (Economou and Gousia (2015). Ciprofloxacin and its related compounds are among the leading broad-spectrum antibiotics for serious gastrointestinal infections such as typhoid fever, lower respiratory infections, urinary tract infections, and gonorrhea.

Eleven-thousand years ago, the domestication of animals brought humans into closer contact with zoonotic infectious diseases. Today, the medication of these same animals has accelerated the evolution of antibiotic resistance (Beceiro et al. 2013; Schroeder et al. 2017). In Chapter 5, we examined the super-urbanization of food animals and its consequences for the amplification and spread of new and virulent infections. This same principle applies to the amplification and spread of antibiotic resistance.

Returning to the tomato, we should note that even the staunchest organic vegan is at risk for the drug-resistant consequences of commercial animal production. The average commercially raised dairy cow produces more than 100 times the feces of the average human. As such, they are potential "factor[ies] for the production and dispersion of antibiotic resistant bacteria" (Marshall and Levy 2011: 719). Multiply these cows by a billion and you have 60 percent of the total biomass of manure from domesticated animals. Include the waste from chickens and pigs and that total comes to about 13 billion tons of manure per year. Much of this waste becomes fertilizer, leaching into groundwater, channeling through irrigation canals, and increasing the risk of contaminating drinking water.

Along with other toxic compounds, fertilizer is rich with many varieties of bacteria. In the absence of antibiotics, manure derived bacteria are often poorly adapted to environments outside the farms from which they originated. But when these bacteria are resistant to the antibiotic residues and toxins contained within the same manure, they have a significant advantage over their microbial competition and will proliferate accordingly. This is also the case for any local bacteria that receive resistance genes from the manure bacteria via horizontal transfer. The result is widespread dissemination of antimicrobial resistance genes across many different ecosystems around the world, including our living areas and food supplies.

6.5 Antimicrobial resistance and vulnerable host populations

In Chapter 5, we examined how poverty, aging, and rising rates of noninfectious diseases increase the vulnerability of human host populations to novel zoonotic infections by lowering the threshold of interspecies spillover and providing reservoirs for the evolution of human-to-human transmission. The same principles apply to antimicrobial resistance.

Although multidrug-resistant bacteria are often described as "superbugs," they are often less virulent and less fit, evolutionarily speaking, than susceptible strains of the same species. This is because many drug-resistance traits often confer a fitness cost to the organism, requiring additional energy and disrupting important cellular processes (Blair et al. 2015; Melnyk et al. 2015). For instance, some bacteria acquire the ability to restrict the entry of certain antibiotic molecules by reducing the permeability of their outer membranes. But decreased permeability often restricts the entry of nutrients as well. Bacterial ribosomes, the organelles largely responsible for protein manufacture, can become "invisible" to the antibiotics that target them because of slight distortions in their structure. But these same distortions also make them less efficient in protein synthesis. And while some bacteria can produce enzymes that destroy certain kinds of antibiotic molecules, this added production diverts resources away from self-maintenance and reproduction. It is even more costly when the bacteria acquire resistance genes via the horizontal transfer of plasmids that must be maintained and replicated as if they were additional chromosomes (Hernando-Amado et al. 2017), In sum, these resistance traits are often a liability in the absence of ongoing selective pressure from antibiotics. Far from conferring super powers, multidrug resistance is often, though not always, a drag for bacteria under normal conditions.

The evolutionary cost of resistance explains three important epidemiological observations. The first is that humans may harbor multidrug-resistant pathogens without knowing it. This phenomenon

was discovered in a study of patients who developed multidrug-resistant *Salmonella* infections after taking antibiotics for other kinds of infections (Levy 2002). It turned out that these patients had already been carrying the *Salmonella* in their intestines, possibly for years. But these *Salmonella* were kept in check by the more competitive microbiota around them, subsisting in numbers too low to cause infection. Once they took the antibiotics, the competition was suppressed and the *Salmonella* populations surged.

The second observation pertains to our earlier discussion about the under-use of antibiotics and the stepwise evolution of drug resistance. Evolution often occurs through incremental changes but these increments are likely to be smaller if the overall change involves additional expenditures of energy and chemical resources. The same can be said for other biological traits, such as human-to-human transmissibility. If the changes needed to invade a human population are expensive, then the invasion may occur in smaller steps; the more cost, the more "chatter" in the form of sharp and sporadic outbreaks. Yet by the same token, these changes are more likely to occur with bigger leaps and at faster rates when the evolutionary steps are less expensive.

We saw this pattern with the delayed emergence of MRSA, which was a rare infection for the two decades after it was first identified in 1961. In the early 1970s, MRSA appeared more frequently in the form of isolated outbreaks among hospitalized patients in the United Kingdom (Newsom 2004). Then in the late 1970s, MRSA found its way into geriatric wards and the outbreaks became more frequent and sustained. By the next decade, MRSA was endemic to long-term care facilities and nursing homes in Europe and North America, institutions filled (and overfilled) with intersecting populations of frail elderly and patients facing the last years of life. Although it has declined in recent years, MRSA is nevertheless a leading cause of drug-resistant infections both in and out of hospitals. About 2 percent of North Americans carry MRSA strains in their nasal passages (Brown 2020).

The story of MRSA brings us to the third observation: antibiotic resistant infections usually appear first in vulnerable populations, where they also tend to spread faster and more extensively (Allel et al. 2020; Alvarez-Uria et al. 2016). We see this in the emergence and spread of MDR-TB and XDR-TB. Ordinary tuberculosis is already a major disease of poverty accounting for the majority of infectious disease deaths in the world's poorest societies (Queiroz et al. 2020). TB is also a major AIDS-defining illness, responsible for a third of all deaths among HIV-infected people worldwide.

TB has long been curable with a combination of three antimicrobial drugs. However, just as the under-treatment of one person can lead to a drug-resistant infection, the under-treatment of the world can lead to many more. Humanity has been missing the window of opportunity for implementing major global treatment programs, resulting in the spread of drug-resistant TB in these same impoverished and co-infected populations. In 2017, it was estimated that 22 percent of the world's TB cases were resistant to one or more antibiotics for a total of 558,000 cases (World Health Organization 2020). Only 40 percent of these infections are treatable with second-line drugs; even then, the additional financial cost is 20- to 30-fold higher than for standard therapy (Kim et al. 2005; WHO 2020).

That said, the cost of not treating these infections may be much higher if they continue to spread. The same can be said for the cost of not "treating" the vulnerabilities from which these infections arise. Recall that in the nineteenth century, TB was the leading cause of infectious disease mortality in all societies, both rich and poor. In the twenty-first century, drug resistance could return TB to its earlier prominence. As with the novel and recurring infections, the key to preventing the rise of drug-resistant infections like MDR/XDRTB lies in addressing their underlying determinants at a global level.

6.6 The persistence of resistance

Is resistance inevitable? One way to answer this question is to observe the continued evolution of drug-resistant bacteria in the laboratory after the removal of antibiotics. Given the biological cost of many resistant mechanisms, we would predict these mutations to revert to their original drug-sensitive forms in the absence of selection pressure. Recent studies support this prediction for eight

pathogenic bacterial species, but only under carefully controlled laboratory conditions when the initial resistance was due to a single mutational event (Melnyk et al. 2015). Outside the laboratory, resistance evolves under complex environmental conditions, the mutations can occur in more than one gene, and the genes can code for more than one trait.

In human environments, many bacterial resistance mechanisms are slower to disappear than the rates at which they arose in the first place. Microbiologists often use the word "persistence" to describe this phenomenon, which they first observed in early laboratory studies of penicillin resistance (Bigger 1944). Even before the first penicillin-resistant infection appeared in a human patient, researchers found laboratory evidence not only that resistance would evolve in the presence of penicillin but that the resistance would persist after the antibiotic was removed.

Several theories have been proposed to explain persistence. For example, at least some resistance mutations appear to arise with little or no cost to the pathogen. This appears to be the case for a form of rifampicin resistance in *S. aureus* and *M. tuberculosis*; the latter pathogen is also capable of acquiring a persistent mutation that confers resistance to streptomycin (Melnyk 2015). Although these no-cost mutations may be exceptions to the rule, they are more likely to occur when the resistance mechanism confers some other advantage under special circumstances; this is the case for certain strains of streptomycin-resistant *Salmonella* that grow more slowly but survive longer in poor nutrient environments (Andersson and Hughes 2011).

Another theory involves compensatory evolution. This occurs when an organism makes up for the cost of a new mutation by compensating with another mutation rather than reverting to the earlier drug-sensitive form. Such mechanisms have been found for mutations that would otherwise decrease bacterial synthesis of important molecules but that additional mutations restore production levels while still conferring resistance. Such compensation has been found in persistently drug-resistant strains of *E. coli*, *M. tuberculosis*, *S. aureus*, *P. aeruginosa, and N. meningitidis* (Hernando-Amado et al. 2017).

Two or more resistance genes may be closely linked together such that even in the absence of one antibiotic, the presence of another antibiotic may tend to keep both genes around. Such is the case for certain strains of *P. aeruginosa* known to cause pneumonia in mechanically ventilated patients. Here, two genes are closely linked, each conferring resistance to a different class of antibiotics such that both persist in the presence of only one of these kinds of drugs (Rehman et al. 2021; Reinhardt et al. 2007). *P. aeruginosa* is also known to regulate at least one of its resistance genes, switching it on and off depending on whether an antibiotic is present (Merker et al. 2020).

This switching is itself a genetically coded trait that is broadly shared by many other animal species in the macro world that must "flex" their physiology in the face of changing environmental conditions. But unlike macroorganisms, many species of microorganisms have the additional advantage of horizontal gene transfer such that they need not even switch their resistance on or off but instead they can lose and regain the resistance genes by transferring to and from other bacteria via mobile genetic elements such as plasmids and bacteriophage.

The persistence of resistance remains a complex mystery, so it is fortunate that that this phenomenon does not apply to all pathogens and antibiotics. There are many instances of declining resistance following the more prudent use of antibiotics (WHO 2020) but there are enough instances to tell a cautionary tale. Even with the best policies, we may not reverse the rise of antimicrobial resistance as quickly or as completely as needed to keep up with our microbial neighbors.

6.7 One Health vs. the resistome

Building on the concept of the microbiome, biologists are beginning to broaden their studies of drug resistance beyond the singular mechanisms that Rene Dubos criticized many years ago. Within the microbiome, they are recognizing a resistome in which a large collection of genetic traits evolve and interact in complex microbial ecosystems that are mediated by medications, non-human animals, and the non-infectious diseases of human hosts

(Checcucci et al. 2020; Crofts et al. 2017). These studies have the potential for translation into clinical practice via more sophisticated treatment regimens that replace simple drug combinations with drug sequences that prevent or reverse evolutionary processes (Merker et al. 2020).

At the macro level, political and global health leaders are also broadening their ecological views with the One Health concept, implementing policies that address not only the administration of drugs in humans but also of food-producing animals and crops in large-scale agriculture and aquaculture, as well as waste and water management (EU Commission 2020; WHO 2015). Yet although many high-income countries have adopted this approach, there are significant barriers to implementation in many low- and middle-income countries (Iskandar et al. 2020; Nadimpalli et al. 2018).

Even with these efforts, the future does not look good for antimicrobial medicine. The genetic adaptations of pathogens have greatly outpaced the technical innovations of their human hosts. Industrial agriculture has permeated our global environment with antibiotics. This and our own consumption of antibiotics has transformed our bodily flora into reservoirs for drug-resistance genes, which can pass these genes to pathogenic organisms. And the most vulnerable of our human communities—the elderly, the impoverished, and the chronically sick—are gateways and incubators for the emergence of new drug-resistant strains of human pathogens. Laurie Garrett, a Pulitzer Prize-winning health writer and trained biologist, predicts that we are heading back to the times of our recent ancestors in what she calls "the post-antibiotic era" (1994). History may prove her right.

That said, even if all our medications become obsolete some day, we can take solace in the lessons of the Second Epidemiological Transition. Knowing that we made our greatest strides in the reduction of infectious diseases prior to the availability of such medicines, we can choose to see the evolution of resistance as a wake-up call for better health practices, programs, and policies. Of course, we should continue to work on new medicines, and we should do everything possible to slow down the process, but we must also apply the ancient and recurring lessons for human health in our current modes of subsistence, settlement, and social organization. If we do this, then resistance may still be inevitable, but it need not be catastrophic.

Notes

1. No longer used as an antimicrobial, Optochin is still used in the laboratory to distinguish *S. pneumoniae* from other streptococci. However, the emergence of Optochin-resistant *S. pneumoniae* may someday render this test obsolete (Pikis et al. 2001).

References

Ackerknecht, Erwin H. 1948. "Anticontagionism between 1821 and 1867." *Bulletin of the History of Medicine* 22: 562–593.

Allel, Kasim, Patricia García, Jaime Labarca, José M. Munita, Magdalena Rendic, Grupo Colaborativo de Resistencia Bacteriana, and Eduardo A. Undurraga. 2020. "Socioeconomic factors associated with antimicrobial resistance of Pseudomonas aeruginosa, Staphylococcus aureus, and Escherichia coli in Chilean hospitals (2008–2017)." *Revista Panamericana De Salud Publica-Pan American Journal of Public Health* 44. https://doi.org/10.26633/rpsp.2020.30

Alvarez-Uria, Gerardo, Sumanth Gandra, and Ramanan Laxminarayan. 2016. "Poverty and prevalence of antimicrobial resistance in invasive isolates." *International Journal of Infectious Diseases* 52: 59–61. https://doi.org/10.1016/j.ijid.2016.09.026

Aminov, Rustam. 2017. "History of antimicrobial drug discovery: Major classes and health impact." *Biochemical Pharmacology* 133: 4–19. https://doi.org/10.1016/j.bcp.2016.10.001

Amyes, Sebastian. 2001. *Magic Bullets, Lost Horizons: The Rise and Fall of Antibiotics*. New York: Taylor & Francis.

Andersson, Dan I., and Diarmaid Hughes. 2011. "Persistence of antibiotic resistance in bacterial populations." *Fems Microbiology Reviews* 35 (5): 901–911. https://doi.org/10.1111/j.1574-6976.2011.00289.x

Armelagos, George J., Kristi Kohlbacher, Kristy R. Collins, Jennifer Cook, and Maria Karfield-Daugherty. 2001. "Tetracycline Consumption in Prehistory." In *Tetracyclines in Biology, Chemistry and Medicine*, edited by M. Nelson, W. Hillen, and Robert A. Greenwald, 217–235. Basil: Birkhauser Verlag AG.

Auta, Asa, Muhammad Abdul Hadi, Enoche Oga, Emmanuel O. Adewuyi, Samirah N. Abdu-Aguye, Davies Adeloye, Barry Strickland-Hodge, and Daniel J. Morgan. 2019. "Global access to antibiotics without prescription in community pharmacies: A systematic review and meta-analysis." *Journal of Infection* 78 (1): 8–18. https://doi.org/10.1016/j.jinf.2018.07.001

Bager, Flemming, Frank Møller Aarestrup, and Henrik Caspar Wegener. 2000. "Dealing with antimicrobial resistance—The Danish experience." *Canadian Journal of Animal Science* 80 (2): 223–228. https://doi.org/10.4141/a99-096

Barnes, David S. 1995. *The Making of a Social Disease: Tuberculosis in Nineteenth-Century France*. Berkely: University of California Press.

Bassett, Everett J., Margaret S. Keith, George J. Armelagos, Debra L. Martin, and Antonio R. Villanueva. 1980. "Tetracycline labeled human bone from prehistoric Sudanese Nubia (A.D. 350)." *Science* 209: 1532–1534.

Beceiro, Alejandro, María Tomás, and Germán Bou. 2013. "Antimicrobial resistance and virulence: A successful or deleterious association in the bacterial world?" *Clinical Microbiology Reviews* 26 (2): 185–230. https://doi.org/10.1128/cmr.00059-12

Berlin, Brent. 1992. *Ethnobiological Classification—Principles of Categorization of Plants and Animals in Traditional Societies*. Princeton, NJ: Princeton University Press.

Bigger, Joseph W. 1944. "Treatment of staphylococcal infections with penicillin—By intermittent sterilisation." *Lancet* 2: 497–500.

Blair, Jessica M.A., Mark A. Webber, Alison J. Baylay, David O. Ogbolu, and Laura J.V. Piddock. 2015. "Molecular mechanisms of antibiotic resistance." *Nature Reviews Microbiology* 13 (1): 42–51. https://doi.org/10.1038/nrmicro3380

Boylston, Arthur. 2012. "The origins of inoculation." *Journal of the Royal Society of Medicine* 105 (7): 309–313. https://doi.org/10.1258/jrsm.2012.12k044

Brown, Kevin K. 2004. "The history of penicillin from discovery to the drive to production." *Pharmaceutical Historian* 34 (3): 37–43.

Brown, Kevin K. 2020. "Methicillin-Resistant Staphylococcus aureus." https://www.cdc.gov/mrsa/healthcare/index.html

Centers for Disease Control and Prevention. 2019. *Antibiotic Resistance Threats in the United States 2019*. Atlanta: US Department of Health and Human Services.

Cerqueira, Francisco, Anastasis Christou, Despo Fatta-Kassinos, Maria Vila-Costa, Josep Maria Bayona, and Benjamin Piña 2020. "Effects of prescription antibiotics on soil- and root-associated microbiomes and resistomes in an agricultural context." *Journal of Hazardous Materials* 400.

Checcucci, Alice. 2020. "Exploring the animal waste resistome: The spread of antimicrobial resistance genes through the use of livestock manure." *Frontiers in Microbiology* 11 (1416): 1–9.

Crofts, Terence S., Andrew J. Gasparrini, and Gautam Dantas. 2017. "Next-generation approaches to understand and combat the antibiotic resistome." *Nature Reviews Microbiology* 15 (7): 422–434. https://doi.org/10.1038/nrmicro.2017.28

Dubos, René Jules. 1987. *Mirage of health: utopias, progress and biological change*. New Brunswick: Rutgers University Press.

Economou, Vangelis, and Panagiota Gousia. 2015. "Agriculture and food animals as a source of antimicrobial-resistant bacteria." *Infection and Drug Resistance* 8: 49–61. https://doi.org/10.2147/idr.s55778.

Etkin, Nina L., and Elaine Elisabetsky. 2005. "Seeking a transdisciplinary and culturally germane science: The future of ethnopharmacology." *Journal of Ethnopharmacology* 100 (1–2): 23–26. https://doi.org/10.1016/j.jep.2005.05.025

EU Commission. "A European one health action plan against antimicrobial resistance (AMR)." (2020).

FDA, US. 2013. *Guidelines for Industry #213*. Washington, DC: Center for Veterinary Medicine; Food and Drug Administration: US Department of Health and Human Services.

Fleming, Alexander. 1945. "Sir Alexander Fleming—Nobel Lecture." Penicillin. Available online: https://www.nobelprize.org/uploads/2018/06

Fu, Jia-Chen. 2015. "The secret project that conquered malaria—and led to a Nobel Prize." *U.S. News and World Report*, October 6.

Garrett, Laurie. 1994. *The Coming Plague: Newly Emerging Diseases in a World Out of Balance*. New York: Farrar Straus and Giroux.

Gilbert, Jack A., Martin J. Blaser, J. Gregory Caporaso, Janet K. Jansson, Susan V. Lynch, and Rob Knight. 2018. "Current understanding of the human microbiome." *Nature Medicine* 24 (4): 392–400. https://doi.org/10.1038/nm.4517

Goldsworthy, Peter D., and Alexander C. McFarlane. 2002. "Howard Florey, Alexander Fleming and the fairy tale of penicillin." *Medical Journal of Australia* 176 (4): 178–180.

Górniak, Ireneusz, Rafał Bartoszewski, and Jarosław Króliczewski. 2019. "Comprehensive review of antimicrobial activities of plant flavonoids." *Phytochemistry reviews* 18: 241–272.

Gross, Cary, and Kent Sepkowitz. 1998. "The myth of the medical breakthrough: Smallpox, vaccination, and Jenner reconsidered." *International Journal of Infectious Diseases* 3 (1): 54–60.

Guy, William H. 1919. "Reactions following the administration of arsphenamin—Report of reaction in a series of twenty-five thousand injections." *Journal of the American Medical Association* 73: 901–905. https://doi.org/10.1001/jama.1919.02610380027009

Hernando-Amado, Sara, Fernando Sanz-García, Paula Blanco, and Jose L. Martinez. 2017. "Fitness costs associated with the acquisition of antibiotic resistance." *Essays in biochemistry* 61 (1): 37–48.

Hippocrates. 400 BCE. *On Airs, Waters, and Places*. Cambridge, MA: Internet Classics Archive.

Hopkins, Janice. 2002. "Old smallpox vaccination may still protect." *British Medical Journal* 325 (7363): 513–513.

Hsu, Elisabeth, and Ronald Barrett. 2008. "Traditional Asian Medical Systems." In *International Encyclopedia of Public Health*, edited by K Heggenhougan, 349–357. New York, NY: Academic Press.

Iskandar, Katia, Laurent Molinier, Souheil Hallit, Massimo Sartelli, Fausto Catena, Federico Coccolini, Timothy C. Hardcastle et al. 2020. "Drivers of antibiotic resistance transmission in low- and middle-income countries from a 'One Health' perspective—A review." *Antibiotics-Basel* 9 (7). https://doi.org/10.3390/antibiotics9070372

Jenner, Edward. (1798) 2020. "The three original publications on vaccination against smallpox." Historic Public Health Articles. https://biotech.law.lsu.edu/cphl/history/articles/jenner.htm

Jones, Williams P., Young-Won Chin, and A. Douglas Kinghorn. 2006. "The role of pharmacognosy in modern medicine and pharmacy." *Current Drug Targets* 7 (3): 247–264. https://doi.org/10.2174/138945006776054915

Kamat, Vinat R., and Mark Nichter. 1998. "Pharmacies, self-medication and pharmaceutical marketing in Bombay, India." *Social Science & Medicine* 47 (6): 779–794. https://doi.org/10.1016/s0277-9536(98)00134-8

Kim, Jim Yong, Aaron Shakow, Kedar Mate, Chris Vanderwarker, Rajesh Gupta, and Paul Farmer. 2005. "Limited good and limited vision: Multidrug-resistant tuberculosis and global health policy." *Social Science & Medicine* 61: 847–859.

Klebs, Aarnold C. 1913. "The historic evolution of variolation." *Bulletin of the Johns Hopkins Hospital* 24: 69–83.

Klein, E. Y., T. P. Van Boeckel, E. M. Martinez, S. Pant, S. Gandra, S. A. Levin, H. Goossens, and R. Laxminarayan. 2018. "Global increase and geographic convergence in antibiotic consumption between 2000 and 2015." *Proceedings of the National Academy of Sciences of the United States of America* 115 (15): E3463–E3470. https://doi.org/10.1073/pnas.1717295115

Klein, Eili Y., Maja Milkowska-Shibata, Katie K. Tseng, Mike Sharland, Sumanth Gandra, Celine Pulcini, and Ramanan Laxminarayan. 2020. "Assessment of WHO antibiotic consumption and access targets in 76 countries, 2000–15: An analysis of pharmaceutical sales data." *The Lancet. Infectious Diseases.* (20): 30332–30337. https://doi.org/10.1016/s1473-3099

Kleinman, Arthur. 1989. *The Illness Narratives: Suffering, Healing, and the Human Condition.* New York: Basic Books.

Lawrence, Roderick, Anthony Capon, and Jose Siri. 2017. "Lessons from Hippocrates for contemporary urban health challenges." *Cities & Health* 1 (1): 72–82.

Lax, Eric. 2004. *The Mold in Dr. Florey's Coat: The Story of the Penicillin Miracle.* New York: Henry Holt & Company.

Lesch, John E. 2006. *The First Miracle Drugs: How the Sulfa Drugs Transformed Medicine.* Oxford: Oxford University Press.

Levy, Stuart B. 2002. *The Antibiotic Paradox: How Miracle Drugs Are Destroying the Miracle.* New York: Plenum Press.

Marshall, Bonnie M., and Stuart B. Levy. 2011. "Food animals and antimicrobials: impacts on human health." *Clinical Microbiology Reviews* 24 (4): 718. https://doi.org/10.1128/CMR.00002-11

McGillicuddy, Timothy J. 1898. "Tuberculosis: Its seed, its soil and its treatment by medical sepsis." *Journal of the American Medical Association* 30 (24): 1395–1397.

McKeown, Thomas. 1988. *The Origins of Human Disease.* Oxford: Basil Blackwell.

Melnyk, Anita H., Alex Wong, and Rees Kassen. 2015. "The fitness costs of antibiotic resistance mutations." *Evolutionary Applications* 8 (3): 273–283. https://doi.org/10.1111/eva.12196

Merker, Mathias, Leif Tueffers, Marie Vallier, Espen E. Groth, Lindsay Sonnenkalb, Daniel Unterweger, John F. Baines, Stefan Niemann, and Hinrich Schulenburg. 2020. "Evolutionary approaches to combat antibiotic resistance: Opportunities and challenges for precision medicine." *Frontiers in Immunology* 11 (1938): 1–7.

NACMF. 2019. "Response to questions posed by the food safety and inspection service regarding salmonella control strategies in poultry." *Journal of Food Protection* 82 (4): 645–668.

Nadimpalli, Maya, Elisabeth Delarocque-Astagneau, David C. Love, Lance B. Price, Bich-Tram Huynh, Jean-Marc Collard, Kruy Sun Lay et al. 2018. "Combating global antibiotic resistance: emerging One Health concerns in lower- and middle-income countries." *Clinical Infectious Diseases* 66 (6): 963–969. https://doi.org/10.1093/cid/cix879

Nelson, Mark, Andrew Dinardo, Jeffrey Hochberg, and George J. Armelagos. 2010. "Spectroscopic characterization of tetracycline in skeletal remains of an ancient population from Sudanese Nubia 350CE-550CE." *American Journal of Physical Anthropology* 143: 151–154.

Newsom, S.W.B. 2004. "MRSA—Past, present, future." *Journal of the Royal Society of Medicine* 97 (11): 509–510. https://doi.org/10.1258/jrsm.97.11.509

Piepenbrink, H., B. Herrmann, and P. Hoffmann. 1983. "Tetracycline flouresences in buried human bones." *Zeitschrift Fur Rechtsmedizin-Journal of Legal Medicine* 91 (1): 71–74.

Pikis, Andreas, Joseph M. Campos, William J. Rodriguez, and Jerry M. Keith. 2001. "Optochin resistance in Streptococcus pneumoniae: mechanism, significance, and clinical implications." *The Journal of infectious diseases* 184 (5): 582–590.

Plotkin, Stanley A. 2005. "Vaccines: Past, present and future." *Nature Medicine* 11 (4): S5–S11.

Rêgo Queiroz, Ana Angélica, Thaís Zamboni Berra, Alexandre Tadashi Inomata Bruce, Maria Concebida da Cunha Garcia, Danielle Talita dos Santos, Marcos Augusto Moraes Arcoverde, Luana Seles Alves et al. 2020. "Effect of social development in reducing tuberculosis mortality in northeastern Brazil areas." *Journal of Infection in Developing Countries* 14 (8): 869. https://doi.org/10.3855/jidc.12196

Reid, Walter V. 1993. "Bioprospecting—A Force for Sustainable Development." *Environmental Science & Technology* 27 (9): 1730–1732.

Rehman, Attika, Julie Jeukens, Roger C. Levesque, and Iain L. Lamont. 2021. "Gene-gene interactions dictate ciprofloxacin resistance in Pseudomonas aeruginosa and facilitate prediction of resistance phenotype from genome sequence data." *Antimicrobial Agents and Chemotherapy* 65 (7): 10–1128.

Reinhardt, Anita, Thilo Köhler, Paul Wood, Peter Rohner, Jean-Luc Dumas, Bara Ricou, and Christian van Delden. 2007. "Development and persistence of antimicrobial resistance in Pseudomonas aeruginosa: a longitudinal observation in mechanically ventilated patients." *Antimicrobial agents and chemotherapy* 51 (4): 1341–1350.

Rios, Jose L., and Maria C. Recio. 2005. "Medicinal plants and antimicrobial activity." *Journal of Ethnopharmacology* 100 (1–2): 80–84. https://doi.org/10.1016/j.jep.2005.04.025

Rodriguez, Vanessa. 2012. "The teaching brain and the end of the empty vessel." *Mind Brain and Education* 6 (4): 177–185. https://doi.org/10.1111/j.1751-228X.2012.01155.x

Rohr, Jason R., Christopher B. Barrett, David J. Civitello, Meggan E. Craft, Bryan Delius, Giulio A. DeLeo, Peter J. Hudson et al. 2019. "Emerging human infectious diseases and the links to global food production." *Nature Sustainability* 2 (6): 445–456. https://doi.org/10.1038/s41893-019-0293-3

Sakeena, Mohamed H.F., Alexandra A. Bennett, and Andres J. McLachlan. 2018. "Non-prescription sales of antimicrobial agents at community pharmacies in developing countries: A systematic review." *International Journal of Antimicrobial Agents* 52 (6): 771–782. https://doi.org/10.1016/j.ijantimicag.2018.09.022

Sams, Erika R., Marvin Whiteley, and Keith H. Turner. 2014. "'The battle for life': Pasteur, anthrax, and the first probiotics." *Journal of medical microbiology* 63 (11): 1573–1574.

Schroeder, Meredith, Benjamin D. Brooks, and Amanda E. Brooks. 2017. "The complex relationship between virulence and antibiotic resistance." *Genes* 8 (1): 39. https://doi.org/10.3390/genes8010039

Scott, Laura C., Nicholas Lee, and Tiong Gim Aw. 2020. "Antibiotic resistance in minimally human-impacted environments." *International Journal of Environmental Research and Public Health* 17 (11): 12. https://doi.org/10.3390/ijerph17113939

US EPA. 2018a. "Final Registration Decision for the Use of Active Ingredient Oxytetracycline Hydrochloride on Citrus Crop Group 10-10." United States Environmental Protection Agency report number: EPA-HQ-OPP-2015-0820. https://www.regulations.gov/docket/EPA-HQ-OPP-2015-0820/document

US EPA. 2018b. "Streptomycin: Section 3 Registration for Citrus Fruits Crop Group 10-10."

United States Environmental Protection Agency memorandum number 449381. https://www.regulations.gov/document/EPA-HQ-OPP-2008-0687-0027.

Ventola, C. Lee. 2015. "The antibiotic resistance crisis: Part 1: Causes and threats." *P & T* 40 (4): 277–283.

von Hippel, E. 1916. "The danger of optochin treatment of pneumonia for the organ of sight." *Deutsche Medizinische Wochenschrift* 42: 1089–1091.

Willcox, Merlin, Drissa Diallo, Rokia Sanogo, Sergio Giani, Bertrand Graz, Jaques Falquet, and Gerard Bodeker. 2015. "Intellectual property rights, benefit-sharing and development of 'improved traditional medicines': A new approach." *Journal of Ethnopharmacology* 176: 281–285. https://doi.org/10.1016/j.jep.2015.10.041

Williams, Keith J. 2009. "The introduction of 'chemotherapy' using arsphenamine—The first magic bullet." *Journal of the Royal Society of Medicine* 102 (8): 343–348. https://doi.org/10.1258/jrsm.2009.09k036

Winau, Florian, Otto Westphal, and Rolf Winau. 2004. "Paul Ehrlich—In search of the magic bullet." *Microbes and Infection* 6 (8): 786–789.

World Health Organization. 2015. *Global Action Plan on Antimicrobial Resistance*. Geneva: World Health Organization.

World Health Organization. 2017. *Antibacterial Agents in Clinical Development: An Analysis of the Antibacterial Clinical Development Pipeline, Including Tuberculosis*. Geneva: World Health Organization. https://apps.who.int/iris/bitstream/handle/10665/258965/WHO-EMP-IAU-2017.11-eng.pdf?sequence=1

World Health Organization. 2018. *WHO Report on Surveillance of Antibiotic Consumption: 2016–2018 Early Implementation*. Geneva: World Health Organization.

World Health Organization. 2020. *International instruments on the use of antimicrobials across the human, animal and plant sectors*. Geneva: World Health Organization.

Zaman, Muhammad H. 2020. *Biography of Resistance: The Epic Battle Between People and Pathogens*. New York: HarperCollins.

The Ancient Determinants of Future Infections

Some histories are so long that we are unaware of their existence. Like continents, we experience them as the immovable terra beneath our feet, even though they continue to shift around and travel the world over great stretches of time. Then one day, a cataclysm occurs: an earthquake, an eruption, a tsunami. We are then spellbound by the unexpected disaster, having overlooked the slower processes that led up to its occurrence. Historians of the Annales School refer to these latter processes as the *longue durée*. Prominent among them, Fernand Braudel argues that "[h]istory may be divided into three movements: what moves rapidly, what moves slowly and what appears not to move at all" (1972: 8).

We have seen these different movements throughout this book. All three can be found in every outbreak we studied; at this moment of publication, COVID-19 presents the most timely example. Moving rapidly, a novel coronavirus suddenly appeared out of nowhere in a large city and then spread throughout the world in a matter of weeks. Moving slowly, large populations of older people struggled for years with chronic non-infectious diseases, only to die from this one particular infection. And not appearing to move at all, the world's poorer societies have acquired the health challenges of the Second Transition while still retaining those of the First Transition, resulting in large and growing populations of highly susceptible hosts for COVID-19 and many other infections. If or when the next new pathogen "emerges" from these populations, there is little doubt that many of us will once again turn the bulk of our attention to the more rapid movements.

With an appreciation of deep timelines, we have identified recurring themes and events that often escape historical attention but have turned out to have profound effects on human health. Nearly all these themes involved transformative changes in the ways that people have adapted to their physical and social surroundings. These included major changes in food production and human reproduction, social distancing, and social hierarchies. Some of these themes were deeply buried in human prehistory, uncovered only by the painstaking methods of the archeologist or physical anthropologist. Others were coded in genomes, marked by molecular breadcrumbs, or displayed in the microscopic interactions between pathogen, host, and vector species. We found widely scattered evidence in the ethnographies of living people and tabulated evidence in the written accounts of historical people. We then traced these themes to epidemiological outcomes, framing human health as broadly as the evidence would allow.

If this book was a simple accounting of human determinants or interesting disease facts, the scope and scale of this project would be too large for a single volume. Instead, we organized these materials around an expanded framework of epidemiological transitions. Each of these transitions provided a common point of focus for many disciplinary approaches, allowing us to ask the same questions with different methods and in very different time periods. In the process of answering these questions, we hope that readers will draw at least two important lessons from this endeavor. The first is that our current disease challenges have ancient precedents. Our first truly emerging

Emerging Infections. Second Edition. Ron Barrett, Molly K. Zuckerman, Matthew R. Dudgeon, with George J. Armelagos, Oxford University Press.
© Ron Barrett, Molly K. Zuckerman, Matthew R. Dudgeon (2024). DOI: 10.1093/oso/9780192843135.003.0008

infections occurred with the rise of acute diseases in the Neolithic, when the lifestyles associated with primary agriculture were first adopted. Antimicrobial resistance has an even longer history insofar as microbes have used these mechanisms to defend themselves from one another for nearly a billion years. Accounting for these timescales, it could be argued there are no truly emerging infections today, only re-emerging ones.

The second major lesson is that the disease determinants of our past are homologous to those of today. Despite radical changes to our environments and lifestyles over the last 11,000 years, the broader problems of subsistence, settlement, and social organization remain essentially the same. Far from solving these ancient problems, our twenty-first-century developments have greatly intensified them with industrial food production, centripetal urbanization, international mobility, and expanding disparities. Yet without an expanded temporal framework, it is difficult to see the recurring patterns. This presents an additional challenge to George Santayana's famous dictum: "Those who cannot remember the past are condemned to repeat it." We must first be aware of our deeper histories before we can hope to remember them.

As we encounter the health consequences of the Third Epidemiological Transition, it is ironic that many of us are paying more attention to the roles of invisibly small creatures than those of the plainly visible people around us. The medical historian, William McNeill, used the terms "microparasite" and "microparasite" to compare the behaviors of disease-causing microbes with the behaviors of disease-causing humans. Both make their livings at the expense of their human hosts, and these parasitic relationships produce our infectious diseases. Yet unlike the blind adaptations of microparasites, which blindly adapt by random change, the adaptations of macroparasites are characteristically intentional, even when they produce unintended consequences.

The primary purpose of this *unnatural* history is to reveal the macroscopic determinants of human infections similar to the ways that early germ theorists once revealed their microscopic determinants. That said, we have not dismissed the germs. Our approach has been one of both soil and seed,

acknowledging the importance of pathogens while stressing their evolution in response to human activities: the ways we feed ourselves, the ways we reproduce and live together, and, for better and worse, the ways we relate to one another.

7.1 Subsistence, then and now

Because of the slow pace of our biological evolution, we are genetically little different than our Paleolithic ancestors. Thus, having examined the protective role of nutrition against human infections today, we can infer the same protective role in our ancient ancestors, foragers who were likely to have diverse diets of wild foods that tended to be high in fiber, low in saturated fats, and replete with essential micronutrients. Notwithstanding the popularity of the Paleo Diet movement today, there is a very good reason why traditional foraging diets often exemplify public health recommendations for healthy eating. For more than 100 millennia leading up to the Neolithic, these were the foods we consumed in our environments of evolutionary adaptation. Despite 11,000 years of radical cultural changes, these are the kinds of diets that are best suited to our physiology. By extension, they are also the best diets to meet the heavy demands of our immune systems.

Intensive agriculture brought an excess of processed carbohydrates into human diets: seed grasses and roots to feed large and growing populations. But the production of these energy-dense foods came at the cost of dietary diversity. Having examined the skeletal record of ancient societies as they transitioned from primary foraging to primary agriculture, we see the health consequences of these dietary changes: increases in the physical markers of nutritional stress, diminished stature, increased mortality at earlier ages, and rising indications of infectious diseases. Unfortunately, we see the same consequences of under-nutrition in far too many populations today who, without exception, carry very high burdens of infectious disease.

The role of nutrition in the emerging infections of the First Transition was underscored by its role in the declining infections of the Second Transition. Improvements in farming and distribution increased the availability and variety of food sources for even the poorest communities of the most affluent societies. While nutrition may not have been the only factor, it is striking that most of the infectious disease declines occurred before the discovery of antibiotics and most vaccines. However, the same could not be said for the infection declines in poorer societies later in the twentieth century, when antimicrobial medicines became widely available. Many of these societies continue to experience food insecurity, the consequences of which are most likely buffered by cheap pharmaceuticals. With the rise in drug-resistant infections, it is troubling to consider what will happen to undernourished populations if these medicinal buffers become obsolete.

In addition to dietary restrictions, the domestication of animals for food and labor brought ancient societies into close proximity with zoonotic pathogens, presenting them with repeated opportunities for spillover into human populations. As these pathogens evolved human-to-human transmissibility, they became humanity's first truly emerging infectious diseases. More recently, these same dynamics have been greatly amplified by the industrialization and massive expansion of commercial agriculture. Our food animals have since became "urbanized," densely stacked under stressful conditions in large-scale production facilities. To make matters worse, commercial food production now includes the inappropriate use of antibiotics as animal growth agents, which is contributing more to the rise of antimicrobial resistance than the human use of these drugs. Consequently, we now have massive and concentrated populations of vulnerable animals with a high risk of becoming reservoirs for novel and drug-resistant infections.

These may seem like distant events to those of us who never encounter the animals we eat. They may seem even more distant to those of us who never eat meat at all. But at a microbial level, all of us are more closely connected to livestock today than at any time in the past. The animals themselves move through international trade networks. Their meat is broadly distributed to markets and stores. And the workers are as mobile and connected as everyone else. Domestic animal waste contaminates ground water, as well as our plant-based foods. Furthermore, the microbiomes of our domestic animals have an even further reach, exchanging genetic fragments that code for resistance and virulence across many different microbial species, including those that peacefully reside in the human gut. Given these dynamics, all of us might as well be farmers and none of us can be purely vegan.

7.2 Settlement, then and now

The earliest form of human settlement was hardly settled at all. For more than a 100,000 years we lived in small, mobile groups that were broadly and thinly scattered throughout the world. Even earlier, our hominin precursors lived this way for more than 4 million years. All told, the large majority of human evolution was spent on the move. This mobility and group-size could not have supported the sustained human-to-human transmission of acute infectious diseases. Chronic infections may well have been a problem, especially the less virulent parasites we inherited from our pre-human ancestors and picked up as "souvenirs" in the course of our travels. Yet most of the human infections we know today would have spread no further than a few human groups.

To have remained unsettled for so long, our ancestors had to keep their group sizes small. They could have accomplished this in at least one of three ways: first, by maintaining very low or zero population growth through relatively balanced birth and death rates; second, by dividing larger groups into small ones; and third, by expanding into new territories. All these strategies would have had their perturbations and limits, and these probably contributed to the crises that preceded the transition to primary agriculture.

Permanent settlement led to major demographic and epidemiological changes in the First Transition. Human and animal populations increased exponentially, both living closely together in a manner that allowed for the sustained transmission of acute infectious diseases. These densities increased even more with the development of towns and cities, which connected with expanding empires and state-level societies through long-distance trade networks. These became the reservoirs and tributaries for pandemic-level infections.

We have seen how changing modes of settlement could have contributed to the mortality declines of the Second Transition. The housing reforms in late nineteenth-century Europe may have helped, but it is more likely that contributions came from the development of water and waste infrastructures to meet the demands of growing urban populations—at least in the economically better developed societies. For the rest of the world, the rapid urbanization of poor societies have presented major opportunities for the incubation and spread of the new, virulent, and drug-resistant infections of the Third Transition. We now live in a world where the majority of 8 billion people live in urban areas, and all our settlements are situated in extensive networks for the rapid movements of people and goods as well as microbial pathogens. Our recent patterns of human settlement have created a global disease ecology.

7.3 Social organization, then and now

A recurring theme throughout this book has been that new and drug-resistant pathogens first enter human populations through their most vulnerable members. This makes sense, given that most of our pathogens originated from zoonotic pathogens that often evolved the capacity for human-to-human transmission in a series of incremental stages. These stages can be even more incremental for the evolution of drug resistance. In the initial stages, successful infection is more likely to occur in vulnerable human hosts, people who are poor, undernourished, overstressed, and compromised by existing infections or chronic non-infectious diseases. Tragically, these people often become the unwilling gateways, or sentinels for novel and drug-resistant infections. They can also become unwilling reservoirs for the growth and increasing virulence of these same infections.

We know that most contemporary foraging societies have social structures that are simpler and more egalitarian than their agrarian counterparts. This is not to suggest that all foraging societies are free from violence or social inequalities. But further social differences and leadership structures are cumbersome and unnecessary for the functioning of small groups, and without these structures there would be little cause for the unequal distribution of resources. This is reflected in the ethnographic record, in which there is a common theme of resource sharing and social sanctions against people having more than their share.

Earlier we examined the physical evidence from burial sites in ancient societies during their transitions from foraging to agriculture. People often die as they lived, and we have seen this reflected in people's graves. In the earlier stages of their agricultural transition, these ancient societies buried their dead with similar artifacts in similar graves. Then, with the intensification of agriculture, differences arise in the quality of artifacts and graves that indicate increasing socio-economic differences. It is not surprising that the skeletons of higher-status people show fewer signs of disease than those of lower-status people. What may be surprising, however, is that these are the first empirical signs of social and health inequalities in the archeological record. We do not have evidence for major inequalities prior to the Agricultural Revolution; it could therefore be argued that such differences have not been a natural constant of the human condition.

The Second Epidemiological Transition presents both positive and negative examples of the ways that socio-economic differences are linked to infectious diseases. We found positive examples within the more affluent societies that first underwent the Second Transition, where declining mortality was often correlated with the reduction of health differences between people of all social classes. These correlations make sense when we consider that infectious diseases had been the primary causes of death and reducing the risk of infection among the poorer classes also reduced the risk of infection for everyone else.

Unfortunately, the negative examples of differences and disease occurred at much larger scales during the latter decades of the Second Transition. While poorer societies also benefitted from declining infections, most of these improvements occurred much later and leveled off much sooner than in the wealthier nations. At the same time, these societies have had to contend with same challenges as affluent societies—aging populations and rapid increases in non-infectious diseases—but with fewer resources to address them.

7.4 Moving beyond the Third Transition

Today, the globalization of human infections into a single disease ecology means that the health risks among the poor are, once again, increasing the health risks for everyone else. While people may debate the "trickle down" effects of the global marketplace, there is no question that human pathogens are "trickling up" at a much faster rate. This reality brings us back to the very first point in this book, that microbes are the ultimate critics of modernity. But criticism should not beget fatalism, nor should the poor be blamed for the shortcomings of larger societies. If anything, our awareness of these global issues should raise our sense of individual and collective responsibility.

An expanded framework of epidemiological transitions can do more than increase awareness. It can inform policies and programs aimed at improving the prevention and advanced detection of human infections. For instance, if we understand the common and longstanding determinants of many infections and other health problems, then we can organize our health efforts on these fewer, upstream determinants instead of dealing with the many downstream consequences after they have already occurred. Denis Burkitt, an Irish surgeon who drew important contrasts between preventable health problems in Africa and Europe, summed up the situation in very concrete terms:

"Western doctors are like poor plumbers. They treat a splashing tube by cleaning up the water. These plumbers are extremely apt at drying up the water, constantly inventing new, expensive, and refined methods of drying up water. Somebody should teach them how to close the tap."

(1979:16).

Closing the tap entails closing the gap in healthy living and healthcare within and between human populations. It entails a redoubling of the positive efforts that brought the Second Transition to many societies until all societies reach similarly low levels of infectious disease mortality. History shows that great gains were had with fewer resources than we have today. Today our global economy has given us more means, and our global diseases have given us more reasons than ever before. Better physical health also entails better fiscal health for nations around the world. Whether for survival, prosperity, or ethics, the same argument should hold sway across a broad spectrum of political philosophies.

Understanding the convergence of disease patterns can also inform greater efficiency in the organization and delivery of health services. A case in point is that the US Centers for Disease Control has recognized the syndemic nature of AIDS, sexually transmitted diseases, tuberculosis, and hepatitis epidemics (CDC 2023). With syndemics in mind, it has recently launched an initiative known as Program Collaboration and Service Integration to bring together divisions and branches that used to address these diseases separately. This kind of program integration is often referred to as a horizontal approach to public health, in contrast to vertical programs that traditionally focused on single diseases like so much water down a pipe (Nichter 2008).

Horizontal approaches minimize redundancies, promote collaborations, and perhaps most importantly, focus more attention on the common determinants of multiple diseases. Inevitably, most of these determinants are social determinants, the same themes we have been exploring throughout this book. Let us hope such programs become globally contagious and that they spread across all manner of health challenges. Perhaps then, we can write about the positive lessons of the next epidemiological transition.

References

Braudel, Fernand. 1972. *The Mediterranean and the Mediterranean World in the Age of Phillip II*. New York: Simon & Schuster.

Burkitt, David. 1979. *Don't Forget Fibre in Your Diet*. London: Collins.

CDC. 2023. "Program Collaboration and Service Integration." Washington, DC: US Centers for Disease Control and Prevention. https://www.cdc.gov/nchhstp/programintegration/default.htm.

Nichter, Mark. 2008. *Global Health: Why Cultural Perceptions, Social Representations, and Biopolitics Matter*. Tucson: University of Arizona Press.

Index

Italic *f* and *t* denote figures and tables